MANAGING CHRONIC ILLNESS USING THE FOUR-PHASE TREATMENT APPROACH

MANAGING CHRONIC ILLNESS USING THE FOUR-PHASE TREATMENT APPROACH

A Mental Health Professional's Guide to Helping Chronically Ill People

Patricia A. Fennell

WILEY

John Wiley & Sons, Inc.

Published by John Wiley & Sons, Inc., Hoboken, New Jersey.
Published simultaneously in Canada.

Limit of Liability/Disclaimer of Warranty: While the publisher and author have used their best efforts
in preparing this book, they make no representations or warranties with respect to the accuracy or
completeness of the contents of this book and specifically disclaim any implied warranties of
merchantability or fitness for a particular purpose. No warranty may be created or extended by sales
representatives or written sales materials. The advice and strategies contained herein may not be
suitable for your situation. You should consult with a professional where appropriate. Neither the
publisher nor author shall be liable for any loss of profit or any other commercial damages, including
but not limited to special, incidental, consequential, or other damages.

This publication is designed to provide accurate and authoritative information in regard to the subject
matter covered. It is sold with the understanding that the publisher is not engaged in rendering
professional services. If legal, accounting, medical, psychological or any other expert assistance is
required, the services of a competent professional person should be sought.

Designations used by companies to distinguish their products are often claimed as trademarks. In all
instances where John Wiley & Sons, Inc. is aware of a claim, the product names appear in initial capital
or all capital letters. Readers, however, should contact the appropriate companies for more complete
information regarding trademarks and registration.

For general information on our other products and services please contact our Customer Care
Department within the United States at (800) 762-2974, outside the United States at (317) 572-3993 or
fax (317) 572-4002.

Wiley also publishes its books in a variety of electronic formats. Some content that appears in print
may not be available in electronic books. For more information about Wiley products, visit our web site
at www.wiley.com.

Library of Congress Cataloging-in-Publication Data:

Fennell, Patricia.
    Managing chronic illness : a four-phase treatment approach / Patricia A. Fennell.
        p. : cm.
    Includes bibliographical references and index.
    ISBN 0-471-46277-2 (cloth : alk. paper)
        1. Chronically ill.   2. Chronic diseases—Psychological aspects.   3. Sick—Psychology.   I.
    Title.
        [DNLM: 1. Chronic Disease—psychology.   2. Chronic Disease—therapy.   WT 500 F335m 2003]
    RA973.5.F46 2003
    616′.001′9—dc21
                                                                                    2003049736

Printed in the United States of America.

10   9   8   7   6   5   4   3   2   1

For Margaret,
who makes it possible.

Contents

PART III   FUTURE DIRECTIONS

Preface

Caritas, Veritas, Fortitudo

This book describes a method for managing chronic illness that employs a Four-Phase Model to assess and treat patients. The effectiveness of the model lies in its ability to address the heterogeneity that characterizes chronic conditions and in its inclusion of the individual's physical, psychological, and social-interactive systems. Although acute illnesses and traumas also involve the totality of an individual's systems, it is rarely as important for the outcome whether they are all addressed or not. With chronic conditions, however, it is essential to consider all the individual's systems. Failure to do so can skew assessment or treatment, rendering potentially useful therapies ineffective because clinicians have not considered the total picture.

Elements of this model came into focus gradually for me in more than 20 years of clinical experience. During my childhood, I experienced medical conditions that would now involve a much broader systems assessment than was used at the time. My experiences then also heightened my awareness of how medicine was practiced and how our society regards people who are ill. Early in my adult career, I worked in hospice, and there, for the first time, I saw in action the kind of assessment and care that I believed all patients, not just the dying, required. Not only were fellow hospice workers openly compassionate, but also I saw clinicians spending time coming to understand and attend to the significant others in a patient's life and coordinating their care with patient care.

Later, in my practice with chronic patients, my colleagues and I saw a large number of clients with a broad range of conditions. By having an extensive population to reflect on, I began to identify distinct phases in the illness experience and the individual's adaptation to it. It became clear clinically that practitioners needed to attend not only to the physical and psychological needs of clients, but also to their family, social, and work relations. Moreover, clinicians needed to coordinate their interventions in such a way that they reinforced each other rather than working at cross purposes. Objectively desirable therapies were not equally effective in certain phases. If clinicians attempted to employ therapies at the wrong time, not only did they fail to produce the expected results, but also clients would often reject the same therapy later, when they would have been able to sustain it and benefit from it. I further found that clinicians tended to experience predictable reactions to clients, depending on the phase the client was in, and needed to carry out a parallel process of personal evolution in the course of treating the chronic patient. It thus appeared that clinicians dealing with chronic illness also went through a phase process.

My experience with chronically ill patients also stimulated my engagement with research in the field. As my ideas took shape, I worked with colleagues to design empirical tests to begin validating what clinical practice has shown to be effective. Empirical testing continues, most recently in Belgium, where the findings indicate that my model is robust.

This book is organized into three parts. Part I introduces readers to phase models and the general setting of chronic illness in our society. It then provides a composite case history along with a brief overview of the Four-Phase process. Part II takes up each phase in detail, using case histories as illustrations and providing reminder checklists for clinicians. Part III analyzes the paradigm shift represented by the model and then discusses a number of research considerations.

Chapter 1, "A New Model for Treating the Chronically Ill," sets the Four-Phase Model into the context of phase theory in general. It then presents the underlying assumptions of the model—the integration of mind and body and the embedded systems of patient, community, workplace, and clinician—and discusses certain conceptual dichotomies that the model attempts to overcome. The chapter analyzes the phenomenon of chronicity and the varieties of trauma that may be experienced by the chronically ill. This is all finally combined into a discussion of the integration assumption of the model.

Chapter 2, "The Cultural Context of Chronic Illness," addresses the social context in which those with chronic illness live. Specifically, the chapter focuses on the health care system: who its actors and agents are, how they act and interact, what their assumptions are, and how medical matters are regarded in the general culture. It then focuses on six potentially traumagenic sociocultural factors in our society: intolerance of suffering, intolerance of ambiguity, intolerance of chronicity, the immediate cultural context of illness, the illness enculturation process, and the media.

Chapter 3, "Introduction to the Four Phases: Betty's Story," presents a brief general description of each phase, which is then dramatized in a composite case history that shows common specifics about how the phase process functions in actuality.

Part II addresses each phase in detail. Chapter 4, "Phase 1: Crisis," sets the frame for the next three chapters. After identifying what constitutes a Phase 1 patient, the chapter addresses in detail the assessment process in all three areas: physical, psychological, and social-interactive. It identifies the clinical goals and treatment issues in Phase 1 and continues with detailed treatment activities for the physical, psychological, and social-interactive areas. The chapter digresses to discuss countertransference and then addresses the countertransferential issues in Phase 1. The chapter closes with a discussion of the role of spiritual-philosophical matters in the Four-Phase process and how these issues present in Phase 1. Starting with the identification of Phase 1 patients, specific case histories are introduced. These continue in the subsequent sections so that readers can see a variety of presentations within the general framework of Phase 1. Each section includes summary boxes and checklists with reminders for clinicians new to the model.

Chapter 5, "Phase 2: Stabilization," follows the same format as "Phase 1: Crisis." Because Phase 2 sees a great deal of work in the area of activity reorganization, the chapter opens with a discussion of the personal energy process (how individuals perform individual actions) and the four general activity categories (activities of daily living [ADLs], personal fulfillment, social, and work). The same case histories from Phase 1 continue in this chapter, but new cases are added to show how the model works when clients first come for treatment later in the phase process. It also discusses the Phase 1-Phase 2 loop, the circling between crisis and stabilization that occurs when clients go untreated or are unable to achieve the insights and skills necessary to move into Phase 3.

Chapter 6, "Phase 3: Resolution," opens with a discussion of the development of meaning, the single most important issue of that phase. The movement toward meaning occurs through interventions facilitating attentive reflection and creative action. The individual patient's sense of meaning is based on a bedrock authenticity, which is also essential to the necessary creation of a "new self." Again, the bulk of the chapter follows the format of the prior chapters, carrying the case histories of those chapters forward and introducing a new one.

Chapter 7, "Phase 4: Integration," begins with discussion of integration as "cure." It notes that this phase process does not conclude—patients will likely undergo future crises—but that successfully traversing the phases gives individuals techniques for achieving integration more quickly. Again, the chapter follows the format of the prior chapters and continues the previous case histories, including those of clients who are unable to attain integration. One new case history is introduced that demonstrates how an individual possessed of insight and meaning may still need phase intervention.

In Part III, Chapter 8, "A Paradigm Shift," returns to general discussion. It notes the distinctive features of the Four-Phase Model: It offers an umbrella framework, addresses the cyclic nature of chronic illness, overcomes common conceptual dichotomies, addresses the ongoing trauma of chronic illness patients, uses countertransference, and includes components concerned with the development of meaning. The chapter then briefly addresses the subject of public policy and chronic illness. It concludes with a discussion of research, which must be predicated on the heterogeneity that exists in chronic illness, including the multiple physical systems involved, the changing manifestations of symptoms over time, and the multiple domains in which changes occur: the physical, the psychological, and the social-interactive. The chapter notes empirical research already accomplished, answers certain questions raised by that research, and proposes areas of new or additional research.

Some years ago, I saw the epigraph that appears at the start of this Preface—*Caritas, Veritas, Fortitudo*—carved in marble on a building scheduled for demolition. I have never forgotten the words, because they sum up completely what is required of those with chronic illness and those who work with them.

Caritas means not only "love," but also compassion. It is a quality absolutely essential for those treating chronic illness patients, but the patients must also have it for themselves. Only when they have compassion for their suffering selves can they move toward the integrated, meaningful life that will make chronic illness only one aspect of it.

Veritas refers not only to "truth," but also to authenticity, which must be the goal of all chronic illness patients. When patients do not achieve authenticity, they must constantly defend structures they cannot support, thereby undermining what health they have. Clinicians treating the chronically ill must also strive for parallel authenticity if they wish to have the credibility necessary to help their patients.

Finally, *fortitudo* is not simply "strength," but also moral courage. Chronic illness is not easy to endure. Achieving Phase 4 does not relieve patients of pain, suffering, or fear. Their lives require a constant exercise of bravery, rarely seen or celebrated by anyone. Clinicians, too, need courage, for it can be daunting to follow the phase process through with their patients.

It is my hope that this book gives clinicians the help they need to assist their patients in achieving *caritas, veritas,* and *fortitudo* and, with them, better, more meaningful lives.

PART I

CONCEPTUAL OVERVIEW

Chapter 1

A NEW MODEL FOR TREATING THE CHRONICALLY ILL

The *Four-Phase Model* (Fennell, 1993, 1995a, 1998, 2001, 2003a, 2003b, 2003c), a method for assessing and treating the chronically ill, addresses the heterogeneity that characterizes chronic conditions. Although phase or stage models are not in themselves new, this particular model offers a robust, flexible, and comprehensive systems approach and applies it specifically to chronic illness. This approach does not separate chronic illness into a number of separate conditions, but it regards certain factors common to all forms of chronic illness as sharing characteristics that can make the Four-Phase Model a particularly efficacious approach.

Chronic conditions represented by the overall term *chronically ill* include:

- Physiological diseases that most of the medical profession considers chronic illness. These include, but are not limited to, conditions such as diabetes, rheumatoid arthritis, multiple sclerosis, lupus, cystic fibrosis, Sjogrens syndrome, chronic fatigue syndrome (CFS), fibromyalgia (FM), and scleroderma.

- A group of conditions that encompasses diseases where the successes of current treatment have extended the patient's life so that the patient lives with the disease in much the same way a patient in the first category does. These include HIV/AIDS, various cancers and kidney diseases, heart disease, stroke, and orthostatic disease.

- A group of conditions for which the Four-Phase Model may provide useful intervention, including addictions, depression, posttraumatic stress syndrome (PTSD), situations involving intractable pain, and postrape and abuse conditions.

Whereas each condition may have specific medical treatments associated with it, which may differ from those associated with other chronic illnesses, the Four-Phase Method addresses what I consider to be the distinctive characteristics of chronicity that make all chronic conditions particularly difficult to assess and treat successfully with current approaches.

NECESSARY PARADIGM SHIFTS

I believe that in order to evaluate and treat individuals with chronic illness appropriately, it is important to adopt a *systemic approach*. First, it is necessary to acknowledge the intimate interplay that exists between the individual's mind and body. Next, the individual, the individual's family, clinician, workplace, social network, and the overarching community must be seen as dynamic, interactive, interdependent factors within an organic whole (T. Wilson & Holt, 2001). The Four-Phase Model considers that a person's body and mind and his or her family, friends, clinicians, colleagues at work, and community at large are essential contributors to a total environment where changes that occur in one part of the system affect all other parts.

The model described in this book addresses several factors often missed in current approaches to care for the chronically ill. It recognizes the existence of the previously mentioned nested set of systems that a patient inhabits and calls attention to several conceptual dichotomies that frustrate successful patient care. It examines the phenomenon of *chronicity* and the varieties of traumatization that can be experienced by the chronically ill. The approach assumes that patients who successfully navigate the four phases will achieve *integration* rather than cure. Because of this changed goal, clinicians engage in a shift of viewpoint and undertake new activities. In addition to ensuring that their patients receive standard medical care, clinicians following this model seek to provide palliation for their patients, guide them toward strategies for dealing with their life situation, and engage with them in discussions of the philosophical or spiritual dimensions of their situation.

The new model defines four broad phases experienced by the chronically ill—crisis, stabilization, resolution, and integration. For each phase, the model describes the events and responses that typically occur in each context of the patient's life—that is, within the physical and psychological self and within the family, clinical setting, workplace, community, and culture at large—and identifies methods of assessment and treatment for that phase. Each phase also addresses the changing experiences of the clinician and provides direction so that clinicians may best incorporate these changing experiences.

The model recognizes that patients may move backward as well as forward among the phases because lapses of insight or new crises of illness or life situation may return the patient to experiences characteristic of earlier phases (Berg, Evangelista, & Dunbar-Jacob, 2002; Chin, 2002; Prochaska, Norcross, & DiClemente, 1994; Sutton, 1997). After patients and clinicians have negotiated the four phases once, however, they have learned to anticipate the experience of relapse in their illness or untoward new experience; and after the initial shock, they know better how to deal with it (DiClemente, 1991). Whereas they must again use the techniques of earlier phases to address the new issues, the time spent moving into resolution and integration diminishes.

Empirical investigation has demonstrated the validity of the four discrete phases. Outcomes demonstrating clinical efficacy have not been completed (Jason, Fennell, Taylor, Fricano, & Halpert, 2000; Jason, Fricano, et al., 2000; Jason et al., 1999; Van Hoof, Coomins, Cluydts, & de Meirleir, forthcoming-a, forthcoming-b).

THE FOUR-PHASE MODEL AND OTHER PHASE THEORIES

The Four-Phase Model takes the increasingly popular construct of stage theory and revises and expands it to define four phases of adaptation that occur in chronic illnesses. The phases are locations along a passage that patients must navigate on the way to defining a new self and a new life. The model describes the events of chronic illness and the responses to it that typically occur at each phase of the illness experience in the context of the individual's life; that is, the model addresses the physical-behavioral manifestations, the psychological manifestations, and those relating to the social-interactive sphere.

It is important to recognize that for those suffering a chronic condition, the alteration in their lives is *imposed* (Chin, 2002). The Four-Phase Model maps a process that, for the most part, individuals do not enter into willingly. This fact distinguishes the model significantly from stage theories that focus on intentional change in the psychological sphere alone (Prochaska, DiClemente, & Norcross, 1992).

Moreover, throughout this process, individuals suffering chronic conditions are subject to experiences in their physical condition or in their social interactive life over which they have little or no control (Onega & Larsen, 2002). It is primarily in their psychological life that these individuals have experiences and can engage in activities somewhat similar to those of stage models such as Prochaska's Transtheoretical Model of Behavioral Change (TTM; Prochaska, DiClemente, & Norcross, 1992; Prochaska & Velicer, 1997a, 1997b; Prochaska et al., 1994).

Once individuals experience the physical and psychological crisis of illness onset, as well as the social responses this sets in motion, their ability to stabilize usually depends on skilled intervention, which recognizes that certain protocols are more successful during crisis and others during stabilization. When intervention ceases at stabilization, however, or does not address the systemic responses of the individuals' social and work world, many of the chronically ill cycle back from stabilization into crisis again and sometimes simply from crisis to crisis (Chin, 2002). In part, this response expresses the individual's own desire to deny the intolerable aspects of chronicity and the ambiguity of chronic illness and return to the former self and way of life. But, in part, it also occurs because of the individual's response to the social pressure of family, friends, and the workplace to return to the precrisis self. Informed clinicians may facilitate movement out of this relapse cycle into the resolution phase by helping patients learn to understand and develop tolerance for chronicity and ambiguity, to grieve for their losses, and to begin constructing a new and meaningful existence in all the domains of their life—the physical, the psychological, and the social/interactive.

Although the phases are sequential, this model, like some others, recognizes that patients may move backward as well as forward; they may exhibit signs of more than one phase simultaneously; and later crises, whether disease-related or otherwise, may propel patients back into Phase 1 (Berg et al., 2002; Prochaska et al., 1994; Sutton, 1997). When patients have successfully progressed through the four phases once, however, the knowledge they gain during the first passage makes it possible for them to process subsequent crises more swiftly and efficiently. This phenomenon has been noted in other stage models (DiClemente, 1991). Patients more quickly understand what is happening to them, know techniques to help improve their situation, and have the skills to seek and utilize necessary clinical help.

Several decades ago, stage theories became a useful method of organizing information in different fields into typologies, categories, or hierarchical constructs (Erikson, 1959; Kohlberg, 1959; Kübler-Ross, 1969; Piaget, 1952). Such frameworks have had a variety of applications (N. D. Weinstein, Rothman, & Sutton, 1998): They help researchers understand how individuals use medical services (Rakowski et al., 1992), they aid in the adoption of preventive behavior (Blalock et al., 1996), and they suggest how to stop unhealthy behaviors (Brownell, Marlatt, Lichtenstein, & Wilson, 1986; DiClemente, 1991; Prochaska, DiClemente, & Norcross, 1992; Prochaska & Velicer, 1997a; Prochaska et al., 1994). By helping to organize research that might seem unrelated or contradictory when not conceptualized from a stage framework, such models offer important heuristic contributions to scientific and social disciplines. In addition, the models suggest new areas and domains of inquiry, as theorists and investigators use these templates to make more precise, targeted predictions (K. S. Berger & Thompson, 1995).

Among stage-theory models, one type posits a pattern of discrete, sequential stages, where each stage contributes to an invariant developmental sequence. The stages progress hierarchically, with each succeeding stage considered a qualitative advance over the preceding one. The new stage is thought to combine aspects of the previous stage with the current stage's new aspects in a more specialized manner (Rest, 1973).

The Four-Phase Model belongs to a second type, which employs stages as a method for arranging information into specific categories. The model employs the term *phase* rather than *stage* because it does not regard the phases as discrete entities, and patients do not necessarily pass through them only once. Phases can, in fact, recur and may overlap, resulting in more than one phase occurring concurrently (Fennell, 1993, 1995a, 1998, 2001, 2003a, 2003b; Jason et al., 1999; Kübler-Ross, 1969).

The Four-Phase Model posits that when coping with the change imposed by a chronic illness, patients and their families progress through phases, similar in nature to those postulated by Kübler-Ross for individuals experiencing the death of a loved one, as they learn to negotiate the illness experience. The model offers a robust design for understanding how all the elements of change in chronic syndromes operate in both the short and the long term.

Like other stage theories that have argued that matching intervention to stage provides the best outcomes (DiClemente, 1991; Prochaska, DiClemente, & Norcross, 1992; Prochaska & Velicer, 1997a; Prochaska et al., 1994), this model indicates what may be expected over time and indicates the best times and ways to intervene to improve the patient's quality of life. Conversely, interventions attempted at the wrong time may prove less effective and may undermine the possibility of the same interventions being effective at a later phase when the patient would ordinarily be responsive to such interventions (Berg et al., 2002; Woods, Haberman, & Packard, 1993).

Finally, the overall goal of the Four-Phase Model is integration of the illness into the patient's life, not a cure in the traditional sense. One distinctive aspect of integration as the final phase is that integration is not a conclusion. Stage models that deal with dysfunctional or addictive behaviors conclude when participants cease using the substance or exhibiting the behavior. But chronic illness patients never leave the phases. The process of maintaining themselves, ideally in the integration phase, is ongoing. It does not reach an end.

Phase 1 of the Four-Phase Model is characterized by *crisis.* Individuals move from the actual onset of the syndrome to an emergency stage. Its severity typically forces sufferers to seek some form of relief. This relief may take the form of medical, psychological, or spiritual help, but sometimes individuals simply resort to a self-administered anodyne in the form of alcohol or drugs. The task of the individual, the family, and the clinician (if present) during this phase is to cope with the hurt, loss, and potential trauma of the new illness.

Phase 2 is characterized by the search for *stabilization.* Patients continue to experience chaos and dissembling about the illness, but often their symptoms have plateaued and they feel a degree of control returning to their lives. Now their struggle is to fit their condition into their lives. The task of the individual, family, and clinician in the second phase is to initiate stabilization and the restructuring of life patterns and perceptions.

It is my clinical experience that without sustained guidance from a clinician, most patients find themselves either perpetually in crisis (Phase 1) or in an endless loop between the first two phases. Each plateau of stabilization recalls the precrisis "normal" life. Patients want to deny that a permanent change has occurred, and frequently those around them in their home and work life want to deny it as well. The potential trauma, stigma, and loss patients suffer as ill individuals offer no incentive to accepting the illness as a permanent condition and learning to cope with it. When they first plateau in their physical symptoms or develop some *modus vivendi* with them, patients can feel a false sense of relief and are usually anxious to return to life the way it used to be. Often, they are also receiving pressure from others to return to former life patterns and activities. This may encourage them to behave in ways that promote a relapse, but equally often patients suffer relapses because that is the nature of their condition or because of a crisis totally unrelated to the illness. With clinical support and guidance, however, patients can be helped to learn from their relapse experiences (Berg et al., 2002; Prochaska, DiClemente, & Norcross, 1992; Prochaska et al., 1994) and, by doing so, make the very important transition into Phase 3.

Phase 3 is characterized by *resolution*. Patients may experience a plateau of symptoms or suffer relapse, but they have learned how the illness behaves and how the world responds. They realize in a very deep way that their condition is chronic—that it will not end in the foreseeable future. The task of the third phase is for patients to develop meaning in their lives and create a new self as they work to accept the chronicity and ambiguity of the chronic illness experience.

Phase 4, the final phase, is characterized by *integration*. Patients may experience recovery, continued plateau of symptoms, or periods of relapse. But they have now integrated aspects of their preillness self with the person each is now. The task in this phase is to continue to find ways to express a new "personal best"; to reintegrate or form new supportive networks of family and friends; to find other vocations, activities, or appropriate employment if they are able to work; and to locate the illness experience within a larger philosophical or spiritual framework. In the most complete integration, patients have validated the realities of their illness, stabilized and restructured their lives, developed meaning, and come to experience a complete life in which illness is only one aspect (Fennell, 1993, 1995a, 1998, 2001, 2003a, 2003b).

Whereas theories of health behavior change are most typically psychological in focus (Prochaska et al., 1994), the Four-Phase Model does not confine itself to the psychological aspects of adjustment to illness (Fennell, 1993; Kübler-Ross, 1969). In each separate phase, it addresses factors proceeding from the physical-behavioral and social-interactive domains, as well as the psychological, and considers problems associated with stigma and illness traumatization. It also examines factors that arise from social and cultural influences (McCahon & Larsen, 2002). Increasingly, researchers in medical family therapy (Doherty, McDaniel, & Hepworth, 1994) and others, such as Wellard (1998) and Henderson (1997), are moving in this direction.

No person exists solely as an illness. At the same time that individuals are navigating the process of an illness—which in chronic illness usually means for the rest of their lives—they are also moving through the developmental and maturation arcs that occur in every life. Simultaneously, they carry out continually changing patterns of activity that include self-care, school, job, care of others, and many other activities. In addition, the personal energy process, which shifts over time and with regard to influences other than health, intersects with the chronic illness experience. These developmental and activity processes are discussed in greater depth in subsequent chapters.

It is also essential in the Four-Phase Model to consider external social and cultural issues because they have a profound impact on the experience of chronic illness. Poverty, violence, discrimination, lack of social support, multiple homes or schools, learning disabilities, and abuse are issues that can make it extremely difficult to negotiate a chronic illness experience as well. Nonetheless, in a fashion similar to the TTM model, the four-phase structure allows clinicians to identify those places and times when it is possible to make meaningful interventions that can permit a patient to escape from an endless loop through successive crises (Prochaska, DiClemente, & Norcross, 1992; Prochaska & Velicer, 1997a; Prochaska et al., 1994). Although the effectiveness of matched interventions and the lack of efficacy of mismatched interventions have yet to be demonstrated empirically, my clinical experience and that of the people trained in this approach initially support the assertion.

Some factors provide positive support for patients. Patients may have always been physically robust before the illness and have had strong recuperative powers. Patients may be psychologically hardy and adaptable. They may enjoy a positive and supportive environment in the form of family, friends, self-help groups, church groups, community organizations, civil rights organizations, and feminist groups. All these social elements can help to integrate those with chronic illnesses into meaningful life with other people.

Some of the salient literature on adaptation to chronic illness focuses primarily on the patient's response to the initial diagnosis (Greer, Morris, & Pettingdale, 1979). The Four-Phase Model describes the experience of the chronically ill over time without being confined to a unidirectional process.

Increasingly, others are paying attention to changes that occur in patients as they continue to live with a chronic illness (Henderson, 1997; J. Lewis, 1999; Rolland, 1987; Wellard, 1998). But even these analyses describe a trajectory for the unidirectional process, whereas the Four-Phase Model incorporates instances of relapse, overlap of phases, and return to crisis. Wellard suggests that the trajectory model may be an error resulting from the deeply ingrained preference of clinicians for achieving cures. In contrast, J. Lewis (1999) suggests that the HIV patients undergoing her "status passages" may move back to a prior status if they experience a remission in symptoms, but at the present time her conception appears applicable only to this specific illness.

Unlike most change theorists, who posit an eventual end to the adjustment process and an end to relapses (Brownell et al., 1986; N. D. Weinstein et al., 1998), the Four-Phase Model views chronic illness as a cyclical experience (Fennell, 1993, 1995a, 1998, 2001, 2003a, 2003b). Even though patients have successfully achieved the psychological and social integration goals of Phase 4, it is possible that relapses or untoward life experiences may return them to an earlier phase. Other stage theorists describe a similar spiral phenomenon in the relapsing behavior of addicts, but their model suggests that relapsers do not cycle endlessly and do not necessarily regress back to the beginning (Brownell et al., 1986; Donovan & Marlatt, 1988; Prochaska, DiClemente, & Norcross, 1992; Prochaska et al., 1994). Instead, they postulate that the addicts learn from their mistakes and can apply different strategies during subsequent attempts to end their addiction (Prochaska, DiClemente, & Norcross, 1992; Prochaska et al., 1994). The Four-Phase Model posits similar learning from past mistakes in the movement through the phases but also asserts that chronic illness patients are never immune from the possibility of being thrown back into a prior phase or into crisis. Following one successful navigation of the four phases, however, such revisitations to earlier phases tend to be partial and of shorter duration than the original progression.

Each different population uses the Four-Phase Model in a different way. For patients and their families, the model helps them to organize a narrative of their experience. Narratives appear to be a very useful coping tool (Neimeyer & Levitt, 2001; Nochi, 2000). The understanding that the narrative gives can reduce fear and anxiety for both patients and their families. The unknown becomes more known and, through the descriptive structure of the phase narrative, patients make sense of their distressing experiences. As ambiguity and chaos diminish, patients gain a degree of coherence about their experiences.

They have a method of validating their experiences, stabilizing and structuring their responses, developing meaning for their experiences, and ultimately developing a full, complete life. The narrative offers roles for patients and their families to assume, giving them a positive framework within which to construct new lives.

For the empirical investigator, the Four-Phase Model provides a template that reconciles diverse phenomena into an integrated, unified construct, potentially permitting a better understanding of the widely divergent experiences of patients with chronic illness. Prochaska, DiClemente, Velicer, and Rossi (1992), authors of the most popular and arguably the most thoroughly researched theory of stage-based behavioral change, have lamented the lack of research on other forms of behavioral change and an analysis of how these forms resemble or differ from their own. Fortunately, the investigation of stage/phase approaches seems to be increasing (Rolland, 1994; Wellard, 1998).

One commentator has noted that clinicians begin working with methods that seem right and valuable—if they do no harm—before they have empirical evidence that demonstrates the efficacy of their approach. He comments that scientific evidence rarely precedes policy and practical developments in the real world (Heather, 1992). Another commentator added that there was no evidence for the effectiveness of Miller's groundbreaking article on motivational interviewing, only a conceptual framework and a practical set of counseling strategies that made sense and could be put into practice immediately (Stockwell, 1992).

In a review article, Prochaska and colleagues allude to the large number of individuals suffering from the problems they address (Prochaska, Velicer, Fava, Rossi, & Tsoh, 2001). With half the population of the United States suffering with at least one chronic illness (Hoffman, Rice, & Sung, 1996), it seems that research resulting in best practice in this area would be of great benefit.

For the clinician, the Four-Phase Model has three specific applications:

1. The model includes phase-specific assessment steps and interventions to help patient and family meet the tasks at hand (Prochaska, DiClemente, & Norcross, 1992; Prochaska & Velicer, 1997a; Prochaska et al., 1994; Woods et al., 1993).

2. It also integrates the assessment steps and interventions into a broad collection of spiritual and philosophical traditions, such as Buddhism and Jungian psychology, as well as with more contemporary therapies.

3. Finally, this phase model provides a framework for using the therapist's or clinician's countertransference experiences.

UNDERLYING ASSUMPTIONS OF THE MODEL

Most of the assumptions of this model are neither novel nor original. The model draws on a variety of approaches and philosophies in clinical care and employs a systems approach.

Body-Mind Integration

The model uses a holistic paradigm based on the concept that body and mind are integrated and that all illnesses involve both soma and psyche to greater or lesser extents. This holds true whether the illness is heart disease, lupus, or multiple sclerosis and whether the initial presentation is of physiological symptoms or of psychological ones. The Four-Phase Model assumes that there are psychological components to physical illnesses and physiological components to illnesses defined as psychological. Clinicians review each patient from the perspective of both body and mind, regardless of the symptoms that brought the patient to the clinician initially and despite the focus of the clinician's primary training. Those trained to treat psychological disease consider physiological problems, whereas those trained to treat physical disease examine for psychological factors. All providers must then ensure that treatment covers whatever is necessary for the entire body-mind system (Doherty et al., 1994; T. Wilson & Holt, 2001).

Throughout this book, the term *clinician* is used to cover a broad range of health care practitioners including medical doctors, psychiatrists, psychologists, medical/clinical social workers, counselors, therapists, and others, rather than repeatedly listing the array of practitioners who might function in a particular context. In some instances where only one or two disciplines would be able to perform the function mentioned, either the particular specialty or the term *clinician* may be used.

The Patient-Family System

The patient is not only an individual body-mind system, but also part of a family (Woods et al., 1993). It is important to note here that the concept of family includes both the patient's biological and marital relatives and any individuals whom the patient considers as his or her family. To be effective, clinicians include the patient's family, however constructed, both in assessment and in treatment. The physiological and psychological symptoms that the patient experiences have a direct impact on the family, and the family's response has, in turn, a direct impact on the patient (Beardslee, Versage, & Gladstone, 1998; Bull & Jervis, 1997; Doherty et al., 1994; Falicov, 1988; Henderson, 1997; Nicassio & Smith, 1995; Travis & Piercy, 2002; Yeheskel, Biderman, Borkan, & Herman, 2000).

The Patient-Family System in the Community and Workplace

Chronically ill patients and their families are inextricably involved in larger communities, particularly in their various places of work. All the mutual interactions that occur between patients and their families also take place among patients, their families, and their larger communities and workplaces. A patient's illness may disrupt work schedules for both patient and family members and may result in lost income, conflicts in relationships both at home and at work, and overall stress. Coworkers, employers, or others in the community may respond in ways that multiply negative social, psychological, and physiological symptoms (Lubkin & Larsen, 2002; Roessler & Sumner, 1997; Satcher, 1992; Satcher & Hendren, 1991; Scambler & Hopkins, 1990; Ware, 1998).

In addition, patients diagnosed with the same chronic illness may have widely varying experiences because they differ from one another as to income level, class, ethnicity, race, sexual orientation, education, and other demographic issues (Anderton, Elfert, & Lai, 1989; W. F. Auslander, Thompson, Dreitzer, White, & Santiago, 1997; Blum, Potthoff, & Resnick, 1997; Heijmans & de Ridder, 1998; Henly, Tyree, Lindsey, Lambeth, & Burd, 1998; J. Lewis, 1999; Penninx et al., 1999; Scambler & Hopkins, 1990; Siegel, Raveis, & Karus, 1997; Woodgate, 1998).

The Patient-Family System and the Clinician

Patients and their families are embedded in the health care system most noticeably through the person of their primary clinician. The clinician is an active part of the health care system, which in turn is an integral part of the patient's family and community system. Along with providing or failing to provide appropriate treatment for the patient, the clinician also defines the patient's condition both for the patient and for the community at large. This definition dramatically affects how the patient will think about himself or herself and how the world will respond to the patient (Anderton et al., 1989; Doherty et al., 1994; Nicassio & Smith, 1995; Scambler & Hopkins, 1990; Tait, Chibnall, & Richardson, 1990).

Embedded Systems and Holistic Assessment and Treatment

Because the different systems interact and have impact on one another, assessment and treatment that focus on the patient alone, apart from all the other systems, may be more susceptible to failure. Each system can reduce, magnify, and sometimes even create symptoms in the patient or in individuals associated with the patient. Patients with difficult problems often have a correspondingly profound effect on the clinicians, their workplaces, and their communities. Problems can continuously transmute and multiply unless clinicians use a systemic holistic approach (Doherty et al., 1994; Nicassio & Smith, 1995).

Many contemporary approaches to medical problems consider themselves *holistic.* The Four-Phase Model uses this term more inclusively than is sometimes the case. Holistic in this model includes more than the body-mind continuum or the importance of philosophical or spiritual factors, though these are obviously important. In addition, this model examines the practical institutions and worlds that affect a patient. It takes into consideration, in both assessment and treatment, a broad range of economic and cultural issues from lost wages and what treatments health maintenance organizations (HMOs) will cover to destructive or misleading attitudes projected by the national media.

Poverty and the Socially Disadvantaged

The poor and disadvantaged suffer disproportionately from chronic illness (Lubkin & Larsen, 2002; Hardin, 2002), yet they have far fewer resources than middle-class people have to help deal with the illnesses. Some middle-class individuals suffer a drastic reduction in income because of their chronic illness and are forced to deal with issues of poverty and lack of access to health care in addition to their illness. Health expenses are the leading cause of personal bankruptcy in the United States, and although many people are devastated by the expenses of catastrophic acute illnesses, many others become impoverished because of chronic illness (Jacoby, Sullivan, & Warren, 2001; Warren, Sullivan, & Jacoby, 2000). Even if poor patients have access to medical care, the services they need may not be available to them. Language and cultural issues may raise further barriers to adequate assessment and treatment. Lack of education may also make some therapies difficult because many interventions require a level of verbal communication that depends in large part on patient and clinician sharing class, educational, and sociocultural backgrounds.

Increasingly, communities are beginning to experiment with new methods of delivering necessary services and support to the chronically ill (Jason, Fennell, & Taylor, 2003); and as chronic illness becomes more widely recognized, public clinics such as CURE, run by Johns Hopkins in East Baltimore, are developing methods of dealing with this patient population. Clinics and public social services recognize the importance of language and cultural assumptions and attempt to get input and assistance from other members of the patient's community. The Four-Phase Model emphasizes the necessity for clinician and patient to form a strong bond that can take place only if clinicians understand or learn about the cultural imperatives in their patients' lives.

CONCEPTUAL DICHOTOMIES

The model presented in this book assumes that previous clinical and scientific approaches have often created conceptual dichotomies in patient care (Riska, 2000; Thornton, 1998; Walter, 2000). These include mind as opposed to body, clinical approaches and realities as opposed to empirical constructs and related findings, *illness* as opposed to *disease,* professional activity as opposed to personal involvement, and clinician as opposed to patient.

Such dualistic thinking has plagued the culture of health care since the Enlightenment. In the Cartesian split of mind from body, physiological, observable, and material things became acceptable objects of medical investigation, whereas psychological, nonobservable, and immaterial things were not (S. L. Baumann, 1997; Bendelow & Williams, 1995; Epstein, Quill, & McWhinney, 1999; Gamsa, 1994; Kirmayer, Robbins, & Paris, 1994; Stuart & Noyes, 1999; Vaughan, 1994). The division included in the province of *mind* everything moral and character-related, leaving medicine to examine only those things connected with the physical being. The actual and observable could be viewed as *real,* or legitimate, whereas nonmaterial processes "existing only in the mind" were *unreal,* and hence not legitimate medical issues. Although in the past 25 years, the health care profession in general and behavioral medicine in particular have made great strides in understanding the interaction of mind and body, the cultural assumption that the two are distinct still subtly or openly persists in much clinical practice.

Body-Mind

Much as the Age of Reason and the Enlightenment helped to establish rigorous scientific analysis, this particular distinction has sometimes served to obscure what actually happens in clinical situations with actual illnesses.

In the seventeenth century, scientists arrived at a territorial agreement with the Church whereby the human body would belong to the province of science, and the less determinable mind and immortal soul would be the province of the Church. Scientists at first regarded the parts assigned to the Church as things that were unknowable by reason, and hence not necessary to their pursuits, and more subtly as things of lesser or diminished importance. What occurred in the mind or soul belonged in the realm of imagination or fancy, whereas physical things were real and could be investigated objectively. Measurable physiological symptoms came to be the only reliable indicators for disease, at least those treated by doctors who were men of science. As scientific and materialist thinking began to dominate cultural conceptions, most people came to share these attitudes, especially about health. Any health issue thought to proceed from a person's mind or soul was in some fashion imaginary or willed, unlike conditions with clear physical causes and symptoms. Inevitably, an imagined or willed illness seemed to many to indicate a failure in the patient's character, if it was not intended fraudulence.

Even after the late nineteenth century, when psychological conditions began to be acceptable as areas of scientific medical study and treatment, they continued to be regarded with suspicion by many in the medical community. Even today, measurable chemical changes in brain chemistry make mental conditions more acceptably medical than conditions for which there are no physical markers. Finally, there is always the possibility that nebulous or irregular symptoms are imagined and may indicate malingering or some other character flaw.

A somewhat negative evaluation of psyche persists in the term *somatization* (Epstein et al., 1999; McCahill, 1995; Stuart & Noyes, 1999). A patient with a psychological condition who manifests physiological symptoms is conceived as having consciously or unconsciously created them from the arena of psyche, whereas a *genuinely* sick person is the innocent victim of physical symptoms caused by completely mechanical or external and undesired agents. Medical personnel frequently determine that patients who manifest intermittent or hard-to-measure physiological symptoms that do not immediately fit into a standard diagnostic category are psychologically ill and creating their physiological symptoms, or somatizing. This is not to say that somatization is without merit as a clinical description. But despite the desire of clinicians to remain objective and nonjudgmental, for some, a *somatized* physical symptom is not in the same category as a *real* physical symptom (Salmon, Peters, & Stanley, 1999).

Chronic illnesses expose the deep flaws of the body-mind split, which is one reason they can make observers so uncomfortable. Despite the fact that today many people, even or especially those in health care, acknowledge that body and mind are inextricably intermixed, the Cartesian split still exists, dividing body from mind and permitting unfortunate and damaging judgments to flourish.

Disease-Illness

A growing dichotomy in the health care field is the one between disease and illness. Everyday language tends to use these two terms interchangeably, but it is useful to distinguish them in a way that will help illuminate an aspect of clinical treatment (Anderton et al., 1989; Durban, Lazar, & Ofer, 1993; Epstein et al., 1999; Ridson & Edey, 1999; White & Lubkin, 1995).

The traditional medical community diagnoses and treats disease. That is, the patient has identifiable physical symptoms (pain, rash, fever, swelling, etc.) that clearly fit established causes (virus, bacteria, physical trauma) for defined sicknesses or conditions (flu, measles, broken leg), and the medical practitioner attempts to return the patient to his or her previous, "normal" state.

Increasingly, however, a growing number of care providers who must deal with more intractable or long-term conditions are seeking to treat "illness" in addition to disease. That is, they try to treat the patient's psychological and social experience and the overall experience of suffering as well as the defined disease. This approach, it can be argued, treats the entire person. It considers the individual's various life experiences in addition to his or her medicalized body. It includes the individual's family system, work situation, and community setting (T. Wilson & Holt, 2001). Within the illness framework, clinicians use the patient's cultural and philosophical or spiritual context, as well as social context, to evaluate that individual's experience of illness. By examining the patient's total experience, the clinician greatly enhances the effectiveness of treatment.

Empirical-Clinical

It has been argued that a gulf separates the people who investigate the causes and treatments of chronic illness and those who actually treat the chronically ill. The disconnect and lack of communication that can exist between empirical investigators and clinicians mean that important new information and understanding about treatment is poorly distributed. This division grows wider as some protocols that have not been empirically investigated have become increasingly popular. This has created even greater distance and, to a certain extent, greater distrust between those who investigate chronic illnesses and those who treat them (Irvine, Phillips, Fisher, & Cloonan, 1989; Ivanoff, Robinson, & Blythe, 1987; Kontz, 1989; Singer, 1995).

Professional-Personal

People educated traditionally in the provision of medical care are usually trained to hold themselves apart emotionally from their patients so that they will be able to make objective, clear assessments and provide effective care. The underlying assumption is that emotional engagement with patients clouds the clinicians' judgment and thereby damages or destroys their effectiveness. Even those who receive psychological training are urged to maintain distance from their patients for the same reasons (Collins, 1994; Durana, 1998; Durban et al., 1993; Hirschauer, 1991; Lang, 1990; Levinson et al., 1999; Ridson & Edey, 1999).

Traditional training often includes discussion of *countertransference*. Clinicians are informed about reactions they may feel in response to patients' issues or experiences, but until relatively recently, they were instructed that having these feelings—that is, experiencing countertransference—was rare and not to be indulged or encouraged. Even today, training in the physiological or psychological domain of medicine tends to assume that emotional distance is the clinicians' most desirable stance (Collins, 1994; Counselman & Alonzo, 1993; Durban et al., 1993; Hirschauer, 1991; Lang, 1990; Levinson et al., 1999; Mitrani, 1993; Ridson & Edey, 1999; Roter et al., 1997). Some change is occurring in this area, which can only be applauded. Many clinicians are now taught that personal reactions to patients do occur regularly and that clinicians should acknowledge and manage their personal feelings.

Not surprisingly, therefore, some patients complain that their providers are impersonal, cold, distant, unfeeling, and fail to communicate with them well (Armstrong, 1987; Barnett, 1998; Lang, 1990; Roberts, 2000). They assert that the providers do not understand them or relate to them or care for them in the broad emotional sense of the term *care*. As a consequence, the patients often do not trust the providers or believe that their treatment will be effective. Patients with chronic problems, who continue to experience symptoms regardless of treatment, often manifest their distrust of and lack of relationship with medical practitioners by shopping for clinicians, going from one to another in an attempt to find someone who will help them and make them feel cared for (Marbach, 1999; Schlesinger, Druss, & Thomas, 1999).

Americans expect clinicians to care for their patients, not simply to assess and treat them, and most traditional medical providers claim that they do care for their patients in addition to maintaining the objectivity demanded by their training (A. O. Baumann, Deber, Silverman, & Mallette, 1998; Harder, Kelly, & Dunkelblau, 1997; Lang, 1990; Roberts, 2000; Roter et al., 1997). Medical personnel say that they strive to act in a warm, caring manner but that it has become increasingly difficult in the current health care environment, where economic market concerns, over which they have decreasing control, continuously shorten the time they may devote to any individual patient (Gordon, Baker, & Levinson, 1995; Harder et al., 1997; Levinson et al., 1999; Ware, Lachicotte, Kirschner, Cortes, & Good, 2000). Health maintenance organizations seek to increase productivity—health care professionals seeing more patients in the same time frame—and, at the same time, they require increased substantiation and documentation of examinations and procedures. In determining how best to serve patients, doctors often feel they have no choice but to focus on measurable assessment and treatment activities rather than on forming relationships with patients, an activity often perceived as time consuming (Fishman, 2001).

Patients continue to insist, however, that they want a personal relationship. When asked, for example, why they seek alternative medical care, most patients include their perceptions that the alternative practitioners are caring and courteous (Hastings Center Report, 2000; Kelner & Wellman, 1997; Neuberger & Woods, 1995).

Another result of restraining personal response to remain "objective" is that patients turn into examples of their disease. They cease to exist as individual human beings of the same sort as the medical practitioner (Levinson et al.,

1999; Mitrani, 1993; Pilnick & Hindmarsh, 1999; Roberts, 2000; Schiller, Crystal, & Lewellen, 1994). Although this may be necessary to help the health care provider endure the horrible news that an assessment may bring, the pain or suffering the necessary treatment may require, or even the annoyance or anger the patient may stimulate in the clinician, separating the patient into a category apart from the medical practitioner ultimately hurts the patient. The patient becomes a different "class" of person from the clinician, one whose pain, suffering, confusion, and terror are not of the same kind or quality as the clinician might feel.

The Four-Phase Model encourages clinicians to consider their own individual natures and their own subjective responses in both assessment and treatment of the chronically ill. The approach asserts that part of clinicians' role is to monitor their own and their patients' subjective needs continuously and to seek to employ these observations and understandings to broaden their assessment and enhance treatment. The more clinicians review their own inner experience and harness their reactions positively, the more they can increase their relatedness with patients and hence their effectiveness (Emanuel, 1995; Howe, 1995; Lazare, 1987; T. Lewis, Amini, & Lannon, 2000). Clinicians must, of course, bear in mind the issues of appropriate boundaries between practitioner and patient and, in some instances, legal issues.

Clinician-Patient

The dichotomy between clinician and patient grows out of the division encouraged between the clinician as a professional and as a feeling individual (Harder et al., 1997; M. Rosenberg & Molho, 1998). All too often this distinction can transmute into the notion that there is an intrinsic difference between those who provide care and those who receive it. The distinctiveness of the clinician is reflected in behavior both on and off professional duty. Some have explained this separateness by arguing that in addition to medical providers' needing to remain objective, they also need to develop and maintain a strong, separate ego to carry out their work. Given the life and death decisions they make, professionals in the health care world, even nurses and technicians, have an aura of special powers. This tends to keep medical providers elevated above patients and isolated from them (Fugelli, 1998; Loewe, Schwartzman, Freeman, Quinn, & Zuckerman, 1998; Mitrani, 1993).

Patients and the public at large have helped to establish medical practitioners on a higher, separate plane because the public wants to believe that their medical providers will always be able to rid them of pain, suffering, and danger. When the medical world fails, as it often must, people generally prefer to blame the patient rather than the doctor and medical science. They prefer to assume that if they were sick, their better attitudes or behavior, in conjunction with the doctor's skill or the pill's efficacy, would produce a cure in them and that failure lies in the patient, not the doctor (Ax, Gregg, & Jones, 1998; Ballweg, 1997; M. S. Bates & Rankin-Hill, 1994; M. S. Bates, Rankin-Hill, & Sanchez-Ayendez, 1997; Epstein et al., 1999; Kirmayer et al., 1994; McCahill, 1995; Morse, 1997; Stuart & Noyes, 1999; Thorne, 1990; Turk & Rudy, 1991).

Not only does this separation damage individual relationships between care provider and patient, but it also hurts the general community (Barshay, 1993; M. S. Bates et al., 1997; Ware, 1998). It leads to unrealistic expectations about prognoses in illnesses and harmful judgments of the chronically ill. In addition, the distance between medical provider and recipient can be further exacerbated by a perception that lack of a caring relationship between clinician and patient is economically motivated (Barnett, 1998; M. S. Bates, 1990; DiMatteo, 1998; Safran et al., 2000; Ware et al., 2000).

At the same time that medical treatment has succeeded in curing an increasing number of acute conditions, the number of chronic illnesses among all age groups has soared. In addition, improved medicine has turned some previously acute conditions into chronic ones (Do Rozario, 1997; Heinzer, 1998). With the average life span in developed nations extending into the 80s and some people living well beyond that, more and more of the general population will eventually experience chronic illness, including health care providers (Barshay, 1993; Elliot, 1996; McReynolds, 1998). All parts of the population will be affected. Children who were ill will survive and become providers. Clinicians who have worked as medical professionals will experience chronic illness and disability and receive care from others, especially in their old age (Barshay, 1993; Counselman & Alonzo, 1993; Durban et al., 1993; Elliot, 1996). One way or another, most people not only will experience a chronic illness, but also will have to help care for someone who is chronically ill. Without doubt, this will increase their understanding of what clinicians are trying to achieve with the chronically ill. Those who receive care and those who provide it will become increasingly interchangeable.

In today's world, the upper-, middle-, and lower-class divisions in health care are collapsing into one increasingly overburdened health care system, and this, too, is bound to affect the quality of care adversely. Yet, it is possible that this very collapse may also help to heal the split between clinician and patient (Casey, 1999; Rauber, 1998; Rosenbaum, 2000).

THE PHENOMENON OF CHRONICITY

The following dichotomies position chronicity in the contemporary cultural context.

Acute versus Chronic Illness

In the history of modern Western medicine, the focus has been on acute diseases, that is, on conditions that have a single clear cause, a specific onset, identifiable symptoms, usually a single treatment, and ultimately a cure (Lubkin & Larsen, 2002). Until about 75 years ago, Americans did not have to consider chronic illnesses very closely because people simply did not live long enough. It is true that in the past some people spent a great part of their lives as "invalids," either with recognized conditions such as gout or dropsy or with unspecified ones, such as often disabling "female complaints." But for most of the population, those who fell sick either recovered—with or without medical assistance—or they died. The same was true for those who were injured. This is no longer true. For the first time ever in history, people are living long enough so that chronic disease is becoming common.

Americans have, as yet, a cultural intolerance of chronic illness. This proceeds in part from Western culture's enduring philosophical split between body and mind. In part, it results from the cultural assumption of health as a normative state and illness as a disruption of the normative (Thornton, 1998). But it also comes about because medical practitioners frequently do not actually observe the ebbs and flows, the relapses and remissions, of chronic illness (M. S. Bates et al., 1997; Epstein et al., 1999; Kane, 1996; Robinson, 1990; Rood, 1996). It is hard to understand the appearance and disappearance of symptoms, especially when clinicians do not actually see them, and it is particularly frustrating, and thus hard to credit, that symptoms keep changing over time. The chronically ill individual often has to report on his or her condition, rather than the symptoms being patently obvious to the clinician or accessible via clinical tests. But self-reporting is subject to question if unaccompanied by other "hard" data. For the most part, only those symptoms observed by the clinician during a medical visit are considered real and then only because they can be observed by the trained, objective clinician. Self-reporting is also suspect because it is tainted by the patient's psychological reactions (M. S. Bates et al., 1997; Heijmans & de Ridder, 1998; McCahill, 1995; Robinson, 1990; Stuart & Noyes, 1999; Turk & Rudy, 1991).

Chronic illnesses, moreover, frequently do not have single clear causes. They do not exhibit simple beginnings, middles, and conclusions. Instead, patients go through cycles of relapse and remission. Chronic illnesses are also frequently hard to treat (Ax et al., 1998; M. S. Bates et al., 1997; Epstein et al., 1999; Mayer, 1999). When a condition does not fit into an acute framework, the system tends to regard it as psychologically based, inorganic, and potentially not legitimate medical business (Ax et al., 1998; Ballweg, 1997; M. S. Bates & Rankin-Hill, 1994; M. S. Bates et al., 1997; Epstein et al., 1999; Gamsa, 1994; Kirmayer et al., 1994; Komaroff et al., 1996; Mayer, 1999; McCahill, 1995; Reis, Hermoni, Borkan, & Biderman, 1999; Stuart & Noyes, 1999). Calling an illness psychological is sometimes simply a way to assert that the illness may not really exist and may, in fact, be an issue of character (Ax et al., 1998; Ballweg, 1997; M. S. Bates & Rankin-Hill, 1994; D. W. Bates et al., 1993; Gamsa, 1994; Kirmayer et al., 1994; McCahill, 1995; Stuart & Noyes, 1999).

Illness as Anomaly versus Illness as Normal Life

In the traditional cultural framework, illness is viewed as unusual or anomalous (Thornton, 1998). In reality, members of all families, workplaces, and communities will experience illness and disability. Illness is just as sure as death and occurs more frequently, a fact society ignores just as relentlessly as it ignores death (Fugelli, 1998). Despite the current awareness that health care is a necessity for everyone and despite the great political debate raging over appropriate forms of health care insurance, health care issues themselves are viewed as something merely possible in life, not as something inevitable (Fugelli, 1998; Ware, 1998). Insurance and hospital promotional materials celebrate their maintenance of *wellness,* not their care of disease. Because Americans consider illness an anomaly, rather than a fact of normal life, they are ill prepared to deal with chronic illness either in themselves or in others.

Given the increasing numbers of people with chronic illness, the culture must come to a new understanding of what is a natural eventuality. Chronic illness needs to become something for which people are emotionally and intellectually prepared and for which they plan, the same way they plan for children or education or retirement. The society needs to develop a language and behavior for open discussion of chronic illness, as well as methods for coping with it (Burckhardt, 1987).

Static versus Dynamic Disabilities

Over recent decades, American society has developed a radically new attitude toward people with disabilities, which it has even solidified into law (Remsburg & Carson, 2002). Wheelchair access that is commonplace today would have been unthinkable in 1950. But the culture, including the world of health care research and care provision, still lacks an awareness that many illnesses are disabling and thus create disabilities (Rolland, 1994) and that disabilities can be dynamic as well as static or unchanging.

Consider a man who has lost his leg. Once his initial physiological trauma is resolved, most people think of his situation as being a fairly static one. Day by day, his disability varies little. Except for secondary physical complications or new forms of technology to assist him, the man's disability will remain the same for the rest of his life.

However, a growing population of the disabled includes what can be called the *dynamic disabled*. These include patients with conditions such as HIV/AIDS, CFS, or FM and, increasingly, patients with lupus, multiple sclerosis, and even cancer. These patients have disabilities, but they are not fixed or static because the patients' symptoms ebb and flow cyclically as their conditions relapse and remit (Bergquist & Neuberger, 2002; Komaroff et al., 1996; Rood, 1996; Ware, 1999). The manifestation of their disabilities can be said to be dynamic.

Some people have combinations of dynamic and static disabilities, requiring clinicians to maintain awareness of both conditions in one individual. In addition, some disabilities can be worsened by physical or social stressors. Stress, for example, is known to exacerbate the symptoms of lupus or multiple sclerosis (Cannon & Cavanaugh, 1998; Gatchel & Gardea, 1999; Ware & Kleinman, 1992). And even though the stress of external events would not change the disability inherent in the loss of a leg, it could well have a significant effect on intermittent chronic pain suffered by the man who had lost the leg.

Clinical Concerns of Chronicity

Most models of Western care approach illness as though it were acute. Protocols for physical and psychological evaluation tend to stress the presenting problem that the patient is experiencing during the clinical visit (Armstrong, 1987; M. S. Bates, 1990; Gamsa, 1994; Macintyre, Ford, & Hunt, 1999; Reis et al., 1999). Symptoms that the patient experiences at times other than the clinical visit may be dismissed as unreal. Patients may even be suspected of fabricating or exaggerating symptoms (Ballweg, 1997; M. S. Bates et al., 1997; Gamsa, 1994; Kirmayer et al., 1994; Marbach, Lennon, Link, & Dohrenwend, 1990; Mayer, 1999; McCahill, 1995; Rood, 1996; Stuart & Noyes, 1999). Such a binary model—the patient either exhibiting symptoms (presumed to occur most of the time) or no symptoms (because they are not seen in the office)—will not support any primary clinician trying to provide quality care to chronically ill patients.

The acute model of disease has recovery as its goal (Cameron & Gregor, 1987; Cooper, 1990). Even when recovery is assumed to include a prolonged rehabilitation period and is thus weeks or months away, ultimate recovery is still assumed. When recovery does not occur and, in fact, the patient's illness is *chronically dynamic* and continues to proceed through cycles of relapse and remission, it is understandable that clinicians may experience each relapse or the unchanged illness state as representative of patient failure. Frustrated medical providers, if they are convinced that their treatment has been appropriate and should be effective, may come to locate the failure in the patient, who may be seen as resisting care, even sabotaging it (Ballweg, 1997; Barnett, 1998; M. S. Bates et al., 1997; Kirmayer et al., 1994; Kontz, 1989; McCahill, 1995; Rood, 1996; Turk & Rudy, 1991). Again, the clinician may suspect that the patient's original symptoms were of psychological origin or perhaps simply reveal a defect of character.

This form of clinical response exists on a continuum of disbelief. Within the acute model framework, once the clinician determines that the patient is not recovering, he or she can relegate the problem to the psychological realm. The patient will then fit conveniently into a schema that begins with denial, moves on to resistance, continues to somatization or conversion, and finally arrives at malingering and moral or character failure (Anderton et al., 1989; Ballweg, 1997; Cameron & Gregor, 1987; Kirmayer et al., 1994; McCahill, 1995; Stuart & Noyes, 1999; Turk & Rudy, 1991).

At the same time, patients treated according to an acute model of care have expectations that are not appropriate to a chronic illness (Benet, 1996; Durban et al., 1993; Rood, 1996; Turk & Rudy, 1991). Most people have been culturally trained to expect an immediate, unambiguous diagnosis, followed by a treatment that provides immediate relief, preferably through the administration of a drug. With the medical advances of the past several generations, patients have come to expect medical miracles. When they don't experience one, they are confused and disappointed. People no longer have cultural expectations of suffering, whether physical, psychological, or social, and they resist and resent any health treatment that requires lifestyle changes. They certainly do not expect to have to change their lives dramatically, let alone permanently (M. S. Bates & Rankin-Hill, 1994; M. Rosenberg & Molho, 1998; Thorne & Patterson, 1998). Understandably, in an acute model of illness, a severely relapsing patient very likely assumes that a relapse after eight years of tenuous improvement is the result of either a personal or clinical failure, when instead it could, in a phase model of chronic illness, be a probability that the patient could plan for.

Although the situation is gradually changing, most clinicians and patients are not yet trained to perform as joint partners in health care (Alonzo, 2000; M. S. Bates & Rankin-Hill, 1994; M. Rosenberg & Molho, 1998; Thorne & Patterson, 1998). Both parties expect that the clinician will find a cause and eventually provide a cure. When both groups are forced to accept new roles in the management of chronic illness—in which the clinician has a decreased level of control and the patient an increased responsibility of management and thus control—the situation can be equally uncomfortable for clinician and patient.

Empirical Concerns Relating to Chronicity

Clinical investigations are also dedicated to an acute model of care. Data are collected from the patient population at a particular point in time, which establish that the patient population has a particular set of symptoms. Even when data are collected several times in a longitudinal study, they still may not capture the characteristic waxing and waning of symptoms in chronic illness. Many patients in a study may not be experiencing all the typical symptoms at any discrete instance of data collection (Armstrong, 1987; Buchwald, Pascualy, Bombardier, & Kith, 1994; Komaroff et al., 1996; McGorry, Webster, Snook,

& Hsiang, 2000; Turk & Rudy, 1991). When the empirical framework takes an essentially binary approach—the simple presence or absence of a set group of symptoms—it does not necessarily capture the chronic illness experience.

Moreover, the acute model fails the empiricist because chronic patients are gathered into one undifferentiated group. Some chronic patients with the same condition offer few usefully similar symptoms or patterns of symptom. The acute model fails to distinguish the distinctly different symptoms and responses that appear in particular phases of chronic illness or disability (Friedberg & Jason, 1998; Jason, Fricano, et al., 2000).

In fairness to the scientific community, as mentioned before, the necessity to develop models of chronic care is fairly recent. At the turn of the century, individuals expected to live 50 or 60 years, assuming that they survived a host of childhood diseases. It was only later in the twentieth century that Americans came to stay alive for such a long time. Thanks to advances in public sanitation, in the pharmaceutical industry, and in technologically driven assessment and surgical procedures, they can expect to live into their late 70s and early 80s.

As the baby boomers, a huge demographic group, continue to age, the percentage of the population with chronic illness can be expected to soar. Furthermore, it is reasonable to assume that members of the aging population will have more than one chronic illness. Thus, it is imperative to develop effective models of chronic care that include protocols for assessment, treatment, and management.

TRAUMATIZATION OF THE CHRONICALLY ILL

Research has drawn attention to the effects of cumulative trauma or adversity, which can result in a spectrum of trauma-related disorders ranging from the more benign (i.e., anxiety) to the severe (PTSD; Alonzo, 2000; Dohrenwend, 2000; Fullilove, Lown, & Fullilove, 1992; Turner & Lloyd, 1995). Individuals who repeatedly suffer traumas that may not meet the diagnostic criteria of PTSD in the strict clinical sense (Scott & Stradling, 1994) may nonetheless experience symptoms that manifest at any point on a continuum of symptomology from severe PTSD to what has been called *subclinical PTSD* (Blank, 1993; Vrana & Lauterbach, 1994). Cumulative adversity and the possible resulting continuum of trauma disorders can impact the patient's ability to cope with the illness experience, the health care system, and other life domains (Alonzo, 2000). Patients may develop impeded responses to their own symptoms and the utilization of health care because of an accumulated burden of adversity. This has been investigated in certain specific medical conditions such as heart patients and cancer patients (Alonzo, 2000; Alonzo & Reynolds, 1996), but clinically it can also be seen as a response to many chronic conditions, which expose patients to various and repeated traumas.

Stigmatization

It also cannot be stated strongly enough that stigma is attached to many chronic illnesses and that this has an adverse effect on the patient as well as those in the patient's world. The medical community, the media, and the public have at times, depending on the illness, variously trivialized, stigmatized, sensationalized, and minimized chronic illness (Ax et al., 1998; Ballweg, 1997; Brody, 2000; J. Lewis, 1999; Marbach et al., 1990; Scambler & Hopkins, 1990; Schiller et al., 1994; Stuart & Noyes, 1999; Ware, 1998). If a person looks healthy, it is difficult to believe that he or she is actually suffering from any illness. In our culture, we expect an obvious physical sign of illness or disability. Without such evidence, people can become suspicious and conclude that the person merely claims to be ill and may actually be lazy, malingering, and vaguely immoral.

Evolving Definition of Trauma

Increasingly, the formal clinical definitions of *trauma* found in the *Diagnostic and Statistical Manual of Mental Disorders (DSM-IV)* are coming under critical scrutiny (Alonzo, 2000; Asmundson et al., 2000; Blank, 1993; Fullilove et al., 1992; Scott & Stradling, 1994; Turner & Lloyd, 1995, Yehuda & McFarlane, 1999). Although there is legitimacy in current definitions, concerns remain, especially in situations concerning, for example, lifelong trauma (Herman, 1999; Mezey & Robbins, 2001). In a paper about survivors of prolonged and repeated trauma, Herman provides strong evidence that current definitions must be expanded to account for a variety of stress-related disorders. As to trauma and CFS, for example, results of a community-based sample study suggest that, in medical practice, when evaluating and treating individuals with chronic fatigue and unexplained somatic symptoms, it is essential to consider coexisting psychosocial and psychiatric issues (R. R. Taylor & Jason, 2000). In addition, some biological abnormalities occurring in individuals with PTSD have occurred in individuals with CFS and FM (R. R. Taylor, Friedberg, & Jason, 2001).

Hence, the current definitions may not be inclusive enough to capture what many clinicians and researchers believe to be genuine trauma experiences associated with chronic illnesses or conditions. Traumas can vary widely, and individuals suffer the effects differently. An individual's history and his or her circumstances at the time of any trauma can further affect the individual's perception of it. Furthermore, the degree to which patients may be traumatized may depend on what others think, feel, and believe about their particular illness. Some conditions generally elicit sympathy and concern, whereas others arouse strong social condemnation and stigma. And, as discussed previously, the accumulation of trauma or adversity also affects individual responses to chronic illness.

Failure to Diagnose Trauma

Research indicates that PTSD is routinely undiagnosed in clinical settings. Clinicians on the primary care level tend not to consider this problem, and they often do not recognize it or differentiate it from other symptoms (Zimmerman & Mattia, 1999). As a consequence, trauma is underreported and not integrated into treatment plans. This situation is changing somewhat for particular medical conditions. Literature is developing as to medical and surgical events triggering trauma sequelae (Scott & Stradling, 1994; Shalev, Schrieber, & Galai, 1993). For example, heart patients can experience trauma symptoms after treatment (Stoll et al., 2000) and, as a result, fail to pursue life-saving interventions in a timely manner during subsequent heart-health events (Alonzo & Reynolds, 1996). Similarly, acute respiratory distress patients can experience trauma after treatment (Schelling et al., 1998). Women can experience PTSD as a result of giving birth (Ayers & Pickering, 2001) and after complicated abortions (Fisch & Tadmor, 1989). A significant literature is developing about cancer and its treatment and traumatic stressors for survivors (Alter et al., 1996; Cordova, Studts, Hann, Jacobsen, & Andrykowski, 2000; M. Y. Smith, Redd, Peyser, & Vogl, 1999), for women in particular (Hampton & Frombach, 2000), for children (Twombly, 2001), and for family members (M. Y. Smith et al., 1999; Twombly, 2001). Controversial illnesses are also being investigated for their potential traumatic effects, including HIV-positive patients (Botha, 1996) and CFS patients (Fennell, 1995b, 2001, 2003c).

Traumas Caused by Illness Onset

The individual's recognition that something is very wrong—the moment when he or she actually experiences the onset of the chronic illness—can be as traumatizing as the actual effects of the illness itself. The specific symptoms of the illness may include pain or infection, severe depression, the inability to walk or speak properly, the inability to read or write, or any one of a number of other physical changes. Because all of these symptoms can result in physical, cognitive, emotional, lifestyle, and social changes that cause additional pain and difficulty for patients and their families, it is hardly surprising that the patient's actually realizing the onset of the illness is frightening, sad, and inevitably accompanied by loss (Alonzo, 2000; Baldwin, 1978; Botha, 1996; Lindy, Grace, & Green, 1987).

Traumas Caused by Family Response

Even though patients may gradually come to terms with their chronic illness and learn productive ways to live with it, their families may not. A patient's changed life may be more than a spouse has bargained for. Parents may simply not want to believe that their chronically ill child is not going to get appreciably better, and children don't like or know how to relate to the changes in a chronically ill parent. None of these reactions is lost on the patient, and each may cause trauma apart from the actual disease symptoms (Cannon & Cavanaugh, 1998; Fisher & Weihs, 2000; Hayes, 1997; Heinzer, 1998; Pless & Nolan, 1991; Scambler & Hopkins, 1990; Ware, 1998). Some families attempt to shield patients from anything that reminds them of their condition or situation. One researcher refers to this as the *trauma membrane* (Lindy, Grace, & Green, 1981). As part of this shielding, families may discourage patients from seeking treatment or from carrying out treatment protocols because these would remind the patient of the unhappy condition.

Traumas Caused by Societal Response

The culture is constructed around an idealized work ethic in which healthy, productive individuals are considered the most socially useful and are valued accordingly. Given this, those who are very young, very old, differently abled, or infirm may be loved, indulged, or even admired but are not seen as contributing to the good of society and thus can be actively devalued. People with chronic illnesses are often unable to engage in economically productive work at their former pace. As a result, these individuals, who frequently have no outward signs of illness or disability, may be perceived as simply trying to escape from doing their fair share or engaging in otherwise self-serving victimization (Bartley & Owen, 1996; M. S. Bates et al., 1997; Henderson, 1997; Plehn, Peterson, & Williams, 1998; Pless & Nolan, 1991; Scambler & Hopkins, 1990; Stuart & Noyes, 1999; Tait et al., 1990; Ware, 1998, 1999).

Accordingly, society's response can be extremely hurtful, and these potentially traumatizing events tend to repeat again and again. Such responses can occur in the workplace, at home among family members, or in any environment or situation where the patient's chronic illness may become an issue (Bartley & Owen, 1996; Cannon & Cavanaugh, 1998; Fisher & Weihs, 2000; Heinzer, 1998; Ware, 1999; Ware & Kleinman, 1992).

The medical community, the media, and the public at large have at times stigmatized, belittled, or sensationalized chronic illnesses such as CFS (Ax et al., 1998; Ballweg, 1997; Brody, 2000; J. Lewis, 1999; Marbach et al., 1990; Scambler & Hopkins, 1990; Schiller et al., 1994; Stuart & Noyes, 1999; Ware, 1998). It was only a few years ago that the term *yuppie flu* was used to stereotype individuals suffering from CFS (Barshay, 1993). If people "look" healthy, it is difficult to believe that they are actually suffering from any illness. In our culture, we expect to see a scar, a crutch, a wheelchair, or some other obvious physical sign of illness or disability (Bergquist & Neuberger, 2002). In the early 1980s, the media called AIDS the *gay plague,* thereby stigmatizing anyone with AIDS as a person who engaged in homosexual (and thus immoral) acts (Kitzinger, 1990). Victims were seen as deserving the punishment of the disease (Nisbet & McQueen, 1993; Schiller et al., 1994; Singer, 1994).

Premorbid and Comorbid Traumas

It is also important to consider traumatic events that are independent of the patient's specific chronic illness but may be confused with it or contribute to the manner in which the patient processes the illness. Premorbid traumas are those that occurred before the onset of the chronic illness (Blum et al., 1997;

Ware & Kleinman, 1992). Examples include childhood incest, assault as an adult, active duty in the armed services, time spent in a war zone, torture, natural disasters, car accidents, and so forth.

Comorbid traumas can include developmental transitions and upheavals, such as the birth of a child, the decision to return to work, and the death of a loved one (Alonzo, 2000; Gatchel & Gardea, 1999; Van Mens-Verhulst & Bensing, 1998). But comorbid traumas may also consist of the illness of family members, caregiving responsibilities, divorce, assault, robbery, or any other unusual life event (Lutgendorf et al., 1995; R. R. Taylor & Jason, 2002). It is important to recognize that trauma can result in some individuals from even a positive situation, such as a new marriage, a longed-for pregnancy, or a new job.

Clinicians also need to recognize and help their patients see that chronic illness may lengthen the processing of life changes such as the death of a loved one because the chronic illness often entails slowed decision making, chaotic thinking, short-term memory loss, the inability of perform activities of daily living, or other cognitive and physical impairments. Avoiding or ignoring issues that arise from chronic illness may confuse both patients and clinicians about, for example, the grief the patient feels when a child leaves home or the misery caused by perpetual pain or exhaustion. Those who provide treatment need to help patients define their experiences on all levels. By separating current external events from emotional and physiological responses to chronic illness, clinicians can help mitigate the disruption surrounding transitional upheavals and the mental or cognitive disorientation associated with the changes wrought by chronic illness.

Finally, it is important for clinicians to recognize that although unrelated to the chronic illness, these other traumas are part of the cumulative trauma package.

Vicarious Traumas

Those who live, love, and work with the chronically ill can also be traumatized (Hayes, 1997; Rolland, 1994; Scott & Stradling, 1994). Like the patient, these people can experience trauma because of the illness onset, their witnessing of the patient's suffering, or their own difficulties because of their changed life. They, too, can suffer from society's judgments and responses to their loved ones. Family members as well as patients have premorbid and comorbid issues. They may be divorcing the newly ill patient, or they may be a patient's child. They may be going through their own developmental crises. They may find that their spouse cannot have children because of a chronic illness. Those associated with the patient also may experience iatrogenic traumatization.

Vicarious traumatization affects clinicians as well (Clark & Gioro, 1998; M. Rosenberg & Molho, 1998). Any clinician can be upset by witnessing the onset of an illness or distressed by the chronic nature of an illness. The inability to cure a patient can produce frustration and despair or anger. It can be argued that all clinicians have their own premorbid and comorbid issues, and all experience countertransference.

Clinicians can also suffer guilt by association and clinical marginalization because of whom they treat (Engel, 1977). Clinicians who treat the poor, the disenfranchised, and the chronically ill report experiences of stigmatization or discrimination by their peers because of treating specific illness groups. One primary care physician reported being warned by her HMO not to take on any more of "those chronically ill patients" (communication to the author). Another physician who was very effective in treating a particular chronic illness group let it be known that she did not want the larger patient community to learn of her effectiveness with these patients. Her HMO had already hinted that she was "misplacing" her efforts and had told the office staff to consider her caseload for such patients closed. Another physician practicing in a popular tourist area was strongly encouraged by local politicians to move his practice elsewhere because he championed the care of a particular group of patients (communication to the author).

Iatrogenic or Clinically Induced Traumas

Iatrogenic trauma is usually associated with a medical response or intervention to a physiological illness (Cuijpers, 1998; Epstein et al., 1999; Kirmayer et al., 1994; McCahill, 1995; Stuart & Noyes, 1999). In addition to including mistakes or unexpected adverse events (e.g., a new illness contracted because of a hospital stay), iatrogenic trauma can also arise from what is normal and appropriate medical care. This kind of medical traumatization may involve the actual treatment itself, and it may also involve frustrating or frightening experiences with the health care system over a period of time (Alonzo, 2000; Alonzo & Reynolds, 1996). This second kind of trauma can affect whether patients continue with medical care or how they respond to it.

In the context of chronic illness, it is also necessary to extend the concept of iatrogenic illness into two other areas. The first is the domain of medical intervention that is not considered procedure-specific, such as informal contact with the patient and the patient interview and assessment (Hampton & Frombach, 2000). The second arena where iatrogenic response is possible is the arena of psychological care (van der Kolk, McFarlane, & Weisaeth, 1996).

All of these potentially traumatizing events interface with one another. They can accumulate over time into a significant clinical concern (Alonzo, 2000).

THE INTEGRATION ASSUMPTION

Unlike medical models that assume an eventual cure, the Four-Phase Model pursues the goal of illness integration. Whether the disease or illness experience is acute or chronic, this model assumes that it needs to be integrated within the ultimate health and quality of life of the patient. Even if a patient is assured of complete recovery and achieves it, the physical and emotional scars of the illness can remain and need to be considered in that person's ongoing physiological and psychological health maintenance. Where a patient suffers a chronic illness and will never achieve a cure, the necessity of integration is paramount, because the patient should not have to experience clinical and personal failure repeatedly with each relapse or illness change.

Immediate disease symptoms (such as pain and fatigue), auxiliary symptoms (such as emotional suffering and loss), traumatization, and stigmatization all need to be approached with the goal of integration. This model conceptualizes that symptom reduction or elimination is one goal, but not the only goal. It is part of an overall effort that seeks to help the patient integrate symptoms into a meaningful, explanatory narrative framework. This approach shifts the expectations of chronically ill patients from unattainable goals to accessible ones and thus makes it possible for both patients and clinicians to achieve success.

PALLIATION

The treatment tools of palliative care are logical additions to the treatment options for the chronically ill. Traditionally, palliation has been applied primarily to the terminally ill and then only to reduce suffering. Medical practitioners do not usually turn to palliation until they have abandoned what are considered active treatment options (Butler, 1996; Marbach, 1999; Stieg, Lippe, & Shepard, 1999).

In current practice, active treatment—treatment aimed at returning the patient's medicalized body to some state considered *normal*—continues, and technological methods are used to assess and treat organic symptoms that can be measured and quantified until the patient is perceived to be gaining nothing from the treatment and hence to be actively dying (Clifford, 1993). At this point, active treatment is discontinued. For some, palliation is offered, often in the form of hospice care. Finally, the patient becomes an object of "care," and he or she is treated as a whole person, not only as a medicalized, diseased body (Weissman, 1997; Weissman & Griffie, 1998).

In the Four-Phase Model, palliation is an active treatment option. In chronic disease, palliation bridges the disease-illness and cure-integration dichotomies. At the same time clinicians pursue specific treatment to eliminate or reduce disease symptoms, they can use the treatment tools employed by hospice and pastoral care providers to improve the patient's overall quality of remaining life. These methods incorporate a variety of auxiliary and holistic approaches, such as family treatment and pastoral care. They are thoroughly acceptable within the hospice setting and have long-established empirical and clinical links with the traditional medical community (Mayer, 1999). Because these methods can distinctly improve the quality of care for chronically ill patients, they might also help eliminate the reasons chronically ill patients seek inappropriate or unproven care.

PATIENT AND CLINICIAN TOGETHER

The Four-Phase Model offers a shared progressive experience for the patient, the family, and the health care provider. The clinician does not treat from outside but is an intrinsic component in the process, which embraces the whole array of embedded issues and worlds the chronically ill patient inhabits. It is a truly holistic, systemic approach. The dichotomy between the patient and the clinician has led to failures in patient care and a great deal of personal suffering (Engel, 1977, 1980; Gallagher, 1999). The chronically ill patient has to negotiate a long and potentially arduous journey to achieve integration about his or her illness. It can be nearly impossible to make this trip without the company and guidance of a care provider who may or may not be able to relate directly to the patient's personal experience of illness but who is invested in the process.

As patients and their families enter the initial phases of chronic illness, clinicians using the Four-Phase Model participate with them, first as assessors and advisors, and then as people who provide treatment. But eventually, if the clinicians truly grasp the heart of the experience, they accompany the patient and the family as fellow travelers. The patient progresses, typically encountering cycles of adversity or suffering and then remission, and the clinician shares the experience. Instead of trying to dampen intrinsic and necessary countertransference reactions as undesirable responses, the clinician continually reacts and feels and pays attention to these responses. By using countertransference effectively, the clinician can actually enlarge and enhance the treatment process for everyone concerned.

The Four-Phase Model also uses the countertransference reactions that proceed from clinicians' negative experiences, including those encountered when professionals practice with a socially marginalized clientele. All of the clinicians' experiences and reactions become useful, compassion-provoking raw material, not only in the immediate patient relationship, but also in the personal and professional growth of the clinician.

When the care provider shares the patient's journey, the treatment can be truly effective (Cameron & Gregor, 1987; National Institute of Health [NIH], 1996). This joining with the patient helps the patient, family, and clinician access the knowledge that suffering is an inevitable part of life but that, nonetheless, the chronically ill can lead productive, meaningful lives that integrate their experience of suffering.

The previous description is an ideal portrait. But it can and does exist in the real world, even within the economic constraints of the current HMO environment. Clinicians who work using the Four-Phase Model must develop relationships with HMOs so that they receive appropriate compensation. They have to explain the benefits of their approach, which is, among other things, cost effective in the long run. Using this approach, patients learn skills and arrive at understandings that reduce their fear, increase their coping skills, and begin to establish them in a new, satisfying identity that has meaning for them. These advances reduce their need to turn to the medical system. This is a practical description, not an ideal. Clinicians using the Four-Phase Model have negotiated with health insurers, and they are paid for their services. Moreover, although the journey taken with a chronic illness patient may occur over a significant period of time, actual visits with the clinician are usually punctuated, occurring consistently during the crisis and stabilization phases, sporadically during the difficult times of the resolution phase, and even less frequently when clinicians are monitoring patient progress with coping skills.

Similarly, I would argue that if public clinics target interventions for their chronically ill patients by phase and address all three systems—the physical/behavioral, the psychological, and the social/interactive—they will achieve better outcomes more cost effectively. By attending to these systems in a patient's life at the appropriate phase, clinics can use their limited resources more effectively. In addition, by intervening with treatments suited to the patient's particular phase—a time when they are more likely to be compliant—clinics can help patients break out of a pattern of repeated crises that usually require more extensive resources in response.

Chapter 2 ————————————————————————————

THE CULTURAL CONTEXT OF CHRONIC ILLNESS

It is stating the obvious to say that chronically ill individuals and their families internalize many aspects of the general culture and that they encounter it externally through a variety of social systems such as the educational system, the legal system, and the workplace. Nonetheless, cultural context is particularly relevant to understanding the experiences of the chronically ill because it encompasses both specifically traumagenic factors and integrative, healing ones. The cultural system with the most salient cultural impact on patients, their families, and their care providers is the health care system.

THE PRIMARY CULTURAL CONTEXT: THE HEALTH CARE SYSTEM

Not only do the various segments of the health care system interact with one another and affect one another's culture, but also the system as a whole affects the larger society in three distinct ways.

Most apparently, the health care system carries out a care and research function that assures the public that an up-to-date medical response will be available to people who come into the system because of physical, psychological, and certain social needs (Berwick, 1989; Gawande & Bates, 2000; Nelson, Splaine, Batalden, & Plume, 1998). The system also has an economic function that affects the general culture. This function is intended to ensure the support and maintenance of health care institutions and their personnel, but it is also arranged so that both institutions and personnel not only support themselves but also profit, often significantly, from their activities (Blumenthal, Campbell, Causino, & Louis, 1996; Campbell, Louis, & Blumenthal, 1998; S. A. Rosenberg, 1996). In addition, the health care system has a largely unacknowledged social function in the culture. It actively participates in society's creation and maintenance of social class, status, and power; hence, it also has an impact on issues of race and gender (Byrd, Clayton, & Kitchen, 1994; Carrasquillo, Himmelstein, Woolhandler, & Bor, 1999; Harder et al., 1997; Phukan, 1993; Ryynanen, Myllykanga, Kinnunen, & Takala, 1999).

How the chronically ill are permitted to navigate the health care system greatly influences their illness experience. This chapter discusses components of the health care system and the impact each has on users. These components include the actual institutions of care; the people who provide the care or support those who do; and the beliefs, attitudes, norms, and rules that determine how users of the health care system are perceived, assessed, treated, discharged, and managed.

Institutions of Care

The institutions of care include, first, the actual edifices and organizations of care provision—the hospitals, clinics, private offices, nursing homes, and so forth. These exist both as physical settings and as bureaucratic organizations. The second institutional group encompasses the governors of care—the professional associations, advocacy groups, government regulatory bodies, and, increasingly, the for-profit "gatekeeper" insurance organizations. The third broad group of health care institutions includes those that provide training and research, such as the medical schools, universities, government facilities, and for-profit companies working in pharmaceuticals, medical equipment, surgical supplies, and so forth.

The physical setting of health care can have a profound impact on patients. Most people have on some occasion had to struggle to find a parking place at the hospital or negotiate its bewildering array of corridors, offices, and acronyms. When individuals are sick or confused or scared, as is usually the case with any patient, not just the chronically ill, these barriers grow proportionally more difficult to overcome (Martin, 2000). And clearing the hurdle of the physical structure only brings the patient face to face with the bureaucratic structure, where an endless array of papers, cards, permissions, and guarantees of payment must be traded before the patient gains access to the doctor or laboratory (Alonzo, 2000; Barnett, 1998; Schlesinger et al., 1999; Tait et al., 1990). Despite the fact that many hospitals and institutions work energetically to ease these problems, the patient courts embarrassment and humiliation at every step of the way, and past difficulties tend to live in the imagination far longer than successes.

Generally, patients must simply accept the illness definitions, treatment standards, and care protocols that the governing bodies of the medical profession set. The descriptions of diseases—their etiologies, symptoms, and treatments—emerge from the experience of the medical profession as a whole, but they are evaluated, judged, and made standard by bodies appointed from within the profession (Cooksey & Brown, 1998; Cullen, 1998). The governing bodies also set standards for practically every aspect of the interface with patients, including matters of ethics, treatment, note taking, record keeping, and how doctors behave with patients. Because these regulations are so explicit and extensive, they actually also define the expected behavior of the patient. It is possible to consider the patient's behavior as the negative space around the defined dimensions of the doctor's behavior. The long process of defining a new disease or syndrome and the one-sided establishment of behavior protocols can have a harmful effect on the chronically ill, as is discussed in further detail later. But as more people, including health care professionals themselves, come to suffer chronic illnesses, perhaps beneficial change will occur more rapidly.

At present, patients try to affect health care most directly through advocacy groups. These groups provide information that participants can give to their sometimes ill-informed health care providers; and they support research, keep members abreast of the latest advances, and press legislators on issues important to their constituency. They may even have an impact on government regulatory agencies, which determine when new drugs come onto the market and set federal research priorities (Aiken, 1997; Rothman & Edgar, 1991).

The health maintenance organization (HMO) system of paying for medical care has introduced a host of new factors into the health care system, which is discussed later in this book. In brief, a perpetual condition of illness, necessitating ongoing visits with clinicians, does not fit conveniently into a profit-driven industry attempting to reduce costs (Barnett, 1998; Druss, Schlesinger,

Thomas, & Allen, 2000; Durban et al., 1993; Roblin, Juhn, Preston, & Della Penna, 1999; Schlesinger et al., 1999; Smith-Campbell, 2002).

The training and research institutions of the health care system have a direct and crucial impact on the experience of the chronically ill. Some emerging or controversial chronic syndromes and illnesses may not even be discussed in medical school, so newly graduated doctors will have to learn about them elsewhere (Durban et al., 1993). Medical students may not receive training in understanding how differently patients experience a chronic as opposed to an acute illness. Even when medical students are cognizant of chronic syndromes, they may choose not to focus on patients with such illnesses for a variety of reasons, including the frustrating nature of chronic illness in general and the social suspicion and stigma that can attach to certain specific conditions (Campbell et al., 1998; Stephenson, Collerton, & White, 1996; S. M. Weinstein et al., 2000).

Research institutions, whether public or private, tend to explore diseases that offer likely opportunities for a cure or have such cultural and media support that they attract funding. Until the advent of advocacy groups, most chronic diseases attracted few researchers. The profit motive operates most strongly in private companies developing new pharmaceuticals and treatment. Increasingly, moreover, frontier areas of medical research are now in the hands of for-profit organizations, which sometimes seek to protect their economic advantage through a secrecy contrary to former commitments to the sharing of breakthrough information (M. S. Bates, 1990; Blumenthal et al., 1996; S. A. Rosenberg, 1996).

System Actors and Agents

Inside the institutions of the health care system are the actual human beings who give and receive care, as well as those who conduct the oversight, determine standards and breadth of care, teach or engage in research, and manage the organizational activities. Participants include patients and their families, doctors, nurses, aides, pharmacists, social workers, rehabilitation specialists, psychologists, advocates and standard setters, academics and researchers, members of government agencies and legislators, receptionists, accountants, hospital directors, and insurance CEOs. It is important to remember that most of these people will take on different roles at different times in their lives. The doctor or the CEO is sure to become a patient, whereas the nurse may become a researcher or the patient an advocate who affects the thinking of legislators (Thornton, 1998).

All the parties have conscious and unconscious attitudes, as well as varying levels of training, skill, and information. All nonpatient individuals in the system have an impact on patients, and patients have an impact on health care personnel, though this receives less comment. Chronic illness makes contacts with workers in the health care system all the more frequent, which increases the opportunities for trauma. This is especially true because the culture at large still has profound suspicions about many chronic illnesses. The effects that the various actors in the health care system have on the chronically ill and that the chronic patient has on health care personnel receive extensive discussion throughout this book.

To complicate the situation, recent changes in the economics of health care have deeply affected the traditional role of the patient (Druss et al., 2000; Managed health care, 1997). Previously, the patient was expected to behave as a passive, unquestioning, grateful recipient of care from a compassionate health care provider who, by virtue of training, occupation, and relative power, occupied a higher social status, even if only temporarily (Cooksey & Brown, 1998; Cullen, 1998; DiMatteo, 1998; Fishman, 2001; Hummel, 2002; Onega & Larsen, 2002). Patients are now exhorted to behave as consumers. Elements of the health care community, seeking some counterweight to balance-sheet medicine, are urging patients to lobby for expanded rights in the health care system (Brink, 2000; Gore, 2000; Reissman, 2000). On the other hand, some health care providers, especially physicians, are now forced to operate openly as business people (Collicott, Gage, Oblath, & Opelka, 1996; Mechanic & Schlesinger, 1996). The new conflicts generated by these changing functions inevitably have an impact on the illness experience of patients.

Health care professionals should get appropriate reimbursement for their services. Some people argue that it is increasingly hard for them to receive proper recompense under any circumstances and that it is particularly hard with services for the chronically ill, who may require innovative or novel services or the provision of services over a long period. It is my experience that third-party payers will pay for the clinical services recommended in this book if clinicians discuss the services with them in advance. The clinician can demonstrate that the efficacy of the treatment and intermittent meetings with the clinician, even though they can sometimes occur over a long time, can ultimately hold down costs.

Once again it is important to note that individuals who are economically and socially disadvantaged suffer chronic illness in disproportionately large numbers compared with the general public (Lubkin & Larsen, 2002). As a consequence, their experience of the social dimensions of chronic illness is likely to be even more difficult, and they have far fewer resources to devote to their care. This can often mean that they are caught in a perpetual experience of crisis (Phase 1) or a repeating loop of crisis and stabilization (Phase 1 and Phase 2) that they often self-medicate with anodynes such as alcohol or drugs. Because clinics serving the disadvantaged are pressed for staff and time, targeted interventions that can help the chronically ill incorporate successful coping skills are highly desirable.

Beliefs, Attitudes, Norms, and Rules

Some of the most important aspects of the health care system are essentially invisible. These include the beliefs that everybody, both inside and outside health care institutions, hold about illness; people's attitudes toward the sick, the infirm, and the disabled; and the norms governing behavior toward such individuals. Beliefs, attitudes, and norms are rarely codified and written down, but rules and regulations about many health care procedures and processes do appear in print (Federal Register, 1999a).

Today, regulations governing professional conduct in professional organizations are being challenged and redefined as the social, economic, and care functions of the health care system come into increasing conflict (M. S. Bates, 1990; Mechanic & Schlesinger, 1996; Ware et al., 2000). Some of the changes further confuse and complicate the situation. For example, rules about a clinician's interaction with patients have become more restrictive as to personal interaction, but at the same time, clinicians are being urged to adopt a more personally engaged manner. Contractual relationships between patients, third-party payers, and clinicians have come under scrutiny as issues arise about care coverage, terms of reimbursement, and a patient's right to choose medical providers. Health maintenance organizations have denominated primary care physicians as gatekeepers, who may be permitted to grant access to specialists only in accordance with insurance company directives. Questions abound about conflicts between a physician's responsibility to inform patients of the best clinical course to follow and the contractual limitations placed on the physician's communications and recommendations by his or her HMO. Patients' rights vis-à-vis HMOs are under discussion at both the state and national level. Health maintenance organizations are coming under increased pressure from patient groups and, consequently, from legislative bodies (Caggiano, Weisfeld, Palace, & Klein, 1997; Rovner, 1999).

Invisible beliefs, attitudes, and norms have major significance because they permeate daily life and because within the health care system, they concern issues of power and authority, "illness etiquette" (Register, 1987), and care procurement and delivery. Strong norms determine how a patient is supposed to go about selecting a provider and how a patient should behave in the presence of a care provider. Because of these norms, for example, the issue of second opinions is fraught with social and psychological difficulties (Hummel, 2002; Onega & Larsen, 2002).

Traditionally, the patient was expected to behave submissively, to accept without question or argument the treatment the doctor ordered. At the same time, strong rules detailed how the doctor was expected to behave toward a patient. The rules acknowledged that the doctor occupied a position of near-absolute authority, but with it came the awesome responsibility of life and death and everything that derived from that responsibility. A change is now occurring in this area. The doctor and the patient are now understood to be in a relationship concerning health care, in which both parties participate and contribute as much as they can toward achieving the goal of the best quality of health in the patient. Nonetheless, old attitudes persist, in part because they concern issues of power and most people relinquish power reluctantly (Bull & Jervis, 1997; Cooksey & Brown, 1998; Cullen, 1998; Inui, 1997; Mechanic & Schlesinger, 1996; Ridson & Edey, 1999). But in part, it must also be said, a new relationship is made more difficult because some patients are reluctant to assume direct responsibility for their health.

In the late nineteenth century, with the remarkable advances in science and the organization of the medical profession, the doctor's authority came to extend beyond health matters and the clinical setting, and this gave the doctor even greater personal and social power in the clinical relationship. Throughout the twentieth century, society reinforced this superior social status by granting the doctor commensurate income and prestige.

Even today, with the gradually evolving participation of the patient in the doctor-patient relationship, when either the doctor or the patient acts outside their prescribed roles, informal censorship usually follows. A fibromyalgia patient, for example, who is unable to obtain medical relief from pain and fatigue, flies into a rage when the doctor explains that he is doing everything possible to improve her condition. The patient feels anger because she believes that the doctor, by failing to return her to health, has not fulfilled what she believes is the doctor's responsibility in the doctor-patient relationship. Or conversely, a patient comes into a doctor's office with a written list of questions and a notebook detailing prior medical treatment. The doctor is annoyed at the invasion of what she perceives as her territory. Along with her primary diagnoses of the patient's physical condition, the doctor "punishes" the patient, perhaps unintentionally, with a psychological diagnosis as an obsessive-compulsive. When questioned later about her diagnosis, the doctor offers the list and the notebook as the only reasons for the diagnosis. But by writing a list, the patient was following the recommendations of many health experts, and the notebook had been created by a relative. Nonetheless, a permanent, and potentially damaging, misdiagnosis has appeared in the patient's records because the doctor felt that the patient had transgressed the proper doctor-patient relationship (Thorne, 1990; Turk & Rudy, 1991).

Issues of illness etiquette extend beyond the immediate clinical relationship between health care provider and patient and into the other social systems in the patient's life. Invisible norms govern how people talk about and behave toward the chronically ill and their families. These are constantly operating within the family unit itself and in the extended family, the community, and the workplace. Norms emerge from cultural attitudes and beliefs, which in turn have been shaped by history, religious beliefs, ethnic heritage, economic and political opinions, and scientific and technological changes. Family members, friends, and coworkers are all unsure about how to address symptoms or disability in the chronically ill individual (Remsburg & Carson, 2002). What are they supposed to say? How much should they help? How much allowance should they make for the illness? The patient is equally confused about how to behave.

Made uncomfortable by confusion, ignorance, and, often, fear, people can revert to outdated cultural beliefs, albeit with modern facelifts. Out of sheer resentment, some people determine that the chronically ill individual is simply trying to exploit a kind of victim's "affirmative action." Others struggle unsuccessfully to fit the chronically ill into the legislated schema of rules relating to persons with physical disabilities (Jordan, Mayer, & Gatchel, 1998). Many people are tolerant of the sufferer or empathize with him or her, but sometimes even they can be made uncomfortable by the unknown.

The etiology of chronic illnesses plays a strong role in subsequent bias and stigmatization. If a specific illness etiology remains vague and little understood, sufferers are more likely judged as exhibiting poor character and possibly malingering (Barnett, 1998; Turk & Rudy, 1991).

In addition, although people with more profound religious or philosophical conceptions of God's purpose or the "just" universe may account for disease and disaster in complex and compassionate ways, some people have difficulty understanding the nuances of such arguments. They tend, either openly or half-consciously, to regard any individual's pain and suffering as a kind of deserved condition, perhaps punishment for immoral behavior. Such people usually define and respond to all illnesses negatively to one degree or another, although they may be more condemnatory of some conditions than others. Cultures with a more differentiated and varied interpretation of pain and suffering tend to have positive as well as negative interpretations of the illness experience (Abrums, 2000; Vaughan, 1994).

American society draws on a large variety of conflicting ideas—some positive, some negative—from numerous cultures (Peters, 1995), but a significant number of people regard the chronically ill as demonstrations of failure or immorality in a just universe. This stance has particular appeal for much of the media, especially supermarket tabloids and sensational TV shows, whose profit-driven exploitation of such judgmental attitudes further reinforces stereotyping and sometimes negative behavior. As discussed later, the media are probably the principal mythmakers of contemporary society and, as such, wield enormous power in the creation of both positive and negative social attitudes.

LEVELS OF DISCOURSE

The beliefs, attitudes, norms, and rules relevant to the health care system manifest themselves on three different levels of "conversation" or discourse—a professional level, a social level, and a mythic or "meta" level. This somewhat arbitrary typology is not intended to be all-inclusive, but should help provide a springboard for discussion and understanding.

Professional Discourse

Professionals in the field of health care continuously articulate thoughts, express attitudes, and engage in discussions about illness. The most formal, codified variety of professional discourse occurs in the context of professional literature, peer-reviewed research, and professional conferences. Typically, professionals are the only participants in such communication.

But professional discourse also occurs on a more informal level in the realm of what might be called *personal communications.* These may be formal in tone and content, as when one professional seeks consultation or data from another, but they may also include the exchange of ideas or opinions that the participants would hesitate to put into print or articulate from a public podium. These less structured exchanges may, in fact, embody some of the most important communications between professionals because the participants feel free to express ideas that contain elements of bias, positive and negative feelings toward patients and illness, and the occasional politically incorrect utterance. Professionals must be able to communicate in this fashion to have normal relationships with their peers and to be able to enjoy their work. Informal personal communications also provide a vehicle for the exchange of new and tenuous ideas, which may over time and through further discussion prove to be scientifically useful. But because this kind of discourse also permits the expression of bias, which aids in the development of negative and inaccurate stereotypes, it can also lead to the stigmatization of certain illnesses and possible traumatization (Turk & Rudy, 1991; Weissman & Dahl, 1990).

Institutions also "talk" with one another. Doctors' offices communicate with hospitals, hospitals with each other, HMOs with doctors and clinics and hospitals. Credit bureaus exchange information with hospitals and insurance companies. Government agencies converse with hospitals, clinics, and HMOs. The Social Security Administration (SSA), for example, exchanges information with doctors and hospitals about the acceptability of disability claims. What the SSA determines as to whether chronic fatigue syndrome (CFS) constitutes a disability in turn affects estimation of the condition in the minds of doctors and society (K. M. Boyer, 1999; Federal Register, 1999b).

Although strong rules existed in the past about disclosure of patient information, increasingly, the requirements of insurers and government agencies are eroding them. In addition, more and more individuals not covered by the formal rules of nondisclosure have access to patient information (Korn, 2000; Rutberg, 1999; Selby, 1997; Woodward, 1995). In addition, employers who purchase medical insurance for employees may have access to medication and other health data of their employees, which would not have been legal in the past (Korn, 2000; Rutberg, 1999; Selby, 1997; Woodward, 1995). Furthermore, the exchange of patient information increasingly travels or is stored electronically—including via the Internet—where it is by no means secure from unauthorized readers. As a consequence, real concern is growing about issues of patient confidentiality and the right of access to information (Korn, 2000; Rutberg, 1999; Selby, 1997; Woodward, 1995). In addition, publicly funded health clinics that serve the disadvantaged may be subject to reporting that might not occur with a wealthier patient and his or her private provider.

Institutional exchanges of information, like those between individual professionals, are essential to the process of providing modern health care. But like individual communications, they can also express biases that can lead to stigmatization and traumatization. And it is vital to note that interinstitutional health care discourse is particularly influenced by the corporate culture and vulnerable to the economic function.

Despite the existence of cross talk between institutions in the health care system, there is almost a complete lack of coordination concerning patient care between these institutions. Cross-institutional conversations exist largely to serve administrative and economic goals, not patient goals. They may work at odds with or directly counter to patient and/or clinical goals. Institutions regard communication dedicated to patient care coordination as an expensive activity that does not enjoy the benefit of reimbursement (Levinson et al., 1999; Woodward, 1995).

Consider the case of the man who learns from his primary physician that his PSA numbers are very elevated, so he sees a urologist about his prostate. After a complete examination, the urologist recommends a biopsy, and the patient is discovered to have cancerous tumors. The patient now sees an oncological surgeon, who operates and prescribes radiation and chemotherapy treatments to follow. The surgeon also prescribes medication to moderate some of the side effects of the after-treatment, unaware that the patient has had difficulties with similar medications in the past. In follow-up examinations, it appears that the cancer has spread. The patient is required by his HMO to work through his primary physician, who also is the professional most aware of the patient's other conditions. But that doctor cannot spend the time and does not have the expertise to take charge and make recommendations in this very specialized situation. Even the urologist and the oncologist will probably work within the protocols established in their local hospitals rather than seeking the best-practice treatment that may be available elsewhere. In part, they may be unaware of the latest treatment, but in part they are also discouraged by the HMOs from moving outside the area where the HMO has established rates and protocols of its own. So who does take charge of managing this patient's overall case? In theory, all the medical personnel are communicating with one another and are fully cognizant of the patient's entire medical history. In reality, no one except the patient is paying attention to the whole picture, and the patient is experiencing such emotional turmoil that he is a poor candidate to act as case manager. Yet to achieve the best outcome, the patient is well advised to research his condition to discover whether he might be better served by treatment not offered locally.

Or consider the case of a newly diagnosed fibromyalgia patient whose inability to work makes it necessary for her to seek disability. Here the failure of communication occurs between the doctor and the disability company. Even if the patient's physician completely agrees that the patient needs disability income, it is highly unlikely that he or she understands the hidden pitfalls of disability claim forms unless the doctor has been through the process many times before. If this is the patient's first experience with a disability claim, she, too, is unlikely to know what kind of documentation she needs. If her physician unwittingly mentions, for example, the existence of a prior illness unrelated to the current claim, that statement alone may be sufficient justification for the agency to deny the patient's claim. If anything in the doctor's notes shows that the patient is physically capable of performing any kind of work, even if it is not necessarily the work she has been doing, that may be enough for the disability company to disallow the claim (Stephens, 1989; Turk, Rudy, & Stieg, 1988).

Patients with any illness can learn that the different institutions involved in health care have widely different ideas about how to treat an illness. Andrew Grove, CEO of Intel, discovered that even with his wealth, intelligence, and social clout, it was difficult to bring about coordination among care protocols. Indeed, the frequently competing or totally opposed ideas confused and upset him and made choice of the best care very difficult.

Such divergence of opinion is all the more common with chronic illness. A fibromyalgia patient, for example, will find that professionals approach this condition from two divergent positions. One group regards fibromyalgia as a condition with a physiological component, but subsequently characterized primarily by somatization. For some reason, perhaps because the patient encountered difficulties recovering, the patient stopped getting better. This group most often treats fibromyalgia with a cognitive-behavioral program. Clinicians use relaxation techniques, guided imagery, behavioral goal setting, but patients are also gradually induced to do more exercise to address deconditioning. Clinicians focus on underlying debilitating emotions, beliefs, and attitudes that the patient is presumed to feel (Bradley, 1989; Bradley & Alberts, 1999).

The other group thinks that the pain of the fibromyalgia patient is pain with a physical genesis and that the patient has difficulty exercising because of that pain. This group considers that fibromyalgia patients may actually have physiologically different pain mechanisms. This group regards the pain as primarily an actual physical experience, whereas the first group emphasizes the interpreted experience of pain. There is a difference between the two, and how patients come to regard themselves may depend greatly on which vision of fibromyalgia the clinician has (Ahles, Khan, Yunus, Spiegel, & Masi, 1991; Bennett, 1993, 1999).

Economic considerations have increasingly turned important health care decisions into adversarial proceedings. Many patients will not receive deserved support or services because the institutions charged with providing them are serving their own economic ends first. Patients quickly learn that many health care-related institutions attempt to limit services in an effort to contain costs and eliminate fraud. If the patient can be judged in adequate health by very strict standards of symptom presentation and hence can be seen as merely complaining about undefined, unrecognized, or nebulous difficulties, the institution preserves its funds, presumably for more deserving cases. With the growth of health care for profit, however, the preserved funds are not necessarily assigned to others who are ill but are returned instead to those shareholders who have invested in the institution. This creates a very difficult environment for genuinely ill chronic patients—by far the majority—who legitimately need to obtain support or necessary services (Bloom, 1996; Halkitis & Dooha, 1998).

In addition, the social functions of the health care system come into play concerning issues of professional status and advancement. Health maintenance organizations do not encourage physicians to spend time getting disability or wrestling with utilization review panels for their patients or working at length with the chronically ill to identify and understand their emerging and receding symptoms. Nor do the doctors see these activities as advancing their practice of medicine. Chronic syndrome conditions that do not yield to treatment do not advance careers. Even when research institutions explore aspects of chronic illness, in many cases, they are not forthcoming with others, who are competitors, about their tentative findings. Hence, the social aspects of the health care system work together with economic concerns as to institutional competition, survival, and profit. As a result, it can be argued that patient coordination and care suffer (Lee, 1998; Mechanic & Schlesinger, 1996; Schlesinger et al., 1999).

Social Discourse

Everybody in the society participates in social discourse about illness, and the "conversation" occurs in a broad variety of social contexts. Both individuals and groups construct a "narrative" for individual illnesses and for general notions of illness as well. Each illness narrative contains the individual's understanding of what the illness is, what happens to a person who has the illness, what happens to those around the person with the illness, and a moral evaluation of people who have the illness. The individual's attitudes—a combination of knowledge, understanding, fears, and hopes—about illness in general colors the specific narrative of each individual illness.

Individual illness narratives grow out of the family's history of how it has treated sick or disabled members in the past. Such narratives are constantly modified and revised as family members fall sick anew or suffer relapses and respites from a chronic illness. Each family member has his or her own individual illness narrative, but the family as a whole also has a collective illness narrative, one that may differ significantly from an individual family member's narrative. With each new or ongoing illness or disability, the family addresses its implications for the individual and for the family, although not necessarily in concert or even in open discussion (McCahon & Larsen, 2002; Travis & Piercy, 2002). Parents, for example, make plans and create strategies to cope with cystic fibrosis in a child. A sister struggles to find a way of dealing with her brother's bipolar disorder. Middle-age children attempt to craft a response to an elderly parent's descent into dementia. A partner deals with the fact that his or her lover will be unable any longer to contribute to the financial well-being of the household.

The typical assumption of American culture today, that illness is a rare occurrence, an irregular condition rather than the ordinary environment of family life, means that most families have not formulated ways to address illness in the family openly and honestly (Anderton et al., 1989; M. S. Bates et al., 1997; Wallander & Varni, 1998).

Even if family members never discuss illness issues openly, however, each member always has a clear sense of how the family responds to physical and mental illness and a clear expectation of how it will respond to future illness. The family's rules and regulations concerning illness may not be codified, but they are rigorously observed nonetheless. The rules shape how a family regards illness in general and how it treats an individual family member who is ill or disabled. They dictate how the sick individual will behave and how family members will discuss and portray sick family members to the outside world.

A family's ethnicity, religious beliefs, class, and race have profound influences on their illness narratives (Berg et al., 2002; Rehm, 1999). Culturewide stereotyping and illness bias also contribute, as do the severity of illnesses experienced within the family and the family's history of tragedy and loss. A working-class Irish Catholic family interprets illness and creates an illness narrative very differently from that of a Midwestern professional Lutheran family or a refugee Cambodian family.

Whereas people learn illness etiquette first within the bosom of their families, social discourse with friends and coworkers further shapes or revises an individual's understanding of illness and rules of illness etiquette. People bring to their conversation the ideas about illness that they learned in their families as well as their take on societywide attitudes. Family members then bring this experience back to the family where it can, in turn, alter the family narrative.

When communities experience devastating upheavals—natural disasters such as storms, floods, or earthquakes—or serious outbreaks of contagious disease, the community is usually either forged into a mutually supportive group or devolves into isolated, fearful, often antagonistic small components. The communitywide experience of such conditions can reinforce or dramatically alter the illness narratives of individual families (Aronoff & Gunter, 1991; Soliman, 1995; Sweet, 1998).

The outbreak of the illness that came to be called *chronic fatigue syndrome* had quite different receptions in different places. In Incline Village, Nevada, despite the evidence of illness in numerous residents, the community as a whole responded negatively to clinicians and their CFS patients. This may have occurred because the illness affected only a minority of the community. It was also an illness of unknown etiology and prognosis, and the local economy was based on tourism. By contrast, in Lyndonville, New York, the same illness afflicted a significant portion of the community, including many children. This rural upstate town reacted by pulling together and rallying behind the local family doctor and his patients. Perhaps because the hamlet did not depend on tourist dollars, the community did not fear financial loss. Perhaps because the doctor and some of the afflicted individuals were important members of the community, the community responded in a largely positive way. Perhaps Lyndonville was simply a coherent, well-integrated community. Whatever the cause, the result for many individuals was a positive impact on individual and family illness narratives (D. Bell, personal communication, fall 1997).

Community-based illness narratives are strongly influenced by culturewide illness narratives. Historically, plagues were often read as divine punishment. The Black Death of the Middle Ages, for example, which killed between a third and a half of Europe's population, was widely attributed to God's wrath at the immorality of humanity. And that attitude had not changed markedly by the nineteenth century when cholera swept Britain. Even today, reactions to AIDS reveal popular preoccupations with the notion of disease as divine punishment. Age-old notions that God sends disease to evildoers created an atmosphere of fear and loathing about illness that has continued to have a profound influence, even after people generally accepted scientific understanding of germs and contagion (Coles, 1984; Swenson, 1988; Thomasma & McElhinney, 1990). Religiously inspired fear and condemnation of illness was countered in the West by a powerful tradition of compassion for the poor, the weak, and the sick in the Judeo-Christian-Islamic faiths. But popular perceptions that the sick had brought their illnesses on themselves were constantly buoyed by theologies that asserted God's ultimate knowledge and control of all that happened in the universe.

American culture also has strong roots in a Calvinist Protestantism. When the Puritans fled persecution in Europe for America, they wanted to both preserve the purity of their religion and survive in a wild, hostile new land. To accomplish this, the leaders maintained a high level of social control and were suspicious and uncomfortable with any behavior that fell outside their strictly defined norms. Although the community believed that God had already predestined each individual to salvation or damnation and that the individual was helpless to change this fate, he or she might possibly discover (and the community could see as well) if this fate was salvation by the individual's continually doing work that was thought pleasing to God. Perpetual work was also necessary for survival. Being idle was thought both to invite corruption and to be a sign of it. Inactivity was avoided at all costs, and illness or disability could easily appear to be the Devil's work. Though the concept has been secularized over the past 300 years, the old Puritan work ethic survives in American culture to this day (Gorgievski-Duijvesteijn, Steensma, & TeBrake, 1998).

Another historical ideal that has contributed to America's culturewide illness narrative is that of the rugged individualist. Here the ideal is the totally independent individual who does not require—who would in fact rebuff—the help of others. By sheer willpower and strength of character, this individual does not allow illness or disability to slow him down. He fights—the ideal is almost always presented as male—against all odds until death, no matter what the physical cost. The true rugged individualist meets sickness and adversity by "pulling himself up by his bootstraps" and pushing on. This particular cultural ideal contributes to many different narratives within the culture, including the capitalist ethic, for example, or the supremacy of individual rights. These aspects of the culture in turn influence America's illness narrative (Burckhardt, Woods, Schultz, & Ziebarth, 1989; Ware & Kleinman, 1992).

In recent years, a number of medical analysts have been concluding that many outbreaks of unidentified sickness are actually examples of mass hysteria. The Centers for Disease Control and Prevention (CDC), for example, were invited to Lyndonville, New York, following that community's experience with CFS, to review the situation. The CDC never returned a report to the community, which later discovered that the CDC regarded the incident as a case of mass hysteria.

A multitude of books have been written in the past few years that express great concern about the rise of what the authors call a "victim" mentality. Citing examples that include the "Twinkie defense," CFS, Gulf War syndrome, sex abuse survivors groups, and so forth, the authors assert that the American populace is becoming mushy and soft. Instead of behaving like the strong, self-reliant men and women who fought for and built America, these sorry individuals expect the government to step in and take care of them. It is interesting, incidentally, that the groups named are almost always genuine victims—of poverty, violence, minority status, illness, or disability. Nonetheless, they are condemned for complaining about their lot and cited as a serious contributory cause of American economic difficulties or the collapse of moral and family values (Hanson, 2000; Hoult, 1998; Stewart, 1995).

Other critics argue that it is America's cultural unwillingness to care for the nation's children, its sick, and its poor that is the true moral outrage, the sign of America's decline as a society. These commentators cite statistics that show, for instance, that despite America's leading position in the world economy, the country offers the poorest health care options of all the industrialized nations (World Health Report, 2000).

Currently, American society's illness narrative is being altered by a number of factors. Among them are the drastically changing nature of the health care system, the nation's decision to let market forces determine nearly all social activities, the increasingly negative view of traditional medicine, the rise in popularity of alternative medicine, disability legislation, and the near-daily appearance of scientific, technological, and medical advances.

The culturewide illness narrative has always contained compassionate and concerned aspects, just as the rugged individualist ideal stood side by side with ideals of community involvement such as barn raisings and volunteer fire departments. Moreover, many groups in society and the ideals that animate them act as positive, integrating forces for individuals otherwise sidelined or disparaged.

But, unfortunately, many Americans still regard illness and disability as moral issues. In addition, the needs of the sick and disabled are perceived as causing an intolerable economic strain because they compete for what are believed to be limited resources (Fries, 1998).

Metadiscourse

The third level of discourse that shapes concepts of health care is what might be called *mythic discourse* or *metadiscourse*. Since the dawn of time, a society's myths were passed orally from generation to generation by storytellers whose tales told the listeners who they were as a people, how they came into being, how they should behave, how they had learned to do all the things they did, in what ways they had gone wrong from some prior golden age, and how they might make things right again. Metadiscourse was further codified in the society's epic poems, heroic adventure stories, and celebrations of magnificent accomplishments. On a darker note, the metadiscourse also included the society's tales of its tragedies, wars, disasters, and illnesses.

In time, many of the myths and stories appeared in writing. At first, only a small minority could actually read or gain access to the written word. Most people still learned their society's myths orally, at the kitchen hearth, on their mother's lap, in the marketplace, in taverns, or at church. But in nineteenth- and twentieth-century America, expanding educational opportunities and literacy created a broad reading public. With this came an explosion of popular newspapers and magazines, which were quickly followed by the arrival of radio, movies, and, finally, television. In this new world, the economically and politically driven visual and print media became the mythmakers of America.

The various forms of media provide America with its news, information, and entertainment, but because of the media's glamour and power, its stories automatically assume the level of archetype, symbolism, and myth. Much of the public assumes that the way the media represent illness and death is fact. Television and Hollywood movies create and enlarge illness and disability generalizations and stereotypes, drawing heavily on current cultural and political trends. What the public perceives as information has actually been created merely to entertain or hold the attention of an audience while the makers simultaneously sell a product or convey a political point of view. How the media represents individuals with, for example, breast cancer, Gulf War syndrome, or addictions, or what the media make of survivors of sexual abuse shifts with every eddy in the cultural climate. The representations lurch from negative to positive and back again, with varying degrees of accuracy. Some of the public, however, believe that each representation is accurate and responds accordingly (G. K. Auslander & Gold, 1999; Dixon & Linz, 2000; Greenberg & Wartenberg, 1990; van der Wardt, Taal, Rasker, & Wiegman, 1999).

Even if a TV movie about a soldier suffering from Gulf War syndrome is largely sympathetic to individuals with that condition and their families, the story is still almost always misleading. The real purpose of the movie, after all, is to tell a dramatic story, one with a distinct beginning, middle, and—perhaps most important—end. Clinicians who treat Gulf War syndrome and those experiencing it know that most patients do not die of the syndrome, that they may or may not give it to their loved ones, but that almost all will experience the syndrome chronically over a prolonged period of time. Such indeterminacy rarely satisfies media producers. The public knows that movies do not replicate real life, but they are taken to represent life, which can generate profound misconceptions in viewers. Thus, this week's movie about Gulf War syndrome, for example, becomes the culturally symbolic boilerplate for what happens to individuals and their families when a member contracts the illness.

The media also serves as a public forum or court in which the issues of the day may be honestly discussed, shamelessly exploited for economic gain, or used as a political football. Most people make little distinction among media presentations but instead attribute accuracy to them all. Issues of illness and disability examined in the media may be treated either with empathy or disdain, but whichever the attitude, the treatment establishes a judgment of the condition that the public accepts. On TV, for example, it makes no difference whether the viewer looks at a health care-related commercial or a news talk show, soap opera, or documentary. How the commercial or program treats the illness can strongly affect what viewers think about it (Dixon & Linz, 2000; Granello, Pauley, & Carmichael, 1999).

As a result, the chronically ill and their families tend to experience an immediate response from their communities after the media suddenly calls attention to their problem. When well-known figures or celebrities such as Betty Ford become associated with addiction problems, or Magic Johnson with AIDS, the public feels enough sympathy with the individual to make their condition acceptable, not only in them, but in others.

But for ordinary people used to anonymity, being regarded, even sympathetically, as a poster child for the condition can make them or their family feel exposed and tokenized. Instead of being an individual with a particular condition, he or she becomes an archetype of all persons with that particular problem. Most individuals with chronic illness find that the media presentation of their condition does even more: It catapults them into the vanguard of a political movement, which is not a role any of them would probably have chosen. As a result of their tokenization by the media and the perception that they are a small minority of the general population, individuals with chronic illnesses are often forced to become spokespeople, which further reduces their sense of privacy and heightens their sense of exposure. The role of spokesperson, they also find, is often one that requires a defensive posture, because they are frequently forced to *explain* their situation rather than describe it.

Special note must be made about profit-driven discourse. Commercials, infomercials, and so-called infotainment news can be particularly problematic for the chronically ill or handicapped individual. Because such infotainment news shows are inexpensive to produce, they are popular with media management and owners. Their content is generated by scans of current events and publications for anything that might attract and hold public attention. If a medical journal, for example, publishes a recent study on a new treatment for multiple sclerosis, the infotainment news show presents the information as a final statement, implying that the producers have thoroughly vetted the information. The show simplifies the information by dramatizing it in the most exciting form possible. Such programs take no account of the fact that peer-reviewed medical studies go through a process of publication and debate within the field before the information is disseminated to the general public. The intended purpose of this process is to excite comment, criticism, attempts at replication of the study, and so forth, and the process often generates modification and changes to the original findings. Such tentativeness and subtlety have no place in an infotainment show, however, which paints in broad, bold, black-and-white strokes.

For their part, infomercials are straightforward attempts to influence the public to buy a product through the creation of an interesting narrative and attractive characters. Despite disclaimers by the program producers, the public is strongly encouraged to accept clearly biased information as fact. Actual product commercials rely less on narrative than on catchy phrases, attractive characters, and stimulating visuals. All three forms of profit-driven discourse use and shape current cultural biases and viewpoints that affect the chronically ill and disabled.

SOCIOCULTURAL INFLUENCES IN CHRONIC ILLNESS AND THEIR TRAUMAGENIC EFFECTS

Beliefs and attitudes inform the perceptions, thoughts, speech, and actions of individuals and groups of individuals. These assumptions proceed from the worldview of the individual or group, which is constructed in part from the three levels of discourse discussed earlier. Whether people are consciously aware of their assumptions or not, these beliefs and attitudes construct their overall sense of who they are—their identities. Everything in the world that individuals apprehend or interact with is filtered through these assumptions. What people perceive as truth and reality are created, almost totally, by their assumptions. All people modify their assumptions continually, based on their experience, but these changes occur for the most part unconsciously. In general, people regard what they perceive and *know* as simply being the truth. It takes conscious self-reflection for individuals to identify their assumptions and critically assess them against other attitudes and against aspects of reality that are verifiable regardless of who is viewing them (Glassner, 2000; Maines, 2000).

As to the concerns of this book, the assumptions of patients, their families, and clinicians are rooted in the illness narratives reviewed thus far, but they also arise from each individual's personal encounters with the world; the experience each has had with nurturing, ethnicity, religious beliefs, family, and community; and how each individual handles and understands the mix of soma and psyche. One person, for example, may have had a chronically ill mother. Another may have professional training that has heightened his or her acceptance of differently abled individuals. In addition, the interaction between individuals in the system subtly or obviously modifies each individual's personal biases, beliefs, ideals, and fantasies.

When individuals engage with the health care system, they encounter the historical, religious, ethnic, class, and economic influences that are peculiar to the culture of the health care system. But perhaps more importantly, they are strongly affected by the particular assumptions of the individuals in the system with whom they have contact.

The health care system has group assumptions constructed from the collective worldview of its members. Care providers, patients, their families, and all the other actors in the system bring individual and group assumptions to all conversations within the system as a whole. These combined assumptions will influence how, for example, the health care system constructs scientific hypotheses or how clinicians interview patients.

It can be argued that any attempt by a professional to remain objective in the face of such influences will be very difficult. Nonetheless, although it requires conscious, open-minded investigation to clarify the motivations that inspire pursuit of any particular current clinical or empirical objective, medical professionals must make the effort. When clinicians are not aware of the personal or professional assumptions that shape their decisions and actions, they put themselves and those they work with at risk (Armstrong, 1990).

POTENTIALLY TRAUMAGENIC SOCIOCULTURAL FACTORS

This work is concerned with six sociocultural factors that can seriously exacerbate patients' experience of chronic illness. If clinicians do not consciously consider these factors and process their own reactions to them, their patients, the patients' families, and sometimes even the clinicians themselves may suffer trauma. Positive influences are also at work in society, and most health care professionals try to perform their jobs competently and respond to patients sympathetically and ethically. The following descriptions focus on negative effects to help clinicians guard against their influence (Fennell, 1995b, 2001, 2003c).

Intolerance of Suffering

Early and medieval Christianity enfolded the concept of suffering into a religious schema where it served negatively as a punishment for sin but positively as God's method of testing and strengthening faith and bringing believers closer to Christ and salvation. When Descartes split the body from the mind/spirit, he also separated the physical aspects of pain and suffering from the spiritual and emotional ones (Jennings, 1985). As far as science was concerned, humans became genderless bodies that responded to stimuli, whether of pain or pleasure. These feelings had no intrinsic meaning, and pain and suffering had no purpose. Medical practitioners following a scientific approach sought to relieve or end suffering by aggressively attacking its somatic manifestations, the only ones that were demonstrably physical and material (Ballweg, 1997; Bendelow & Williams, 1995; Gamsa, 1994; Stuart & Noyes, 1999).

Mental and spiritual suffering, which are nebulous and subjective from the scientific point of view, remained the province of religion or philosophy. Increasingly, as science became the privileged new approach to knowledge and understanding, religion was relegated to a peripheral cultural role in Western society. In addition, the containment that religion had provided for suffering—whatever meaning could be ascribed to it—was sidelined also. But religious attitudes did not die out altogether, even among convinced materialists. They were simply pushed to the margins of cultural influence, where they continued to nurture now often unconscious attitudes among the population at large (Bendelow & Williams, 1995).

Despite Descartes, however, suffering inextricably involves both body and mind/spirit (Jennings, 1995). It is impossible to separate physical suffering from mental and emotional suffering. Moreover, scientists quickly discovered that it was impossible to measure physical suffering objectively. Inevitably, they had to rely on an individual's self-reporting, which was not only subjective, but varied enormously according to the individual's background and circumstances. Although flawed data on pain had to be used in day-to-day medical practice, it was sufficiently subjective to discourage researchers, until recently, from investigating pain and suffering in general (Armstrong, 1990; Ballweg, 1997; Stuart & Noyes, 1999; Turk & Rudy, 1991).

Suffering is a ubiquitous human condition, with certain identifying characteristics. It increases in relation to how uncontrollable it is or how uncontrollable the sufferer believes it will be and how long it will continue. When suffering persists, people experience a profound sense of helplessness and also of hopelessness (Jeffrey & Lubkin, 2002; Onega & Larsen, 2002). They feel that their bodies are running out of the physical resources that combated the pain. They perceive their suffering as intolerable and at the same time as interminable. Ambiguity about their prospects produces anxiety about the future, which further exacerbates their suffering. Moreover, with suffering comes a loss of physical, cognitive, and emotional viability and hence a greatly diminished sense of self. This loss produces debilitating grief at the same time the individual needs to engage in the difficult readjustment to his or her new condition (Bendelow & Williams, 1995; Do Rozario, 1997).

Chronicity and ambiguity deeply affect the sense of suffering. People can often endure more severe pain if it is acute—that is, if it is pain that lasts, or they believe will last, only a short duration. In a sense, suffering comes into existence when pain, even mild pain, persists and shows no indication of ever ending.

Generally, modern Americans ascribe no positive value to suffering. It is mysterious, enigmatic. They do not understand it; they regard it as frightening and many times as meaningless. Usually they expect and demand aggressive action on the part of medical practitioners to end the suffering immediately. Americans do not want to suffer themselves, and they may experience difficulty being around others who are suffering. It can make them unhappy to see others suffer, and they may also fear suffering. It reminds them that all life is fragile and people are easily hurt or disabled. Witnesses to suffering cannot help but think about their own death or possible future suffering (Barshay, 1993).

When the person suffering is someone an individual loves, the witness is often compassionately engaged, especially if the suffering does not persist for a long time. But long-term suffering strains even the most loving of relationships. People who are suffering and those witnessing their suffering feel grief and often shame. But contemporary society frowns on public expression of such feelings, especially among men. Both sufferers and witnesses are prevented from relieving themselves and finding recognition and acceptance of their powerful emotions. Instead, they are forced to push the feelings underground, from which they can often reemerge in behavior destructive to self or others. It is important to remember that trauma can occur to witnesses as well as sufferers when appropriate expressions of grief are closed off (Ballweg, 1997; Barshay, 1993; Stuart & Noyes, 1999).

Clinicians, whose profession puts them in constant proximity to people who are suffering, protect themselves against reactions of avoidance, anger, and despair by doing precisely what science advocates and the public desires. They locate a cause for the suffering as quickly as possible and provide appropriate treatment to end it. If, however, they cannot find the cause or if the suffering persists even with treatment, some clinicians can become frustrated and even angry. Their personal fears begin to emerge. In self-protection, some may conclude that the suffering cannot have a physical genesis, but must proceed instead from psychological causes (Jeffrey & Lubkin, 2002). These carry an implicit judgment of characterological failure, causing the sufferer to experience iatrogenic health care in the form of blame (Cameron & Gregor, 1987; Kontz, 1989; Stuart & Noyes, 1999).

When clinicians are frustrated because they cannot perform "competently," this can be quickly communicated to patients. So, too, is their preference for clear physical symptoms. Patients receive negative reinforcement for accurate reporting and subsequently limit the information they provide clinicians to acceptably physical or "real" events. In addition, because some clinicians also subtly encourage only good news or reports of progress and improvements, patients adapt and thus censor how they describe their illness experience.

The ongoing diagnostic controversy that surrounds many chronic syndromes can become a traumatic issue when encountered in a health care provider's office. The medical community tends to be skeptical of certain chronic conditions. Some have become politicized, and controversy over them can range from etiology to diagnosis to treatment. The very existence of some conditions as medically recognized diseases continues to hover in professional discourse. This also may cause clinicians to convey to patients the notion that the patients are at fault and that their condition indicates characterological inferiority or defect or even deliberate malingering (Cameron & Gregor, 1987; Kontz, 1989; Stuart & Noyes, 1999).

Patients develop a fairly predictable set of responses to such attitudes. They think and worry more about their disease after a visit to the doctor. They feel confused about their identity and what is "real." They do not know whether they are sick, well, or crazy. The intensity of the diagnostic controversy erodes patients' ability to determine what is helpful and what is not, who is trustworthy and who is not. Patients go to clinicians hoping for answers or at least solace but come away feeling confused, blamed, frightened, and vaguely immoral or "bad." As a result of these experiences, many patients experience more anger and sadness and decide to avoid health care providers entirely (Ballweg, 1997; McCahill, 1995; Stuart & Noyes, 1999).

The pressure not to disclose their real condition causes many chronically ill people to avoid intimacy, sometimes most especially with those who have been their intimates before the illness. To prevent rejection, they misrepresent how they truly feel and start trying to "pass" as healthy people (Saylor, Yoder, & Mann, 2002). They feel forced to construct a falsely "normal" public persona and share their more genuine private persona with fewer and fewer individuals. They go into the closet much in the same manner as gays and lesbians to protect themselves from stigmatization. The pressure of this dual existence, with its concomitant rejection of self, loss of esteem, and depression, can lead to further avoidance of intimacy, increased isolation, substance abuse or alcoholism, marital problems, and sometimes suicide (Biordi, 2002).

For individuals who have participated successfully in the mainstream culture until their illness, chronic illness can expose them for the first time in their lives to social abandonment and rejection. To make matters worse, it occurs for reasons beyond their control. In this regard, racial minorities and the economically deprived are less likely to suffer this particular effect because they have already experienced it time and time again. For them, chronic illness is just one more instance of unfairness in an unfair world.

Ultimately, the greatest harm caused by the culture's intolerance of suffering is the violation of the social contract. People who have worked hard to perform as good partners, parents, workers, and friends suddenly find that something beyond their control has turned them into second-class citizens who are easily dismissed and barely tolerated. Vows that an individual's partner will be loyal "for better or for worse" frequently become meaningless. The health care profession, to which people always believed they should turn in such situations, not only fails to help them but may even imply that their suffering is their own fault (Alonzo, 2000).

Intolerance of Ambiguity

Most people in Western culture are also intolerant of ambiguity. They dislike the not-yet-known or the unknowable, and they avoid—even fear—complexity or chaos. They want issues to be clear and straightforward and solutions preferably simple. The prevalence of science and technology in today's culture has contributed to this cultural intolerance by elevating quantitative systems of knowing and simultaneously devaluing qualitative and subjective systems of knowing. In today's cultural system, all that is true or real is observable, measurable, and ultimately knowable. Anything that does not yield to these criteria is suspect. People continue to have doubts about situations or problems as long as the situations remain ambiguous.

In terms of the soma/psyche dichotomy, it is the physical body that is knowable, whereas the psyche is unknowable and, hence, suspect. The cultural elevation of the quantitative and allegedly objective above the qualitative and subjective has contributed to the view that ambiguous situations or problems are potentially dangerous and possibly immoral and, therefore, should be avoided. Ambiguity generates a sense of powerlessness. If a person does not know what something is, he or she cannot take action, which further heightens powerlessness. With ambiguity, a person is often rendered impotent. No matter how horrible a disease may be, if it has a clear cause, known symptoms, and an acknowledged, even if deadly, prognosis, it is often more bearable for the sufferer, family, friends, and clinicians than a condition of unknown origin with an unclear prognosis (Armstrong, 1990; Ballweg, 1997; Bendelow & Williams, 1995; Stuart & Noyes, 1999).

In today's society, those suffering chronic illnesses must endure the ambiguity of their condition without the aid of spiritual and psychological devices, which used to be part of Western culture and are commonplace in other traditions such as Buddhism. Whereas modern Western society's aggressive determination to eradicate physical suffering keeps it from falling into the kind of quietism or indifference to suffering that can characterize some cultures, it has also lost familiarity with philosophical and spiritual conceptions of suffering and the meaning and solace they may offer.

People in contact with the chronically ill are sometimes frightened by them simply because their condition is ambiguous. They fear potential contagion or contamination. This may be an atavistic survival instinct on the part of humans as a species, but even when science has clearly identified modes of disease transmission, people still fear contamination, as AIDS has shown repeatedly (Kitzinger, 1990). If the etiology of an illness is unclear, perhaps it is easy to catch. If the prognosis is unclear, who knows what might be in store if they caught the disease. People are adrift along a continuum of the unknown, from the origin of the illness to its outcome (Armstrong, 1987; Barshay, 1993; Kahn, 1995; Scambler & Hopkins, 1990).

Flooding in to alleviate the anxiety caused by ambiguity comes the notion of the just world and deserved punishment. People automatically begin to distance themselves from those who are suffering, especially if the cause is ambiguous. By specifying to themselves how they would have avoided the situation, solved it differently, or responded differently, people create a comforting belief that they can avoid personal tragedy by using farsighted protective action. This rationalization creates a false sense of calm and control over the uncertainty of living. As a defense mechanism, it supports the illusion that the people are invulnerable to illness, disability, and mortality. It also facilitates the unfortunate, yet somehow comforting, blame of the victim. Perhaps individuals with a chronic illness have actually brought it on themselves, or perhaps they are lazy or faking, trying to get out of work or responsibilities. Perhaps they are immoral or flawed in some other way, which makes the disease an appropriate retribution.

The intolerance of ambiguity may produce a sense of powerlessness in the chronically ill and then guilt, depression, and grief (Onega & Larsen, 2002). As ordinary participants in the culture at large, some chronically ill individuals internalize the message that they have probably caused their problem by some personal action and, therefore, deserve their condition. They suffer in addition because they feel, sometimes correctly, that they are a burden to those they love. Rejection and abandonment are not false fears, but realities all too often a part of the lives of the chronically ill.

Clinicians can also experience profound powerlessness when they treat the chronically ill. It is frustrating when knowledge accumulated from years of study, hard work, and experience produces no measurable or meaningful effect in their patients. Human nature, unfortunately, often makes it preferable to blame the patients rather than continue to experience a sense of incompetence and failure.

The most serious harmful effect arising from society's intolerance of ambiguity is that the chronically ill are openly or subtly held responsible for their condition, an attitude which the chronically ill usually share. As a consequence, they suffer strong feelings of guilt, depression, and grief.

Intolerance of Chronicity

Americans do not like chronicity; it upsets the society's action- and achieve-ment-oriented culture. The society prefers illnesses that are acute because, although they disturb personal and organizational output, they do so in a pre-dictable manner. Heart disease, appendectomies, and medicated depressions return individuals to the workplace in a fairly timely manner. But problems or illnesses that do not have a distinct beginning, middle, and end and are not easily treatable run contrary to a perceived notion that health problems will respond to powerful drugs or advanced technological intervention. Chronic illnesses, with their unclear etiologies, courses, and outcomes, are frustrat-ing, potentially expensive, and, consequently, devalued.

The medical profession focuses on achieving cures—that is, returning pa-tients to essentially the same status they had before the disease. The public has come to expect cures, especially in the past 50 years, with the amazing progress of science in pharmaceuticals and the technological tools of diagno-sis and treatment (Armstrong, 1987; Stuart & Noyes, 1999). When medicines or other treatments do not return the patient to normal, both clinician and pa-tient experience a sense of failure and both feel varying degrees of responsi-bility for it. Because chronic disease is not amenable to cure and the patient does not achieve a return to "normal," both clinician and patient can repeat-edly suffer powerful feelings of failure (Ax, Gregg, & Jones, 1997; Banks & Prior, 2001).

Many people do not understand chronic illnesses at all, particularly the fact that these illnesses are chronic; that is, they do not go away. When people see improvement in a chronically ill friend, family member, or even in them-selves, they believe this change is the start of a long, slow climb back to total health or "normalcy." A single relapse may cause only disappointment or sor-row, but several relapses or even prolonged failure to return to normal can generate annoyance and anger in those who are not sick and varying degrees of self-loathing in those who are.

Family resources are often insufficient to support the chronically ill properly, and society provides little help. Chronically ill adults may find it difficult to continue to earn money at the same rate as they did before or sometimes to earn any money at all. They may need help—sometimes only periodically, but other times constantly—to carry out the basic activities of feeding and clothing and sheltering themselves (Hardin, 2002; Lubkin & Larsen, 2002). Many partners of chronically ill individuals simply cannot adjust to the new situation and divorce the ill spouse, leaving that individual with even fewer resources to manage his or her illness (Joung, van de Mheen, Stronks, van Poppel, & Mackenbach, 1998).

Moreover, the chronically ill are once again punished—that is, people are annoyed with them, avoid their company, or desert them—if they take proper care of themselves. This includes patients' acknowledging how they really feel and what they actually can do. Instead, the chronically ill are rewarded for unhealthy self-care, for behaving as though they were feeling well. When the strain of operating so counter to reality becomes too much, some react by withdrawing altogether. Sufficient social isolation and depression eventually lead some to commit suicide.

The failure of chronically ill patients to return to normal can cause them to experience identity confusion (Saylor, Yoder, & Mann, 2002). Are they a person attached to an illness or an illness attached to a person? In their experience, clinicians and others in their social world regard them almost wholly in terms of their illness, as though they no longer had any other attributes. At the same time, and often as a consequence of the multiple traumas they may have suffered, the chronically ill themselves can become totally absorbed by their illnesses. They may attend obsessively to their disease to the exclusion of all other interests. This obsession is, perhaps, the most important harmful effect caused by society's intolerance of chronic illness. It is also the most insidious, because even when patients are finally ready to branch out from their preoccupation, society—and sadly sometimes clinicians as well—keep regarding them solely in terms of their illness.

Immediate Cultural Climate Concerning Disease

Every illness—whether tuberculosis, atherosclerosis, lupus, or AIDS—is born into a specific cultural climate concerning disease that is made up of all of society's currently existing illness intolerances. An illness that emerges for the first time today, for example, is born into a society that has experienced and formed attitudes about AIDS and multiple sclerosis. Social attitudes are also influenced by the new economic environment of medicine, in which people fear that costly new diseases may prevent the HMOs from covering their own medical needs adequately. Society's attitudes toward disease in general are continuously evolving (Cooksey & Brown, 1998; Cullen, 1998). This is not the same environment as 1950 (Armstrong, 1990; A. Wilson, 2000).

How society regards illness in general and an individual's specific illness in particular makes a significant difference to that individual's experience. But no matter how socially acceptable an illness has become, the individual, simply by having it, is marked as being outside society's primary defining group, the healthy (Bendelow & Williams, 1995; Thornton, 1998).

The public also tends to perceive the chronically ill as damaged goods. They become social examples of what the public does not want to have happen to them. The experiences of the chronically ill can mark them permanently as separate and different.

Illness Enculturation Process

Every disease has a history, a chronology during which it is recognized, assessed, researched, and treated. Concomitantly with discussion in professional discourse, new illnesses become part of general social discourse as well, but social understanding of an illness usually lags well behind medical understanding, especially in popular media presentations. Nonetheless, it is through this process that disease is culturally constructed and becomes a form of social reality (Armstrong, 1990; Clarke, 1994; Jason et al., 1997).

When an illness first appears in a culture, it is regarded with skepticism and fear until the society has investigated the phenomenon and decided how to respond to it (P. Lewis & Lubkin, 2002). Initially, patients are often shunned or treated as immoral as well as sick, as happened with AIDS. To acquire multiple sclerosis in 1950 was entirely different from contracting it today. Over time, the patterns or effects of a disease come to be recognized, and social fears are put into perspective. Eventually, the disease becomes integrated into the cultural consciousness, or enculturated.

The enculturation of a chronic illness usually works to the benefit of those who suffer from it. When a syndrome first attracts attention, those exhibiting its symptoms and the people they approach for help are puzzled by the problem at best and disbelieving at worst. Neither the sufferers nor clinicians have adequate language to describe the condition. They are forced to rely on terms appropriate to other conditions, which can easily misrepresent the situation. If a person lacks the language to describe something, its reality is a constant matter of question.

Besides lacking language or even metaphors to describe the new experience, both patients and clinicians lack models for assessment and treatment.

Again, they rely on approaches that have been useful for other illnesses, but in the case of chronic illnesses, old approaches are almost always unsatisfactory. Assessments do not adequately capture the nature of the symptoms or the way they are expressed over time, and treatments fail not only to produce cures, but even improvements in quality of life.

After an illness first appears, there usually follows a period during which the health care profession struggles to determine its "authenticity" and describe its etiology and symptoms. This is never a matter of "pure" science. Political and economic issues always cloud the investigation, sometimes by outright denial of funds or social support and sometimes more subtly through pervasive cultural attitudes that affect researchers just as they do all other members of the society.

During the enculturation period, the media are free to say anything about a new condition and make any evaluation of people who "claim" to be sick with it. Given the predispositions of the culture, the responses are often disbelief in the condition as an actual physical illness, ridicule, annoyance, and condemnation, with the obvious attendant effects on those suffering with it. Only bleeding hearts or the professionally compassionate are sympathetic. The ill are stigmatized and distrusted.

As the disease achieves description and acceptance in the medical world, it gradually becomes more acceptable in the society at large. Patients who develop a chronic condition now have vocabulary to describe their symptoms—to themselves, to family, to employers, and to medical professionals. Clinicians have either become familiar with the condition or can readily find professional literature discussing it. The public comes to believe that those suffering with the condition have a genuine illness.

Media

The media function as a forum for public opinion and judgment. They are the vehicles in which professional and social discourse converge and are thoughtfully repackaged for purchase. In the repackaging process, the media exert their own particular influence on the development of social discourse. They can create or enlarge stereotypes that appeal to and reinforce cultural prejudices. The media make public judgments, they publicly determine roles and worth in society, and they organize public ridicule or support (Kirkwood & Brown, 1995; Saylor, Yoder, & Mann, 2002).

When the media reinforce cultural prejudices, targeted groups are publicly judged, and scapegoating (which can be a manifestation of the just world notion) occurs. Public assignment of social role and subsequent worth can be clearly spelled out in black and white as the chronically ill and their families read the latest popular description of their illness on the pages of supermarket tabloids. Patients may be supported or ridiculed, but whatever the case, their personal problem has been identified, evaluated, and socially scripted for all the world to see. The effect of having a personal tragedy so publicly exhibited, even if no one ever mentions it to the sufferer, can be harmful.

Media presentations invade privacy directly as well. People who hear about irritable bowel syndrome or fibromyalgia on TV, for example, remember that a fellow worker has missed work because of this sickness. Suddenly, that individual loses whatever health privacy he or she had. All that person's fellow workers become instant experts on the condition. If the media has construed the condition as ridiculous or self-generated, the individual can suffer negative public judgment and find life at work more difficult.

But even if the condition has been treated with sympathy, the individual's privacy is transgressed. Because TV discussions rarely convey the nuances of living with a chronic condition, the individual faces misinformed sympathy, which is very hard to address successfully. In addition, the individual with the chronic illness knows that what is sympathy now may quickly turn to scorn or ridicule or anger if some other TV show or tabloid article presents a negative or derogatory story.

The reality that a chronic illness makes sufferers liable to public judgment about their character and their morals increases their social isolation. It is nearly impossible to ignore broadly held public judgments about themselves, so the chronically ill may withdraw from social contact. Although they may have had strong, supportive social connections before the onset of their chronic illness, subsequently, these are frequently eroded. When the chronically ill come from deprived or disrupted backgrounds, especially where issues of poverty or race are involved, the situation can be even worse, and the individuals will have fewer resources to help cope with the situation. With the attendant loss of privacy, the chronically ill report increased fear and anxiety, magnified feelings of grief, and a lowered sense of worth.

Chapter 3

INTRODUCTION TO THE FOUR PHASES: BETTY'S STORY

It is often easier to absorb the details of a multidimensional model if the reader has a broad general grasp of the whole, yet it is hard to keep generalities in mind unless they are anchored by specific examples. To provide an overview that incorporates concrete elements, this chapter examines Betty's story, a composite case history that includes typical manifestations for each phase in the Four-Phase Model. Each phase is broken down into the physical/behavioral domain, the psychological domain, and the social, interactive domain.

A NOTE ON DEVELOPMENTAL LIFE PROCESSES

It is very important for clinicians to remember that as the chronically ill traverse the four phases that lead to integration of their illness experience, these phases occur simultaneously with developmental and maturation processes and are influenced by them. In addition, patients' changing patterns of activity at home or at work affect the experience of chronic illness, as does their changing level of personal energy. All these nonillness processes, cycles, or arcs are affected by matters other than health and, at the same time, have a profound effect on health (Carter & McGoldrick, 1988; Henderson, 1997; Lubkin & Larsen, 2002; Mercer, 1989; Newby 1996; Nicassio & Smith, 1995; Peters, 2002; Rankin & Weekes, 1989; Register, 1987; Rolland, 1987; Rosman, 1988; Woodgate, 1998).

Developmental transitions and upheavals tend to compound the suffering of the chronically ill, so it is most important for clinicians to help patients separate experiences directly attributable to the chronic illness from those caused by other intense situations that are happening simultaneously, such as the death of a loved one, the decision to return to work, or the birth of a child. Clinicians also need to assist patients to distinguish the grief they may feel, for instance, as parents when a child leaves home, from the grief they feel because of the severe restrictions imposed on them by chronic bone-numbing pain, cognitive confusion, or perpetual exhaustion. In addition, such non-disease-related factors can precipitate illness relapses in Phase 2 and subsequently; thus clinicians need to remain alert to these events (Carter & McGoldrick, 1988; Henderson, 1997; Lubkin & Larsen, 2002; Mercer, 1989; Newby, 1996; Nicassio & Smith, 1995; Rankin & Weekes, 1989; Register, 1987; Rolland, 1987; Rosman, 1988; Woodgate, 1998).

BETTY'S STORY

Discussion under each phase section begins with a general description of each domain, followed by what happens specifically to Betty.

Phase 1: Physical/Behavioral Domain

The physical functioning of a person with a chronic syndrome in Phase 1 occurs in three stages. Although illness onset can occur suddenly, more typically, patients go through a coping period when they experience some combination of symptoms, which they try to ignore or which may remain below consciousness. Over time, the coping period gives way to an onset stage in which symptoms more insistently demand the patient's attention. This onset stage usually climaxes in an acute incident. Patients may point to a particularly pernicious illness, a trauma, or a surgery as the trigger that precipitates the acute emergency stage.

The acute stage can continue for days or weeks, if not months or sometimes years, depending on the severity of the syndrome and the quality of support available to the patient. Crisis terminates with a diagnosis and/or the beginning of a personal recognition of a set pattern of symptoms.

Betty is a married White woman in her late 30s. She has two children, Lisa, age 13, and Michael, age 11. Bob, her husband, is a computer hardware troubleshooter, which often requires him to work out of town for one or two weeks at a time. Betty works part time at a bank in the suburb where the family lives.

Over the past several weeks, Betty has been increasingly distracted by a number of physical symptoms that are beginning to frighten her because they are interfering with her life and her work. She has episodes of tingling and weakness first in one leg, then another, and then in her arms. It goes away, but then it comes back again. She also has strange sensations in her body, again a kind of tingling, but it's hard for her to describe. She is exhausted much of the time, but what seems very strange to her is that she sometimes has trouble walking. Betty has never been sick with more than occasional colds, so she rarely goes to the doctor. She does not think her situation is very different from that of many of her friends, because all the working mothers she knows are always tired, too. She just keeps trying to carry on with her regular activities, snatching whatever moments she can to nap or, at least, rest.

Betty is just entering Phase 1. Physically and behaviorally, Betty is in a coping stage. Even though she does not feel well much of the time, she is generally able to ignore her symptoms, to push them out of her consciousness, and to continue her regular activities.

Eventually, however, Betty's condition deteriorates enough so that she cannot ignore it, and she enters the onset stage. Unlike many chronic patients, for whom a particular incident—a flu virus, a car accident—triggers onset, Betty simply experiences an ever-diminishing level of functioning. When she realizes one day that she is physically incapable of walking up a full flight of stairs, she goes to see the doctor.

Her doctor listens to Betty describe her symptoms and gives her a quick physical examination. They talk a bit about her situation at work and at home. The doctor tells Betty that she has nothing physically wrong with her. What with the many demands of her job and family life, it sounds as though stress may be causing her difficulties. He also thinks that she is mildly depressed, but not enough to require medication. The doctor recommends that Betty relax, try to get enough sleep, cut back at work, and perhaps join an exercise class to help relieve her stress.

It is often suggested to chronically ill individuals, especially women, that they are misinterpreting their experiences and are actually suffering from depression. They may continuously receive these messages while they suffer the symptoms of their illness.

Betty wants to follow the doctor's suggestions, but she does not dare cut back on work because the family needs the income from her job. And she cannot see how to fit an exercise class into her already-tight schedule. Her symptoms get worse. She is now having trouble driving because she feels so weak. Her difficulty walking has become noticeable to her best friend at work, and she is extremely fatigued much of the time.

Betty is now entering the acute emergency stage. She goes back to the doctor, who refers her to a neurologist, and he orders a complete physical. For months, she is examined and tested and generally shuttled about in a diagnostic limbo. It is not until almost a year later that she is given a tentative diagnosis of multiple sclerosis (MS). Even now, the doctors are not really sure it is MS because plaques do not show up on her MRI. The specialist ordered a spinal tap, but it is ambiguous. Not all doctors agree on the factors determining MS. Betty's history is largely suggestive because she does not have the typical hallmark findings—MS plaques and abnormal spinal fluid.

But having a diagnosis, even a tentative one, makes an enormous difference to Betty because it finally gives her a way to understand and describe her experiences to herself and others.

Phase 1: Psychological Domain

Many patients, especially those who experience a lengthy onset, use denial as an appropriate coping mechanism. Because of the lack of recognition and support from the health care community and from the society at large for the vague and varied symptoms of chronic illness, patients initially collude with others in the denial of their symptoms in an effort to continue their daily lives. As their condition continues to deteriorate, this denial gives way to intrusive feelings of fear, self-hatred, despair, and disorientation. As patients physically begin to move into the crisis stage, fearful ideations may intensify when compounded with feelings of shame and loneliness. Patients are typically receiving conflicting advice and disbelief from professionals during the crisis phase. They do not know how to describe their condition to themselves, let alone to family, friends, and coworkers, and have increasingly painful experiences caused by emotional isolation, fear of others, mood swings, confusion, and an absence of useful information.

During Betty's lengthy coping and subsequent onset stage, she uses denial as a coping mechanism. Denial particularly comes into play after her physician tells her that she is mildly depressed and suffering from the stress of a woman's life today. She colludes with her doctor, her husband, and people at work because it makes it possible for her to live her daily life.

But as Betty's symptoms worsen, other feelings begin to obtrude. Like all people, Betty has constructed two selves while growing up—a private persona and a public persona. And like everyone, Betty reveals more or less of her private persona to individuals in her life depending on how intimate she is with them and what particular situation she is in. As Betty's condition continues to deteriorate, Betty finds that her private persona begins to impinge on her public persona in ways that she cannot control. One day at a staff meeting at the bank, Betty suddenly bursts into tears, embarrassing herself, her superior, and her coworkers. This behavior is not the self that Betty recognizes. She is not the sort of person who cries in public. She is greatly ashamed of herself and begins to wonder what could possibly be wrong with her. She cannot bear her loss of self-control.

Betty's shame and self-hatred occur at the same time she is feeling increased fear and despair. Could she actually be dying or perhaps losing her mind? She knows she feels terrible physically and is getting worse, but maybe something is also wrong with her mind. She feels shock, even dissociation. It is important to remember that no one has yet given Betty's situation a label. No one knows what is going on.

Betty has no way to express how she is feeling and when she tries, the people she talks with can only make up explanations and suggestions for improvement based on their own personal experiences, not on an understanding of what is happening to Betty. Betty feels increasingly isolated because she fears what is happening to her and what other people will think of her. She's particularly afraid to talk to the person who used to be closest to her—her husband, Bob. Betty and Bob have already been having marital difficulties because of conflicts over money and the amount of time Bob is forced to be away from home. Betty feels that Bob, by default, gets out of his fair share of home and child care duties. She cannot quit her job to stay home full time because the family cannot do without her salary financially. In any case, she likes her job, which she does very well. She has received much praise at work, especially from her superior, and she and Bob have both been hoping that she will get a promotion. The new position would bring in more money but would require that Betty work full time.

In part because of her pain, her fears, her lack of useful information about her condition, and her growing isolation, Betty now begins to suffer mood swings. Half the time she is in tears, she says, and the other half she is furious. Bob has tried to be sympathetic, but now he is getting annoyed. The children act scared of her and disappear whenever possible. Even Betty's coworkers find her snappish and distracted, whereas she used to be pleasant and cooperative.

Phase 1: Social/Interactive Domain

Patients find that as they can no longer hide or disguise their chronic illness symptoms, some friends, acquaintances, coworkers, and health care providers see them as crazy, lazy, or immorally evading work, which increases burdens for others. They continue to receive these inaccurate and painful messages at the same time they are suffering from their symptoms. The disbelief and discomfort of health care providers, the shock and suspicion of friends, and rejection by society, together with the debilitating aspects of the syndrome, can lead to the initial isolation of chronic illness sufferers within their disease. Patients may become cautious or fear expressing their physical pain and emotional discomfort, expecting further rejection or negative stereotyping. They withdraw emotionally from others. Physical limitations may further hinder efforts to reach out for social contact.

Thus, three critical issues become evident during Phase 1:

1. The patient can be traumatized by the physical, psychological, and social impact of the chronic illness in the emergency stage of Phase 1.

2. Friends, family, and clinicians experience shock, disbelief, aversion, and life work shifts in response to the acute phase of chronic illnesses and, as a result, are often vicariously traumatized.

3. As a result of their vicarious traumatization, together with internalized attitudes toward disease, others begin to queue up on a continuum that extends from suspicion to support in response to the patient. These social responses are often very negative, if not stigmatizing, and cause further secondary traumatization in the patient.

Depending on the maturation of the organization that the clinician works in (that is, the level of supervision and support) and the maturation and premorbidity and comorbidity of the patient's social network, ongoing traumatization will be propagated or minimized. A healthy social network can allow the disruption of work and social exchange that emergency stage events bring while serving as a container and buffer for the individual experiencing the entry into the chronic illness free fall of the acute phase. A healthy health care organization provides support and supervision to health care providers who experience the daily grind of treating chronic suffering so they can return to their work fresh and avoid vicarious traumatization, subsequent burnout, and inflicting unintentional iatrogenic traumatization.

Many of Betty's psychological mechanisms and reactions result directly from what is happening in her social/interactive life. During the coping and onset stages, Betty's family, friends, and coworkers respond in various ways to what they see of her experiences. Although she is in denial, they notice only that she is tired much of the time and sometimes misses work. For a while, they are sympathetic. She is a hard worker, and her female coworkers particularly have strong personal understanding of how hard it is to juggle a job, home, and children. As Betty accomplishes less and misses more work, however, they become critical. They have difficult lives, too, but they manage to come to work, and they accomplish their assigned tasks.

Betty's children think that she is acting strangely. She does not behave like the mother they are used to. Bob finds her unpredictable and emotionally extreme. He is used to hearing Betty say she is tired, but when she complains about tingling and weakness in her limbs and trouble with walking, Bob is genuinely worried and urges her to go to the doctor. The doctor's diagnosis of stress seems reasonable to Bob, and he makes an effort to help more by staying in town or taking only short jobs away from home. But that cannot go on forever, and Betty does not seem to change. He thinks she could do much more if she tried, but she seems just to complain or sleep.

During the acute emergency stage, while Betty is being examined and tested extensively, Bob sometimes wonders whether anything is actually wrong with Betty. Maybe it is all in her head. Some of her coworkers feel that way, too. Maybe Betty is having a kind of nervous breakdown.

Finally, Betty gets her diagnosis, however tentative, of MS. Although this gives her the relief of a name and an explanation, she now finds that the illness has put her squarely on the forefront of a cultural debate. Caught in a mesh of divergent popular beliefs about her partially understood disease, Betty finds that some of her friends and coworkers—even some of the medical personnel she sees—regard her negatively. For the first time in her life, Betty begins to experience rejection by society at large. She becomes very cautious about expressing her fears or revealing her pain because she does not want others to withdraw from her. Not only is she afraid of other people now, but her physical condition itself interferes with her reaching out socially to other people.

Unfortunately, Betty's home life was already stressed before the onset of her illness, and her illness has exacerbated the situation. At the bank, Betty's immediate supervisor is very sympathetic because the supervisor's sister, with whom she is very close, has fibromyalgia. The supervisor has a good grasp of Betty's problems and wants to help. Upper levels of management, however, think that Betty should probably be replaced, and it is unclear how effective the supervisor's advocacy will be. On the medical front, Betty's primary physician has become very involved with her case and would like to spend more time on it, but the HMO permits only fifteen minutes per patient visit. The doctor cannot spend the time he would like talking with Betty, but he must focus on assessment and treatment of her acute physical symptoms, which are what the HMO regards as the only "real ones," that is, chargeable ones. The doctor cannot discover in depth how Betty is feeling or how she is coping with the whole illness experience.

Phase 2: Physical/Behavioral Domain

As Phase 2 starts to unfold, patients proceed physiologically from the emergency phase to the plateau phase. During this period, symptoms are stabilizing and assume a familiar cyclic pattern that the patient is beginning to recognize. This in turn helps orient the patient cognitively and psychologically.

During Phase 2, Betty attempts to create order from chaos. Her physical symptoms stabilize. They do not disappear, but they rarely go outside a pattern that she is beginning to recognize. She knows that if she climbs a set of stairs in the morning, she will not be able to do so again later in the day. If she drives for more than 10 or 15 minutes, she will become fatigued and weak. Although life is very difficult, Betty has identified a set of parameters around which she can function. Her health care professionals discuss a few of these parameters with her, but, for the most part, Betty discovers them on her own. To some extent, her new-found knowledge also orients the people around her.

While in Phase 2, Betty suffers two physical relapses, during which her symptoms suddenly become more severe. In the first episode, her doctor consults with the neurologist Betty saw earlier, who recommends that she be put on a trial of medication. Both times, she eventually returns to a plateau of stabilized symptoms, which she recognizes and can negotiate.

Phase 2: Psychological Domain

After the initial diagnosis is made, individuals have a sense of immense relief. Finally, their experience has a name that demystifies some of the disturbing uncertainties about their symptoms. Some of the ambiguity and chaos is removed through the symbol of diagnosis or, if they have not received a diagnosis, at the very least, a recognizable symptom pattern.

During Phases 1 and 2, patients accumulate experiences of stigmatization, rejection, and iatrogenic traumatization. As a result, patients and their families censor how much they say and to whom they say it. Patients engage in "passing" for well. This in turn results in social withdrawal in general, specifically from those who wound them. These adaptations can be a healthy part of the stabilization effort if the patient turns to others of like kind who have successfully adapted and to nontraumatizing professional resources.

Unfortunately, the respite that an initial diagnosis often provides is short-lived because patients quickly realize that this new label or symptom pattern does not include a precise etiology of the condition or a definitive treatment option. As a result, they may become embroiled in a period of service confusion and searching for doctors who they hope will cure them. This behavior is part of the natural seeking process of Phase 2. Patients are attempting to exert some healthy control over the traumatic losses and disempowerment they experienced in Phase 1. Such searching is part of their normal effort to stabilize through learning and analysis and acquiring helpful resources. But confusion, urgency, and desperation intensify as patients make these medical rounds and encounter a multitude of conflicting opinions. A significant number of patients report a general lack of support and guidance from health care providers, if not outright hostility, when they attempt to learn more about their illness experience, and this further adds to their confusion, despair, and traumatization.

Concurrently, patients are caught up in limit rejection and boundary confusion. They can no longer perform as they used to, but because of familial and community pressure, they attempt to maintain former roles and schedules and repeatedly fail. Resultant feelings of guilt and shame heighten patients' increasing sense of failure, worthlessness, and anomie. Patients discover that formerly easy tasks such as climbing stairs, shopping, or cleaning have to be renegotiated because they are no longer able to complete them or can accomplish them only sporadically. Patients feel like children, not completely confident about how their body, brain, or emotions will behave in any given situation. These continually changing physical and psychological parameters, as well as internal and external pressures to maintain a self-image that no longer exists, create a cycle of daily failure and subsequent confusion about limitation. As patients and their network struggle with boundary confusion, they become increasingly cautious in the presence of others.

Unlike many people with a chronic illness, Betty actually receives a diagnosis. Initially, she feels enormous relief. Finally, she has an explanation for why she has difficulty walking, why she has this strange tingling and weakness, why she becomes so fatigued, and why she has such extreme mood swings. Her uncertainties also lessen as she begins to recognize her symptom pattern. Furthermore, diagnosis gives her a way to learn about her condition, so that she can exert a semblance of control over her life again. She reads everything she can about MS and seeks out others with MS so that she can discuss her situation in a supportive setting.

But Betty quickly learns that the diagnosis does not explain how her illness started or what is going to happen in the future, so ambiguity returns. No one seems to know what to do to cure her. No one can make her symptoms stop, and no one seems willing or able to tell her how she is supposed to live her life under these conditions.

Like most people in this country, Betty grew up believing that if she worked hard and told the truth, everything would come out all right in her life. But here she is, working extremely hard to get better, telling the truth when she talks to family members and friends and clinicians, and yet she finds a significant amount of the time from a significant number of people not acceptance, but rejection. In fact, she is sometimes being blamed. So Betty has become very cautious. She carefully censors what she says and to whom. Whenever she possibly can, Betty acts as though she is well and nothing is wrong with her.

Betty decides to avoid such secondary wounding by withdrawing from any social contacts that may bring negative judgments on her. Instead, she tries to get in touch with other people with MS and advocate for those with MS because they will not be hurtful and they will understand her situation.

She continues to read and research her condition and seeks other sources of emotional sustenance to make up for the losses she has suffered elsewhere.

Because her medical outcome is uncertain and Betty still believes that cure must be a possibility, she suspects that her health care professionals are not adequate to deal with her problem. She collects the names of other doctors from friends and new MS acquaintances and attempts to find a professional who will offer her better treatment and, she hopes, a cure. This behavior erodes the relationship she established with her primary care physician, who regards her actions as dysfunctional.

Because Betty finds little guidance and meets with confusing responses and even outright hostility as she tries a number of doctors, she attempts alternative treatment. A practitioner of shiatsu massage listens to her with enormous empathetic patience. Betty's cousin urges her to try acupuncture. A coworker swears that a complicated vitamin and supplement regime returned her bedridden niece to full functioning and could do the same for Betty.

Betty has lost a sense of her boundaries. Because she seems to others to have returned to "normal," a false appearance that she helps to create by her "passing" behavior, Betty is being encouraged, even urged, by family and employer to return to her former roles and schedules. But Betty cannot do this without serious repercussions. She has trouble getting up in the morning. Her husband has to make the children's school lunches. She can no longer serve on committees at work because she can just barely keep up with her regular obligations. Nothing about her body or her emotions or her mind acts the way it did in the past, yet Betty keeps trying to behave as though she were the person she used to be. Despite her efforts, Betty fails daily at what she attempts, and daily she feels guilty and ashamed. Increasingly, she feels worthless.

Phase 2: Social/Interactive Domain

Patients encounter increased conflict as friends, family members, and some care providers lose patience. Most of the existing support system urges patients to "get back to normal." Without an acceptable diagnosis and/or a rapid course of treatment, the persistence of symptoms continually frustrates the support network. Part of the frustration expressed by the social network stems from their own experience of vicarious secondary wounding or traumatization. The lifestyles and work habits of spouses and parents are dramatically altered in response to the chronic illness: They have witnessed the suffering of the patient in addition to their own and other family members' suffering, and they have experienced the guilt by association of societal stigmatizing responses. This societal marginalization of those who associate with or care for the stigmatized and thus marginalized is also experienced by clinicians, who, as a result, selectively reveal to their peers and supervisors their treatment of, and reaction to, marginal populations such as those with chronic fatigue syndrome or post-traumatic stress disorder. Not considering all members of a patient's network in the treatment and support effort can result in vicarious traumatic manifestations such as drinking, avoidance, or abuse, and subsequent normalization failure or patient and network breakdown.

Betty experiences growing conflicts with family, friends, and some of her medical care providers as they lose patience with her failure to become symptom-free or to adjust to her illness in a manner that allows her to return to her former functioning. Although she has a diagnosis, such treatment as she receives does not produce rapid, let alone complete, improvement. At one point when she could not walk at all, Betty's doctor put her on a course of medication. She improved, but she still has periodic difficulties, and the persistence of her symptoms frustrates everyone.

Bob has told Betty that she is no longer the person he married, and this is not the life he signed up for. She has got to change if their marriage is to continue. Betty can tell that her coworkers are annoyed and believe that she could function a lot better if she just pulled herself together and put her mind on the job. One of them knows an MS patient of higher functioning and tells others at work that she cannot understand why Betty doesn't manage as well as her friend does. Betty is not imperceptive. She knows that people think she is not trying hard enough. To make matters worse, a close friend with deep religious convictions has urged Betty to pray, saying that if Betty has a sincere desire to get better and asks for God's help, God will cure her. Betty does not share her friend's convictions, but deep inside she fears that maybe she is sick because she is somehow unsatisfactory in God's eyes.

As Betty goes through cycles of relapse and remission, all the people in her life experience them as well. They become as exhausted by the process as Betty does, and they are traumatized just as she is. Bob has lost the wife he married and the life he had, and his new life is not at all what he wants. Their son, Michael, has always liked school and done well, but now his grades are beginning to suffer. Lisa is behaving badly at home, and she has taken up with a troubled crowd at school. Betty does not know whether this is just a part of adolescence or whether Lisa and Michael are reacting to her health problems and her squabbles with Bob over money, the division of labor at home, and her condition.

Betty's family are not mean-spirited. They are sad and scared to see this person who is very important to them suffer pain, confusion, and unhappiness. Outside the house, they suffer a kind of guilt by association. Lisa's friends sometimes treat her as though she is as weird as her mother, and Lisa once saw one friend imitate the way her mother sometimes walks. Bob's boss is clearly concerned about whether Bob will be able to fulfill his job obligations, given the demands of Betty's illness. Some secretly wonder whether MS might be catching, and just for safety's sake, many keep their distance.

Even Betty's doctor is affected by the stigmatization of her illness. By and large, careers are not made by treating the chronically ill, and few health insurance organizations encourage doctors to engage in the extensive dialogue over an extended period that chronically ill patients require.

Because normalization failure is so common in Phase 2, it is not unusual for either the chronically ill or those around them to turn to anodynes such as alcohol or drugs and for people in the social network to engage in avoidance or abuse of the chronically ill individual. Any of these factors or even a totally new factor can produce a new crisis in the chronically ill, which returns them to Phase 1. Bob's mother dies and the entire family must deal with that trauma. Later, Betty has a high fever during a bout with flu, which triggers a severe relapse.

Without informed clinical guidance, many chronically ill people become caught in a repeating cycle of Phase 1 and Phase 2. Each new crisis produces new wounding and secondary wounding. With luck, following each crisis, the patient manages to arrive at a plateau of manageable symptoms until the next crisis sends the whole system into chaos again. Some people, particularly those on the margins of society who have almost no sources of support, never escape Phase 1 but are buffeted from crisis to crisis, relieved only by alcohol and drugs.

Betty is not in that position. She has some warm and loyal friends. Her supervisor persuades the bank management to let Betty take a position with fewer hours. And a new social worker affiliated with Betty's doctor becomes involved in helping Betty cope with MS.

Phase 3: Physical/Behavioral Domain

In Phase 3, individuals with chronic illnesses often maintain a continued plateau, but relapses can occur. If a relapse takes place, it is sometimes in response to the typical cycling of the syndrome, or it may be triggered by persistent attempts to engage in precrisis tasks, roles, and pursuits—that is, to behave as the "normal" people they were before the onset of the chronic syndrome. True entry into Phase 3 comes, however, when patients recognize that they cannot perform as they have in the past and recognize relapses, if they occur, as the normal cycling of their chronic syndrome.

In Phase 3, Betty enjoys long periods of stabilized symptoms, sometimes even improvement, but she still has relapses. Most of these are simply in the nature of the illness. As Betty comes to comprehend the nature of chronicity and the ambiguity inherent in her condition, she lets go of her search for an elusive cure and works instead to integrate her illness into a new life.

Phase 3: Psychological Domain

Patients in Phase 3 experience an increasingly internalized locus of control and an increased tolerance of ambiguity and chronicity. They are also increasingly aware of the effects caused by social attitudes and stereotypes. They begin to have compassion for themselves. All of this occurs, however, because they suffer a secondary emotional crisis or grief reaction when they understand that their lives have really and permanently changed. They now realize that they are not the same as they once were, and they will never return to the person they considered themselves to be. They begin to wrestle with the reality that they "can't go home again."

As a result, they feel demoralized and devalued. They see that they can no longer sustain the life roles of parent, worker, lover, or friend as they once planned them. They question what good they are, who they are, and why they should continue to exist. This begins the process of mourning their precrisis self.

This appropriate, necessary grief reaction—what might be called the "dark night of the soul"—is obviously a tenuous time. Individuals can be lost to their own understandable withdrawal, fall victim to predatory providers of not-so-helpful care, or succumb to their own despair and thoughts of suicide.

For patients, their families, and their caregivers to survive this difficult time, meaning has to be developed.

Meaning is established through three transformational steps or intervention processes:

1. The allowance of suffering as opposed to its rejection and the subsequent rejection of the suffering self
2. Development of a compassionate response to the suffering of the rejected, sick, stigmatized self
3. Development of respect for the actual act of suffering—that is, for the time spent in the tunnel, not for the light at the end of it

This process creates a respect for the new self. To carry out this lengthy, frightening activity usually requires that patients and their families borrow from the wisdom and faith of the care provider. With this help, they can, in the pit of their grief, begin to consider another way to be in the world, through role and identity experimentation or overtly creative endeavors. The process helps patients develop meaning for their experiences, and it creates an opportunity to begin integration of aspects of the precrisis self with the new emerging respected self. This is a time of profound and intense exploration, which often includes spiritual or transcendent aspects.

Twice in Phase 2, Betty suffered severe relapses brought about in part by her repeated attempts to do all the things that her precrisis self did. Throughout that time, she wanted to be her former self, and everyone around her wanted her to be that person, too. But repeated relapse has taught her that she cannot sustain the roles that she had always thought she would fulfill as spouse, parent, worker, or friend, or at least not in the way she used to imagine. Betty comes to understand that her life has changed entirely and forever.

With the help and encouragement of her new MS friends and the social worker, she explores and expresses the grief she feels for the loss of her old self and she mourns the end of that life.

At this point, all the major existential questions come into play. Betty wonders, "Who am I?" "What good am I?" "Why did this happen to me?" "Why should I live?" "Is there any value to my life?" During this painful period, she struggles to locate a meaning for her existence. Betty is very vulnerable. She could be lost because of her own very considerable social withdrawal. She could fall victim to cynical and predatory providers. She could give way to despair and attempt to kill herself.

But Betty is fortunate. Her new friends and the social worker help Betty navigate the difficult course between necessary grieving for her past self and foundering in clinical depression. She learns not to reject her new suffering self, but to have compassion instead. This is not an easy task because Betty is constantly receiving messages from people she knows telling her that if she stays the way she is, if she remains ill, they no longer want her among them.

To move forward from grief and mourning, Betty tries to discover meaning for what has happened to her and locate a way to live in the future. She begins to engage in philosophical or spiritual thinking to come to a new place. Betty starts by learning to respect the person she is now—not the person she might become, but who she is right now.

As is typically the case, Betty does this through a creative act, which becomes an act of meaning development. She decides to write a journal describing her experiences. Other people she knows have done things as various as taking up cooking or becoming MS advocates—even remaking their wardrobe and hairstyle. One friend of hers actually made a movie. In the process of composing her journal, Betty recreates herself—she integrates herself and begins to discover meaning in her experience.

Betty draws heavily on both the social worker's personal support and encouragement and on a variety of wisdom traditions that seem to speak to her. Betty is not religious in the traditional sense. In fact, she regards herself as an atheist. But since she has consciously begun thinking about the basic issues of life and meaning, she has discovered aspects of Buddhism and Celtic philosophy that resonate strongly with her personal vision of what is significant in life.

Phase 3: Social/Interactive Domain

For the most part, patients undergo even greater loss. They may experience some integration of new friends and supporters, but, inevitably, important significant others and clinicians give up and friends disappear. Patients experience abandonment, isolation, and stigmatization. Not enough can be said about their increased realization of, and experience with, this engulfment in stigma; it weighs heavily on the patient and the family and clinicians who remain attached to the patient. With support, as patients are experimenting with new social and vocational roles and developing a growing respect for their experience, they may choose to break the silence of engulfment in a variety of demonstrable ways. Some may choose to confront those who reject them or minimize their experience. This is part of the integrative process, part of experimenting with new ways of being in their new life.

The role of the clinician is never more crucial than in Phase 3, and never is the clinician's own support and supervision more crucial. Working with chronic illness patients and their families can evoke strong reactions in the treatment provider. It is not uncommon for experienced clinicians to feel disbelief, frustration, sadness, and fear in response to the chronic suffering of patients. If their reactions are not processed and modulated effectively, clinicians risk burnout, unintentional further traumatization of patients, and missed opportunities for effective interventions.

The strides Betty makes in her psychological evolution during Phase 3 do not occur in a benignly static social environment. In fact, she endures a considerable blow when she and Bob agree that they must divorce. At first, Betty worries terribly about how she will manage. She still has a job at the bank, but she has always been on Bob's health plan. As part of the divorce settlement, he agrees to keep her and the children covered. As time passes, Bob demonstrates that he will continue to meet his financial obligations to her and the children. He is also good about having the children regularly, which gives Betty needed quiet time and reduces her anxiety that the divorce will cause harmful distance between the children and their father. Betty knows that in this divorce experience, she is much more fortunate than one of her friends with MS who kept custody of her children, but lost her home when she subsequently lost her job.

Encouraged by an MS friend, Betty explicitly asks Lisa and Michael for help at home. She is surprised to find that Lisa responds enthusiastically, especially to cooking. Michael is good about drying dishes and putting dirty clothes in to wash if he is reminded, but recently he has gotten restive about living with "a bunch of women." Betty, who could not have endured letting him go two years ago, feels confident enough about his basic attachment to her so that she is planning to let him spend his next school year with his father.

At the bank, Betty feels competent to deal with her present job requirements, and her coworkers have gotten so used to her condition that they have more or less forgotten it. Her confidence was further bolstered when the social worker offered to conduct a workplace consultation on her behalf. Betty decided that it was not necessary at the time, but she felt she had someone on her side if she should need it.

Betty knows, however, that her job security depends almost entirely on her supervisor, and she has begun investigating other part-time work she might do, perhaps at home. The social worker has also reminded Betty that she is eligible for disability if she is unable to work, and she has been inquiring among her MS friends about this as well.

In any social arena now, Betty refuses to pretend or to keep silent about her MS. When people react badly or seek to label or stigmatize her, she may confront them about their bias. She has been surprised at how empowered such behavior makes her feel, and she is even thinking about becoming formally involved in advocacy work. With the end of her marriage and the inevitable loss of some old friends and acquaintances, Betty has been forced to consider new roles and to seek new friends. Despite the fact that this experience has been amazingly painful for Betty, she has survived it. She is surprised to find how positive the process has turned out to be and how much she likes her new self.

As Betty freely acknowledges, it would have been very hard for her to navigate this passage without the devoted and informed help of her care provider—the social worker. Not only did this woman affirm the realities of Betty's trauma and illness, but she listened and counseled sympathetically as Betty traversed the process of finding her new self. She suggested a number of books that she thought might help Betty think about the philosophical issues involved and put her in touch with a former hospice worker, who helped Betty discover what issues had bedrock significance for her.

Phase 4: Physical/Behavioral Domain

Phase 4 may see continuous plateau, improved well-being, or possible relapse. In any case, patients who have reached Phase 4 recognize the cyclic nature of chronic illnesses and no longer regard relapse as a failure. It is simply another cycle to be integrated. This understanding manifests the true nature of recovery for the chronic illness patient, which is integration of the illness into the patient's ongoing life.

For the most part, Betty experiences continuous plateau and occasionally she enjoys periods of distinct improvement. But she has also had three relapses, one severe and two lesser ones. Betty now realizes that relapses happen, and she no longer regards them as some failure on her part. She even knows that she may one day have a terminal episode. But short of death, which will happen to everyone eventually, she intends to try to reintegrate herself after each relapse experience. Betty comprehends that integration is the "recovery" she should strive to maintain.

Phase 4: Psychological Domain

In Phase 4, patients have achieved a true integration of the precrisis self with the newly claimed respected self who has suffered and endured. This achievement is maintained through a daily commitment to the allowance of suffering, to meeting it with compassion, and to treating it with respect. Integration is not a "cure," but consists of small daily acts of bravery in the presence of stigmatization, rejection, or the pains of the illness itself. This standing with the self turns suffering into conscious suffering and prevents neurotic suffering. Patients project and live up to a new "personal best." The experience transcends the original trauma of Phase 1 and is built on the stabilization of Phase 2 and the development of meaning in Phase 3. Typically, patients choose to continue to pursue their emotional and spiritual/philosophical growth.

Chronically ill individuals in Phase 4 have only occasional need for clinical help. When a serious blow knocks them back into Phase 1, they may turn again to a helpful clinician to speed the process of integrating the experience into their lives, and frequently they keep in touch to review maintenance protocols. But for the most part, they can manage living with their chronic illness by themselves.

Betty maintains her new self by consciously recognizing who she is now and by standing with herself. This does not mean that life has become easy. Sometimes Betty cannot climb stairs at all. Sometimes she is so debilitated she must use a wheelchair, which she hates. She can still become mentally confused, especially if she overextends. Nearly every day, she experiences some difficult moments of stigmatization, rejection, and even her own pain. But she speaks out against bias and has learned to endure the symptoms of her illness. She has created a new ideal self and takes pleasure in seeing how well she can live up to it.

Betty finds that a constant, active, conscious consideration of meaning and purpose enriches her life and places her experiences, both positive and negative, in a context larger than herself. She still finds great solace in Buddhist conceptions of suffering, but she has also discovered a new trove of wisdom in the material discussed by a Great Books group that she has joined.

Phase 4: Social/Interactive Domain

Because of the formation of a new self, Phase 4 often brings patients new friends and sometimes new partners. The hope is that through intervention patients may also be reintegrated with alienated family members, friends, and lovers. Patients frequently, through personal reorganization, turn to new sources for socialization and support and to alternative opportunities for self-gratification in purposeful ways. They may seek to modify their schedules, change jobs, or find an entirely new type of work. Some obtain disability benefits and, if physically possible, use this period as a chance to retool for an alternative type of employment. Some spend their available "healthy time" with educational and support organizations or in political activism. Others have undergone intensive personal examinations and have applied themselves to spiritual paths. These transformed individuals have taken control of their illness and their lives by constructively defining their own experience. Through this effort, they can make a profound positive impact on the encompassing organism of family and community to which they are inextricably bound.

Betty continues to nurture the new friendships she began establishing in Phase 3. She also sought out her younger sister, from whom she had been estranged as an adult, and the two have found they enjoy the openness and honesty of their new relationship as much as they like reminiscing about their childhood. Betty's frankness about her condition and her refusal to accept derogatory estimations make it perfectly clear to people who she is now, and some admire her for it and see the truth of her self-assessment.

Betty is about to change her job. While she worked at the bank and when she was at home sick, she became adept with computers, so she has decided to take a position running an MS web site and chat room. Although Bob has remarried—an event that threw Betty into an emotional crisis—he is intrigued with her new job and enjoys discussing it with her. Relations between the two are better than they have been for many years.

Betty even dares to contemplate entering a meaningful sexual relationship again. One of her MS friends remarried recently, which gives her hope, and she has met a man she likes very much in a monthly writing class. Because of his encouragement, she sent part of her journal to an MS newsletter.

Betty knows that crises and disasters happen all the time in life. She worries a great deal about her children. A friend of Michael's was just arrested for stealing a car, and she thinks that Lisa may have had a pregnancy scare. One of her MS friends took a terrible turn for the worse and will probably not survive. This scares Betty terribly because she knows the same could happen to her. But Betty is learning to separate those things she can control from those she cannot. Although it is a continuous effort, she endeavors to exert herself in the things she can affect and to endure with grace those she cannot.

PART II

THE FOUR PHASES

Chapter 4 ———————————————————

PHASE 1: CRISIS

During the first, or crisis, phase of the Four-Phase Model, chronically ill individuals experience a gradual or abrupt onset of the illness. For most patients, it suddenly or eventually culminates in an acute emergency that drives them to seek professional intervention to obtain relief.

Typically, patients attempt to obtain medical help, but they may also approach a psychologist, a social worker, a member of the clergy, or some other

---

PHASE 1
Course of Illness

Physical/Behavioral Domain
  Coping period—symptoms interpreted within the normal
  Onset period—symptoms recognized as beyond the normal but bearable
  Acute/emergency period—symptom severity demands assistance

Psychological Domain
  Loss of psychological control
  Ego loss
  Intrusive shame, self-hatred, despair
  Shock, disorientation
  Disassociation, fear of others, isolation, mood swings

Social/Interactive Domain
  Others experience shock, disbelief, revulsion
  Vicarious traumatization
  Responses dependent on family/organization maturation
  Suspicion-support continuum

---

meaningful counselor. The first professional contacted may carry out an extensive evaluation in an attempt to address the problem, or that professional may refer the patient to another who seems better suited to treating the situation. Clinicians may, therefore, conduct the initial assessment, or they may receive chronically ill patients by referral, in which case they should analyze all the data gathered by the referring party and make sure to coordinate any treatment program.

Typically, primary care physicians find it difficult to spend the time necessary for full assessment and treatment of chronically ill patients (Gordon et al., 1995; Harder et al., 1997). For the most part, doctors assess and treat the most pressing somatic problems and then refer these patients to other clinicians for the more in-depth psychological and social systems examinations. The referral clinicians may be nurse practitioners or physicians' assistants working in the primary care physician's office, or they may be psychologists or social workers with independent practices. Whatever the case, it is important to the successful assessment and treatment of the chronically ill for all the clinicians involved in a case to work as a team, to share information, and to be cognizant of and coordinate their own tests and therapies with those ordered by the other clinicians (Carbone, 1999; Fennell, Levine, & Uslan, 2001; Levinson et al., 1999; van Eijk & de Haan, 1998; Wagner et al., 2001).

Increasingly today, most clinical practice requires such a team framework. With the exponential increase in medical, pharmaceutical, and technical information, it is very difficult for one professional to hold in mind all the pertinent or potentially pertinent information about his or her patients' conditions and potential therapies. Whereas the situation of the chronically ill foregrounds this issue, it is now crucial in acute disease as well. Clinicians must not only rely on the expertise of others to treat patients, but also make it their practice to check with other clinicians involved with the same patients to make sure that all recommended treatments work together rather than counteracting one another.

In this sense, public clinics that serve the economically disadvantaged are actually well designed to address the problems of chronic illness because they usually include a collection of professionals who function as a team. Moreover, they are liable to have well-established connections with social workers who are already addressing systems issues that involve the patients. Often, these clinics are also more sensitive to minority racial and ethnic cultural contexts. Because many clients of public clinics suffer from chronic ill-nesses, the phase assessment and treatment model discussed here might prove effective for the patients and easier to implement in clinics than in some private practice situations. I must note that the cases discussed in the following chapters concern the middle-class patients in my personal prac-tice, but this phase method has been applied to good effect by others who treat disadvantaged patients.

When clinicians see chronically ill patients for the first time, the patients may conceivably be in any phase, although they are usually in Phase 1 or Phase 2. Most patients seek help during their first emergency crisis in Phase 1. If life circumstances make that impossible and the patients weather the ini-tial storm, they may reach a plateau of symptoms and a degree of relief on their own. In that case, they may not seek aid until Phase 2 of their illness ex-perience. It is also possible that patients experience Phase 1 with an initial clinician but have attained Phase 2 stabilization by the time a referral clini-cian sees them.

IDENTIFYING PHASE 1 PATIENTS

Urgency

Patients in Phase 1 are typically overwhelmed by a sense of diagnostic and treatment urgency (Fennell Phase Inventory; Fennell, 1998; Jason et al., 1999). They want to be fixed immediately, to have their painful condition removed as quickly as possible. Their sense of urgency usually includes an overwhelming need to identify their condition and what caused it. They desperately want to name the problem under the assumption that this will provide some degree of control over it.

Locus of Treatment outside Self

Patients in Phase 1 are also firmly convinced that the locus of treatment and cure exists outside themselves. They believe that the ability to do anything about their condition lies wholly in the hands of others, most typically the clinician.

PHASE 1
Identifying Characteristics

Urgency
Locus of treatment outside self
Self-pathologizing
Intrusive ideations and denial
Ego loss
Low tolerance for ambiguity

Clinical Goal
Trauma and crisis management

Clinical Summary
Bond
Affirm
Teach
Observe
Safety plan

Self-Pathologizing

At the same time, however, most Phase 1 patients engage in a high level of self-pathologizing and self-blame. Occasionally, they may also blame others for their condition, but self-blame is dominant. Thus, patients feel simultaneously out of control, yet totally responsible and filled with a presumption that they are bad or defective simply because they are sick with whatever illness they have. They are frightened and pleading, but sometimes angry and blaming as well.

Intrusive Ideations

Intrusive, repetitive—even obsessive—negative ideations, particularly of dying, are very common in Phase 1 because of the multiple traumas these patients have suffered and are suffering (Alonzo, 2000; Klein & Schermer, 2000; Matsakis, 1992; van der Kolk et al., 1996). Terrified already by what is happening to them, the persistent ideations further frighten patients and reinforce both their sense of urgency and lack of control. Intrusive ideations can often alternate with a numbing cycle where denial is in operation as a method of coping. In the denial state, patients can be emotionally flat or distracted and out of touch with the troubling content of their lives. But many patients are anxious, even extremely anxious, and this anxiety may alternate with deep depression, which can fuel negative and suicidal ideations.

Ego Loss

Phase 1 patients often demonstrate ego loss. Their physical difficulties diminish their sense of the self's integrity, and their inability to perform their customary roles erodes their social self-esteem. As the public self they have built up from childhood is worn down, primitive aspects of the personal self erupt unbidden in public, further shaming the patient and reducing self-esteem. These outward ego losses are matched by an inner loss of ego. Phase 1 patients can experience a dissociative state (Alonzo, 2000; Kauffman, 1994; Klein & Schermer, 2000).

Low Tolerance for Ambiguity

Phase 1 patients are characterized by a very low tolerance for ambiguity. The unknown is unmanageable and hence completely beyond their ability to accept.

These identifying aspects of Phase 1 patients are suggestive rather than exhaustive. Depending on the clinicians' professional specialty, it is likely that they will encounter other repeated and defining manifestations to indicate Phase 1 placement. Clinicians unfamiliar with phase placement may find it helpful to employ the Fennell Phase Inventory (Fennell, 1998; Jason et al., 1999).

Examples

To give these general statements reality, consider the following cases.

Urgency

Kim was a 44-year-old White woman in the process of completing a graduate degree, whose urgency for identification and treatment related directly to her overwhelming need for symptom relief. She suffered almost constant pain, particularly in her back, because of degenerative disk disease. In childhood, she had also been diagnosed with restless legs disease, and those symptoms had persisted into the present. They made her feel that all her nerve endings were exposed, and she sometimes simply wanted to tear off her skin. The restless legs had disrupted her sleep from childhood, but now, with her persistently powerful back pain, she found it impossible to obtain needed rest. She was becoming increasingly unfocused and clinically anxious. **Kim** was a patient whose physical urgency was a powerful drive for seeking help.

Lewis was a 37-year-old, Black high school math teacher whose urgency arose out of his intense, repetitive ideations. These were sexual in nature, and he feared that they indicated he might eventually harm someone. He was almost indifferent to his physical manifestations, an assortment of tics, which eventually proved to be Tourette's syndrome.

Sophia was a 33-year-old Black biologist whose urgency proceeded from the intense ego loss that illness onset brought. An immigrant to the United States, she had always been first in her class at school and had earned a doctorate in biology from one of the nation's most prestigious universities. She had an excellent job in industry, where she devoted all her time and effort to her work. She regularly received glowing job reviews and was advancing rapidly until she was stopped abruptly by totally debilitating exhaustion. Unable even to get out of bed or dress herself on many days, **Sophia** was forced to take sick leave so frequently that she finally asked her supervisor to recommend a doctor. The supervisor directed her toward a practice that worked for their common employer. These clinicians determined that nothing was wrong with **Sophia**. She later saw other doctors, who diagnosed chronic fatigue syndrome (CFS). At the same time, she discovered that her work evaluations had suddenly became highly critical and derogatory. Apart from the pain and exhaustion of her illness, **Sophia** suffered enormous urgency concerning who she was now that she could no longer perform intellectually and was no longer admired and valued for the effort that largely defined her self-image.

Everett was a 63-year-old White man when he suffered a disabling stroke. The stroke was treated as an acute episode, and **Everett**'s life was saved. But after an initial exposure to rehabilitation, his HMO determined that he had achieved a plateau and further treatment would not be cost effective. **Everett**, who was still paralyzed on one side, had not learned how to live, and his urgency related to his inability to tolerate the ambiguity of his disabled condition. His doctors had not precluded the possibility of further improvement, but they could not tell him how to bring it about.

Christine was a White nurse in her early 40s when she entered treatment. Her urgency was almost entirely social. **Christine** came from a large ethnic family, in which she was the oldest daughter. Not only did she function as a second mother to her younger, though now adult, siblings, but when her father died, she took over many household repair activities that he had usually performed. She enjoyed her position greatly. Since her siblings had grown up, she had become the person who organized the frequent family get-togethers. When she suddenly fell ill with multiple sclerosis (MS), she was unable to work, let alone accomplish her traditional family activities. Although she was not diagnosed immediately, she suffered less from the ambiguity of her situation than some patients because as a nurse, she was more attuned to the ambiguities that are actually inherent in medical practice. She did suffer enormously, however, because of her family's reaction. They regarded her illness as a failure and an insult to them personally. One sister even refused to allow her children to visit with **Christine**, even though she had been their favorite aunt. A fellow nurse, who later married **Christine**, was the only person who seemed willing to help her negotiate a period when she was bedridden most of the time. Her isolation from her family was the primary problem that plagued **Christine**, and the solution to the problem, she felt, lay entirely outside herself.

Locus of Treatment and Cure

All five of these patients saw the locus of treatment and "cure" to be outside themselves. This is partly because even before seeking help, they had been doing everything they could think of to manage. After requesting medical help, they cooperated as completely as they could with all tests, procedures, and protocols. From their point of view, there was nothing left for them to do. All help had to lie in the hands of others. Moreover, they all believed that in the various divisions of labor in society, the health care profession had the obligation and expertise to effect the cures they sought.

Intrusive Ideations

The most dramatic sufferer of intrusive ideations was **Lewis**, who believed that his insistent dramatic fantasies might ultimately translate into inappropriate or seriously antisocial behavior. He saw no connection between other physical manifestations and the persistent scenes of his imagination. But **Lewis**'s sense of disconnect between his ideations and his physical symptoms was actually unusual. Most chronic patients suffer from intrusive ideations of inadequacy and despair. They sometimes fantasize their suicide as a solution to their apparently hopeless situation.

Sophia, for example, kept imagining the disappointment of her family (although they were, to a person, supportive), the critical comments of colleagues, and the uselessness of her life henceforth.

Christine kept thinking of herself as a bad person. If she were worth anything, she would be able to get up. She would be able not only to care for herself but also to fulfill the expectations of her family.

Everett's mind, too, perpetually played out minidramas of how useless he was, how incapable of any action of, or even the appearance of, a proper man.

Wracked by pain and tired beyond the ability to think, **Kim** frequently imagined suicide. Finding no relief in the treatment she had received so far, she could not imagine any release from misery outside death.

Denial, the reverse side of intrusive ideation, however, was there as well, particularly in **Christine** and somewhat in **Sophia**. Whenever symptoms abated with these patients, they regarded themselves as returned to normal. They attempted to accomplish the full range of their past activities. When the inevitable relapse came, they still tried to believe that this was simply a temporary moment of difficulty or, even worse, a failure on their part to try hard enough. Here, **Christine** suffered more than **Sophia** because **Christine**'s family reinforced every moment of denial and deprecated any claim that she was actually sick. **Sophia**'s family, on the other hand, although they were at a distance, believed that she was seriously ill and urged her to take care of herself. A sister even traveled to this country to help her. In **Sophia**'s case, it was her own self-estimation that was stimulating her negative ideations.

Ego Loss

All five patients suffered serious ego loss, but more strongly in different areas.

Obviously, **Sophia** lost her central defining self when she could no longer perform her job, the embodiment of her intellectuality, and her lifelong academic superiority. She also suffered ego loss from stigmatization at work. People whom she had trusted to value her on the basis of their previous attitudes suddenly ceased to value her at all, even beyond the level of work proficiency. Her ego was diminished, as is true for all patients, by her physical pain and her exhaustion, but it was her mental anguish that caused her the most grief.

Kim, on the other hand, suffered ego loss almost wholly in relation to her physical pain and distress. Exacerbated by her sleeplessness, her totally raw nerves defined what remained of her diminished self.

Lewis found himself becoming potentially monstrous. Whatever meaningful self he had been was being devoured by his fear of what he might be becoming.

Everett believed he had ceased completely to be the self he had been. Only a return to his previous functioning would return him to the person he believed was his only self.

ASSESSMENT: PHYSICAL/BEHAVIORAL DOMAIN

It is important to remember throughout this book that the original changes that chronic illness patients experience are imposed on them. They are not a matter of choice or intention. Moreover, as patients navigate the four phases, new changes are imposed as well as changes they choose to make. This situation is unlike that described by several current stage models of behavior change. These models also focus almost wholly on the psychological (Prochaska & Velicer, 1997b; Prochaska et al., 1994). The Four-Phase Model, on the other hand, encompasses all three systems that affect the patient's life: the physical/behavioral, the psychological, and the social/interactive. Each of the three systems can have a profound impact on the other two, and the interrelationship of these three systems changes over the course of the phases. Clinical practice has shown that successful intervention and treatment in any one system depends a great deal on accurate assessment in all three systems. Failure to assess a patient's family situation accurately, for example, may make recommended physical interventions ineffective because family members encourage or demand noncompliance (Berg et al., 2002; Woods et al., 1993).

Medical Review

Clinicians need to make a thorough assessment of the patient's physical and behavioral status, beginning with an in-depth medical review. Using a team approach, medical practitioners must make sure their examinations consider

---

PHASE 1
Assessment

Physical/Behavioral Domain
    Medical review
    Activity level review
    Physical benchmark
    Neuropsychological review
    Sleep assessment
    Other assessments

Psychological Domain
    Phase placement
    Psychosocial assessment
    Initial trauma assessment
    Psychiatric evaluation
    Personal narrative (combined assessment and treatment)

Social/Interactive Domain
    Family and couples evaluation
    Work evaluation

---

the psychological and emotional dimensions of patients' problems, even if this means referring patients to other clinicians. Conversely, psychologists or social workers first seeing the chronically ill must make sure that patients receive a complete physical examination. In other words, it is essential that clinicians learn how the particular condition of chronically ill patients manifests itself in both the patient's soma and psyche. Teamwork is key here. Practitioners with different expertise must not only share information and test results, but also actually read and understand the information to make sure that recommended therapies are coordinated.

Examples

With patients like **Kim** and **Lewis**, it was extremely important to coordinate with their doctors. Both patients had nebulous conditions, which suggested a number of different possibilities and a number of different treatments. I recognized from other physical symptoms and behaviors of **Lewis**'s and deduced from his family's physical history that he might be suffering from Tourette's syndrome. In conjunction with his doctor, I arranged for a complete evaluation by specialists in another city, who confirmed Tourette's and identified obsessive-compulsive disorder as well.

Everett's condition was perhaps the best known and understood of the five, but it was still important for all members of his health care team to know what the others were recommending as therapy.

Christine and **Sophia** required close medical attention because their physical conditions were constantly fluctuating at the time they first came to my office. **Christine**'s medical background, however, gave her the advantage of greater knowledge and quicker access to information resources, whereas **Sophia** was completely mystified initially by her condition. Moreover, MS, **Christine**'s illness, has greater acceptability in the medical world today and more agreed-on therapies, whereas **Sophia**'s CFS still meets with disbelief among some health care professionals and the treatments are not as clearly defined.

Activity Level

In addition to using the reports from the other members of a patient's team, the principal clinician can assess precisely how patients feel and their activity level through the use of activity logs and body charts (Furst, Gerber, & Smith, 1985, 1997). An activity log chronicles in fine detail the activities patients carry out during the day and the degree of difficulty, pain, and/or exhaustion they experience as they accomplish these daily actions. Patients then use this log or list, along with a detailed picture of the human body, to describe what they think about each part of their body. The clinician may prompt them to address parts of the body that the patients overlook. Patients begin with a discussion of how their brain feels and what their thinking ability is like. As they move downward through the eyes, ears, mouth, teeth, and so on, clinician and patients examine how much dryness or pain or dizziness they feel, how often they feel it, and under what circumstances.

Discussion with patients about the activity log and the body chart helps clinicians establish the activity threshold level of their chronically ill patients. This issue is rarely discussed with chronic illness patients unless a specific rehabilitation program has been ordered. And even rehabilitation programs usually address only very specific activities that would include, for example, raising arms above the head or walking up a flight of stairs. With the chronically ill, however, clinicians need to understand a much broader range of activities. They need to determine in some detail how patients go about all of their daily business—not only self-care, but also cooking, cleaning, laundry, getting to work, and so on. It is important for clinicians to know how patients accomplish all of the activities that patients regard as their responsibilities.

Physical Benchmark

Not all individuals start from the same physical benchmark (Anderton et al., 1989; Armstrong, 1987; Frosch, 1990; Vacha, 1985; Wellard, 1998; Willan & Humpherson, 1999). Clinicians need to assess the physical activities level of their patients in the context of each patient's premorbid "constitution." Clinicians can elicit this information about the past as they discuss the current situation. Some patients will have been very active physically in their preillness life. They may have enjoyed sailing or rock-climbing or hiking or daily jogging. But others will have never done much more than walk from a parking lot to a store. One mother of small children will habitually have run up and down stairs without noticing it, while another will have been perpetually exhausted by her kids well before her illness. One person will have regularly slept eight or nine hours a night, while another will usually have slept only five or six.

What patients were and believed they were before becoming sick constitutes a major aspect of their identity. Determining their physical benchmark contributes significantly to understanding how patients are experiencing their current situation and helps in developing strategies for productive, meaningful coexistence with it.

To capture the original benchmark and the current activities, clinicians should elicit detailed descriptions of regular activities that patients accomplish over the entire waking period. Conversation about activities takes place in connection with the body chart and the activities log, and information about the premorbid benchmark is gleaned at the same time, for example, what patients do in the morning or if the patient is still working, what the patient used to do on arriving at work before he or she became ill. Particularly when patients show a high level of activity before the illness, the clinician can explore what other things they did outside the daily round. But even in the ordinary activities of a week, it usually becomes clear that some patients were energetic, constantly on the move, and lively, where others were quieter, more placid, or always harassed and exhausted.

To establish patients' activities levels, clinicians may want to administer scaled activity measurements such as the Medical Outcome Survey (MOS-SF-36; Friedberg & Jason, 1998; McHorney, Ware, Lu, & Sherbourne, 1994; McHorney, Ware, & Raczek, 1993) and fatigue scales such as the Fatigue Severity Scale (Krupp, 1989) and the Multidimensional Assessment of Fatigue (Belza, Henke, Yelin, Epstein, & Gilliss, 1993). Friedberg and Jason recommend that clinicians who employ fatigue scales use at least two for each patient to help overcome deficiencies that exist in the separate scales.

Some clinicians may prefer to rely on extensive individualized questioning. If so, they begin by identifying kinds of activities. For example, a set of questions about food shopping might be:

"Do you do your own grocery shopping?"

"How often?"

"Do you shop by yourself or with assistance?"

"What did you do in the past?"

Clinicians may wish to group patient answers into categories because the distribution of a patient's activities will become an important intervention strategy in Phase 2. Broadly, activities fall into four kinds:

1. Activities of daily living (ADLs), such as personal physical care, laundry, food purchasing and preparation, housecleaning, and so on
2. Activities related to personal enrichment or fulfillment, ranging from playing golf or taking bike rides, to reading or attending concerts, to taking courses or attending religious services
3. Activities involving all family and social activities
4. All activities related to work or employment

It is important when discussing current activities with patients to determine whether they actually complete the tasks they say they assign themselves.

Finally, clinicians should ask their patients to describe in detail the structure of a typical day's actual activities. If the patient's narrative is too general ("I got up, ate breakfast, went to work, came home, had dinner, watched TV, went to bed"), the clinician interrupts to ask clarifying questions, such as:

"What time did you get up?"

"Did you shower or bathe when you got up or do you usually do that sometime later in the day? Did you wash your hair while you were showering?"

"Did you make your breakfast? Did you make breakfast for anyone else? What do you usually have to eat?"

"How did you get to work? How long does it take?"

"Did you take lunch, or did you go out to buy lunch? Who makes your lunch if you take it to work?"

In other words, clinicians are seeking information on the amount of activity hour by hour. Where there are obvious omissions, clinicians need to ask about them. These include things like showering, hair washing, cleaning the house, washing dishes, answering bills, and sexual activities.

During the activities assessment, both the content of the interview and the manner in which patients share the information provide valuable information. Moreover, in addition to the obvious information about how patients perform physically at the current time, clinicians gain psychological insights about how aware patients are about what they are doing daily and social systems insights into how patients interact with their home and work systems, particularly in the context of this new situation of illness stress.

Examples

Assessing activity levels was a particularly important component in the cases of **Sophia**, **Christine**, and **Everett**. For the two women, it helped begin to define the reasonable limits that they needed to set to any single day's activity. It also called attention to whether they were engaging in activities across the four activity areas or whether they were overly committed in one or two.

In **Sophia**'s case, it was immediately clear that her life had been very active in the past intellectually. She had expended most of her energy on work-related activities, devoting only the minimally necessary time to ADLs. Her personal fulfillment activities were almost entirely conflated with work, with one extremely important exception—her spiritual life. Social life with her family was attenuated by distance, but the emotional bonds were strong and supportive. **Sophia**'s friendships, however, were almost wholly work-related.

With **Everett**, the activity evaluation helped begin to indicate to him how much he was actually doing, as opposed to the hopeless inactivity he thought characterized his current life. It became apparent that before his stroke, **Everett** had been a very active person physically, who enjoyed doing yard work, keeping the house in repair, and going camping with his family. He had never considered daily self-care activities, most of which he could once again accomplish, as being activities at all. Nor had it occurred to him that friendly conversations with neighbors or discussions at the dinner table constituted important activities.

Neuropsychological Review

When clinicians feel there may be neurological concerns, they may decide to order a neuropsychological review to capture neurological functioning as well as psychological and cognitive information. In some cases, neuropsychological reviews may also be necessary validating documentation for later disability or insurance claims. For this or any other kind of testing, however, clinicians first should ask themselves whether the test will make any difference in actual treatment of the patient (Burke, 1990; I. K. Smith, 2001). At what point, in other words, do they have enough information to conduct proper care and guidance? When does any further testing simply constitute the pursuit of technological possibility over the guiding and defining of practice?

Examples

It was important in the cases of both **Kim** and **Lewis** to carry out neuropsychological reviews because of the clinical input such reviews would provide. But it was perhaps equally important to order them for **Sophia** and **Christine** because both women would almost certainly need to apply for disability. **Everett**'s poststroke disability at the time he entered my practice was sufficiently clear and clinically acceptable to preclude the need for testing at that time. It was probable, however, that later, as his functionality changed, it might become necessary to order testing for a variety of reasons, including the maintenance of his disability status.

Sleep Assessment

A significant number of chronically ill individuals have unsatisfactory sleep patterns (Buchwald et al., 1994; Korszun, 2000; Krupp & Mendleson, 1990). Usually, they have trouble falling asleep, or their sleep is broken. Even if they sleep for a normal period of time, they do not wake refreshed. It is also important for clinicians to remember that people dealing with strong reactions to stress use up enormous numbers of calories and may require more sleep than others. Chronic illness patients benefit greatly from coming to understand these issues and being taught better sleep hygiene. Given the costs associated with formal sleep studies evaluations, it is sometimes sufficient for clinicians themselves to discuss this with patients or for the patients to have an interview with a sleep studies specialist rather than an entire evaluation.

Examples ———————————————————————————

Of the five, **Kim** most desperately and immediately needed a sleep assessment and introduction to improved sleep hygiene. But **Christine** and **Sophia** also had disrupted sleep patterns due to their conditions, and they needed to learn how to maximize their rest. **Lewis**'s plummeting self-esteem was causing his sleep to suffer, but that was more related to his fear than to a sleep disorder per se. **Everett** had not learned to adapt his sleep pattern to his changed physical life, but again this was probably more a question of sleep education than an actual disorder.

Other Assessments

During assessment, clinicians may also wish to use ancillary services such as physical therapy or occupational therapy to expand the assessment picture, but this is usually not helpful until patients reach Phase 2. Although many chronic illness patients are in a deconditioned state and suffer from other disorders that impact them physically, Phase 1 focuses on containment—that is, helping patients to reduce their fears, their anxieties, and their overwhelming urgency. Once they have achieved sustainable and operational ADLs and have thereby regained a small sense of control over their lives, it is then usually a better time to investigate the efficacy of physical or occupational therapy.

ASSESSMENT: PSYCHOLOGICAL DOMAIN

Phase Placement

The initial assessment of the patient's psychological condition takes place when clinicians evaluate the patient for phase placement. Where patients are on the phase continuum suggests what kinds of interventions will work most effectively and how best to develop a relationship with the patient.

Patients engage with and respond to treatments best when these interventions fit with the phase the patients are in. When interventions do not take phase into consideration, patients may become noncompliant or even sabotage treatments. They may not be ready for the interventions and sometimes are not even capable of them. Sometimes the significant others in their lives are so unsupportive that patients become noncompliant. In addition, the failure of an ill-timed intervention may taint the intervention in a patient's mind so that even when the patient could benefit from it at a subsequent phase, he or she does not wish to try because it did not work the first time. Other stage theories also call attention to the desirability of matching intervention and stage and inutility of mismatching them (Prochaska, DiClemente, Velicer, & Rossi, 1992; Prochaska & Velicer, 1997b). There has been some empirical study of the need to match stage and treatment, but the results have been inconclusive so far. On the clinical level, however, the benefits of matched treatment and the inutility of mismatched treatment have been clearly observed.

Clinicians not only assess new patients for phase placement, but also continuously monitor patients for changes in phase placement.

Examples

All five patient examples—**Kim**, **Lewis**, **Sophia**, **Everett**, and **Christine**—clearly indicated Phase 1 placement.

Psychosocial Assessment

In addition to reviewing the physical medical history of patients, clinicians should conduct a general psychosocial interview, which will give them an up-to-date profile of the patient's cognitive, emotional, and social symptoms. It is important to assemble as much personal and health information from the patients, families, and social networks as is reasonable, including information relating to any preexisting psychological conditions such as substance abuse, depression, trauma, and so forth.

Just as clinicians try to establish what the individual patient's physical "constitution" was before the illness, they want to explore what kind of emotional character the patient exhibited before the illness (Kraft, 1999; Lambert & Lambert, 1999; Low, 1999). Some individuals are people who might be called emotionally "hardy" (Craft, 1999). They are not thrown by untoward events, and they deal calmly with stress. But many normal, healthy people are easily upset or confused by stress or unusual events. In addition, just like the population at large, both emotionally hardy and emotionally sensitive individuals have pre- and comorbidity issues that affect their psychological response to chronic illness.

Examples

Before his stroke, **Everett** had been normal to hardy in his physical life, and he had had a relaxed, rather laid-back personality. He rarely took on more than one task at a time and worked issues through slowly and without much heat. His anger, frustration, fear, self-loathing, and despair after his stroke came as a total surprise to himself, his family, and his friends.

Sophia had led an average-normal physical life before her illness, but emotionally and psychologically she was enormously energetic and capable of complex multitasking. This led some individuals to comment that she had brought her condition on herself because she had overdone everything, but actually she had simply behaved like her peers and they were not sick. The kind of relaxed, bland, nonaggressive personality that some people thought should be comfortable for **Sophia**—because it is satisfactory for many people in the world—would have been a wholly inappropriate way to understand **Sophia** because it did not represent at all her personal benchmark personality.

Kim had enjoyed only a few years of physical good health as a child until she contracted restless legs, with its attendant sleep problems. Emotionally, she had always been tense, high-strung, and fragile, but she also had developed a good deal of insight. With the onset of her degenerative disk problem, she became increasingly anxious, but she had also developed skills for dealing with anxiety. So whereas **Kim** had an emotional benchmark of fragile, she also had acquired rather remarkable coping skills on her own.

Christine was very hardy physically and emotionally before her illness. She had extremely high energy levels and was capable of dealing with many issues at one time. The change in her life could not have been more extreme, but her experience as a nurse had educated her sufficiently so that she was not completely surprised by what was happening to her.

Lewis had had an average-normal core physical life before entering my practice. A highly intelligent and perceptive man, he had, over his lifetime, learned how to obscure his rather extensive array of tics so that they were largely unnoticeable to the casual viewer. He had grown up in a poor farming family in the South, but largely through the efforts of the pastor of his church, **Lewis** had been encouraged to excel in school. His drive and self-discipline had propelled him through high school, and he was the first of his family to attend college. His professional career as a high school teacher was a source of great pride to **Lewis** and all members of his family. Emotionally, **Lewis** appeared to be normal-average except for very subtle but powerful concerns with, for example, finishing items on a list or being a stickler for rules. He was, however, capable of accomplishing a number of tasks at once and of responding to change, surprise, or upset with reasonable calm. Fairly early in treatment, I learned that **Lewis** had sustained great and repeated emotional traumas as a child and had been suffering from posttraumatic stress syndrome (PTSD) in addition to his Tourette's.

Initial Trauma Assessment

Trauma assessment is essential (Saigh & Bremner, 1999; van der Kolk et al., 1996). By the time chronic illness patients reach clinicians, the patients are suffering the trauma of their illness and trauma caused directly by the illness onset. Even when the illness begins very gradually—as, for example, in a person with Sjogren's syndrome, who notices only that her eyes are increasingly dry and gritty and that her mouth is always dry—it causes patients pain and suffering apart from their symptoms when they finally recognize and acknowledge that things are not what they should be. In some patients, the onset can be obviously and dramatically traumatic—the MS patient who suddenly cannot walk or see properly or the CFS patient who literally cannot get out of bed.

In addition, individuals with chronic illnesses may have preexisting or coexisting traumas that tone or shape their behavior in the present condition.

Moreover, today's culture almost always engenders some degree of trauma and stigmatization in people suffering a chronic disease. Family members, coworkers, and employers have very likely expressed disbelief or fear about the patient's condition and may also have been dismissive or contemptuous.

It is important for clinicians to probe for possible iatrogenic trauma. Many of the chronically ill have experienced disbelief and condemnation from medical personnel, which is particularly damaging because patients have approached these people with the expectation of receiving help. Iatrogenic traumatization is not only hurtful in itself, but usually causes patients to censor or modify what they report to clinicians, thereby destroying the accuracy of the clinical picture.

It is also possible that patients may be experiencing concurrent life crises, such as marital difficulty, a teenage child's pregnancy, or other concerns that are neither strictly transitional nor developmental in nature. The psychosocial assessment provides contextual information about patients, which clinicians need to help patients distinguish between natural reactions to life problems and chronic illness manifestations.

In Phase 1, however, clinicians conduct trauma assessments to locate only the most obvious traumas that are having the most profound impact. Again, containment is the issue in Phase 1. Once a degree of control and manageability have been reached, at the start of Phase 2, patients are ready to examine trauma issues more extensively and completely.

Examples _____

All five cases suffered fairly obvious traumas. It is particularly worth noting, however, that **Christine** was completely preoccupied with the painful traumas she suffered because of her family's reaction to her illness. Although she acknowledged the pain of her condition and the losses it occasioned her personally, she tended to dismiss these issues before the overwhelming pain of shunning and condemnation by her family. She had suffered some iatrogenic trauma, especially before her diagnosis, but that, too, she absorbed, because as a nurse she regarded those kinds of clinicians as idiots who shouldn't practice medicine in the first place.

Sophia, on the other hand, probably suffered workplace and disease trauma just about equally. But she also experienced an unusually severe degree of iatrogenic traumatization because the original clinicians she saw had a vested interest in finding her basically healthy and either malingering or personally overextending herself.

Psychiatric Evaluation

Depending on information gathered in the physical and psychological assessments, clinicians may wish to conduct or order a medication evaluation and/or a full psychiatric evaluation. The Structured Clinical Interview for DSM-III-R (SCID) (Robins, Helzer, Cottler, & Goldring, 1989) is recommended.

Examples

It was important, because of the overlap between **Lewis**'s physical and neurological condition, to order a psychiatric evaluation. **Lewis** was very high functioning for most people with Tourette's, so it was important to get as many angles of vision on his condition as possible. It also seemed likely that he might need medication to manage his intrusive ideations and to help with his sleep.

Because **Kim** was experiencing more and more periods of anxiety, it was desirable for her also to receive a full psychiatric evaluation.

Personal Narrative

Clinicians should ask patients to give them a personal life story. This is actually both an assessment and a treatment tool because it is the first telling of the patient's narrative, the life's journey that will be reevaluated and retold as the patient works through the phases.

Clinicians may suggest that patients break their life story into seven-year segments and include in each seven-year period all the physical, emotional, social, and environmental issues that the patient felt were most important during that period. It is fruitful to suggest that patients employ whatever materials they feel best express the significant aspects of their lives. The "document" produced most often takes the form of writing, but it may also include materials such as photographs, spreadsheets, artistic productions, or records of meeting the patient's children, and so on.

Patients may well be intimidated by the request for a narrative or irritated by it. Clinicians can help reduce or defuse tension before it arises by articulating and demonstrating with gestures that the narrative can be a few short notes on index cards or a tome of material. With some populations, it may be necessary for clinicians to draw out the story orally. Clinicians need to assure patients that they will pay close and complete attention to the patient's story, regardless of how it is told.

Ultimately, as noted previously, the personal narrative becomes one of the defining therapeutic activities for patients in the Four-Phase Model. Clinicians will work with patients to help them read and rewrite their stories in ways that lead to increased understanding and more meaningful lives. At the start, however, the patient's personal narrative provides clinicians with invaluable initial information. It also helps to develop a close relationship between clinician and patient.

Clinicians must take a respectful and egalitarian stance in creating the personal narrative. It provides them with an extremely rich lode of information and, at the same time, gives patients an opportunity to express their experiences without intermediation. The experiences are not fitted into a standard medical history format or typical psychological or social categories, but represent the patients' own hierarchies, evaluations, and understandings. Used correctly, the personal narrative infuses the patient-clinician relationship with a degree of humanity and equality, which can help to dissolve some of the social, historical, and status impediments to honest exchange between patient and clinician. The process of composing the narrative also shows clinicians how the patients organize their thinking, how they structure their personal story, and how they express the aspects of their lives that are most meaningful to them. How patients respond to the task also alerts clinicians to the patients' engagement with or resistance to the therapeutic process.

ASSESSMENT: SOCIAL/INTERACTIVE DOMAIN

The Four-Phase Model places great importance on understanding and working with the social systems of chronic illness patients. Family, friends, neighbors, coworkers—the patients' social world—exert a strong influence on how patients understand their condition and how they behave concerning treatment and coping (Lubkin & Larsen, 2002; M. E. Travis & Piercy, 2002; Woods et al., 1993). This social world is in turn affected by patients, often significantly. Over the course of the phases, moreover, the effects of patients' illness on the social world and the interactions of that world with the patients change. It is a dynamic system that must be examined in each phase.

It is also essential to consider patients' sociocultural characteristics—age, race, marital and family status, ethnicity, economic condition, and so on—when assessing and treating chronically ill individuals (Agnetti, 1997; Rumrill, Millington, Webb, & Cook, 1998; G. Sumner, 1995).

Family and Couples Evaluations

The social/interactive domain divides broadly into two subcategories: home life and work life. It is almost always desirable at some point during assessment for clinicians to conduct couples or family evaluations. Clinicians need to meet together with patients and either their partners or members of their families, however patients construct the concept of family. In the Four-Phase Model, family includes any particularly significant others in the patient's life, whether blood kin or housemates, neighbors, fellow parishioners, and so on. Because partners and families determine the most immediate environment for patients, their attitudes and understandings have significant impact on the ability of patients to improve.

Examples

Christine was the patient suffering most obviously and extensively from social trauma, related in her case to her family. Even her husband, who had cared for her during her initial siege of illness and married her in full knowledge of her illness, was beginning to have difficulties by the time **Christine** came to me. Despite her family's almost pathological treatment of her, **Christine** desperately wanted to reintegrate with them. Moreover, by her account, approximately half of the friends she had before her illness dropped her after she became sick. It quickly became clear that, for **Christine**, the social arena would require a great deal of attention.

Sophia, on the other hand, was blessed with the appearance of a younger sister, who not only took over most of the housekeeping and cooking, but also accompanied **Sophia** to the doctor and helped her to organize her increasingly scattered thoughts about what she wanted to ask her physician. A living embodiment of family affection, **Sophia**'s sister also, by making her long trip to help **Sophia**, demonstrated the strength of the family's spiritual life. This further reinforced **Sophia**'s already strong personal belief in a benign God who had a purpose for her and who would help carry her through her time of darkness.

Work Evaluation

The work environment can also dramatically affect patients' ability to progress. For those patients who can continue to work even though they are ill, the activities they regularly perform at work during the period they are being

PHASE 1
Checklist for Assessment

Physical/Behavioral Domain

_____ 1. Has the patient received a complete medical review, including a medical history and a list of prescription and OTC medications currently in use? List findings.

_____ 2. Has the patient received a detailed screening on activities over the course of two weeks? Have symptoms also been recorded in detail and in relation to activities?

_____ 3. Has the patient provided enough information to establish a current physical benchmark? What levels of activity can the patient carry out at the present time?

_____ 4. Was it desirable for the patient to undergo a neuropsychological review? If so, what were the results?

_____ 5. Has the patient undergone a sleep assessment? If so, what were the results?

_____ 6. List any other physical assessments.

Psychological Domain

_____ 1. What indicators place this patient in Phase 1?

_____ 2. What psychosocial assessment instruments were used to evaluate the patient? What were the results?

_____ 3. Have you made an initial assessment of the patient's traumas, including especially physical and emotional traumas relating directly to the condition, preexisting and coexisting traumas, and cultural and iatrogenic traumas (stigmatization, disbelief)?

_____ 4. Was a psychiatric evaluation performed? If so, what were the results?

_____ 5. Has the patient begun to construct a personal narrative?

It is important to remember that this narrative need not be written out formally, but can be any materials that capture, in seven-year segments, the patient's experience of family, friends, school/work, sex/partners, health, hopes/plans, and troubles/fears. It is also important to remember that this ongoing narrative serves as both an assessment tool and a treatment intervention.

Social/Interactive Domain

_____ 1. Have you conducted a family and/or couple evaluation? What were the results?

_____ 2. Have you conducted a work evaluation? Are there issues with the patient's employer or fellow workers?

assessed may be draining their energy unnecessarily. In these cases, physical therapy may help retrain or recondition patients so that they can perform their jobs less stressfully. At some point, it may also become desirable for clinicians to conduct a workplace evaluation or consultation. Clinicians may need to assess what job requirements are actually placed on patients and whether these can or need to be modified to accommodate patient needs. Under the Americans With Disabilities legislation, many employers have obligations to make certain rearrangements for people with a broad range of disabilities, and many are actually eager to cooperate in making such accommodations.

Example

Sophia was still technically employed, although she had not been able to go to work for several weeks before seeing me. It became clear that she was going to need help in getting disability because her employer seemed intent on building a case against her illness as a legitimate disability.

CLINICAL GOAL AND TREATMENT ISSUES IN PHASE 1

The overarching clinical goal during Phase 1 is trauma and crisis management.

The treatment issues or presenting problems are essentially those that identify patients as being in Phase 1. These include, most importantly, the patients' diagnostic and treatment urgency. Another significant issue is the intrusive ideation/denial cycle. Patients feel that the illness originates completely outside themselves and that diagnostic and treatment control exist entirely outside themselves. At the same time, they are self-pathologizing and experience a strong sense of cultural shame because they feel that they are somehow responsible for bringing the condition on themselves. They usually experience significant ego loss and possibly dissociation. They are highly intolerant of the ambiguity of their situation and want the clinician to remove that ambiguity as soon as possible.

It is important for clinicians to understand that the following treatment interventions and those for the subsequent phases are suggestive rather than exclusive. Many of the recommended activities are ones already being carried out by clinicians. While providing some new treatment approaches, the Four-Phase Model functions largely as a new organizing and strategizing paradigm, under the umbrella of which clinicians employ the interventions that they feel work most effectively in their practice. It is a question of strategy and tactics. The strategy involves comprehending the chronic illness experience in a new way, which involves all the systems in the patients' lives and allows clinicians to understand what general kinds of interventions are necessary and effective at each phase and what kinds will be ineffective until later. My particular assessments and interventions—the tactics—may be helpful to some readers, but the essential issue for clinicians is to embrace the new clinical and empirical strategy that this paradigm presents for chronic illness.

TREATMENT: PHYSICAL/BEHAVIORAL DOMAIN

Multidisciplinary Team

Successful treatment of the chronically ill involves a team of clinicians. One doctor usually has oversight of the patient's physical condition and recommends other specialists in physical medicine, as the illness requires. In addition, one clinician works on the highly individual psychological and sociological aspects of the patient's condition. All participants need to act as a team. They need to inform one another about their findings and coordinate care recommendations. As a consequence, one clinician should be designated as the team manager. Often, given the time and economic constraints on many clinicians, the team manager is a nurse practitioner or physician's assistant working in the practice of the primary care physician (Carbone, 1999; van der Eijk & de Haan, 1998; Wagner et al., 2001). It may also be the clinician working on the psychological and sociological aspects. It is essential that whoever takes the manager's role keep all team members informed about changes in the patient's condition and alterations in physical or medications protocols. It is also the manager's job to query any seemingly contradictory orders and to report any deleterious side effects of protocols. The team needs to work with respect for one another and respect for the manager.

Medical Protocols

Clinicians such as social workers or psychologists need to know what medical findings have been made and what protocols have been ordered. They need to understand the patient's prior medical history, especially because premorbidity and comorbidity problems can dramatically affect the patient's experience

---

PHASE 1
Treatment

Physical/Behavioral Domain
  Multidisciplinary team
  Medical protocols
  Physical structural/behavioral goals
  Restructure activities of daily living
  Physical safety plan

Psychological Domain
  Relationship establishment
  Illness/trauma affirmation
  Education to illness phases
  Introduction to process and content
  Introduction to the observing self
  Introduction to identification and differentiation
  Education about ego loss and dissociation
  Assertion of positive values, humor
  Establishment of psychological behavioral/structural goals

Social/Interactive Domain
  Family trauma care
  Family case management
  Health care system management
  Workplace/employer intervention
  Clinician advocacy

---

of the chronic illness. Doctors may order short-term physical treatments or medications to address a particularly acute presenting problem, but generally, physical treatments for chronic illness are palliative or lifestyle management ones. Psychologists and social workers, for example, need to coordinate with doctors if they learn from their meetings with a patient that an exercise program the physician recommended for stress reduction is actually compromising the patient, who is already committed to as much physical activity as is sustainable at that point.

Physical Structural/Behavioral Goals

Clinicians work with patients to structure their lives in a way that permits them to carry out recommended physical protocols. These behavioral goals for physical activities may include setting up systems to ensure that patients take their medications, understand recommended changes in diet or nutrition, and develop reliable methods for incorporating these into their lives as they are actually lived. Clinicians also help patients establish manageable exercise levels and teach them sleep hygiene techniques to make their sleep as restful and restorative as possible.

Restructuring the Activities of Daily Living

During the crisis, and usually the chaos, of Phase 1, it is frequently desirable for clinicians to try to simplify patient activities as much as possible to make the patient's life functional. In Phase 2, many patients are physically and psychologically capable of expanding this activity level significantly, but in the containment effort of Phase 1, it is best to simplify the patient's life as much as possible (Fennell, 2001).

Using the activity threshold levels reported during assessment, clinicians work with patients to establish realistic activity patterns. Reassuring the patients that these new activity routines are not permanent changes, but simply ones instituted now to protect and increase their functioning in their present situation, clinicians teach patients to stretch out jobs, reorganize them, or eliminate them (Fennell, 2001; Furst et al., 1985, 1997). Activity restructuring in Phase 1 focuses on the ADLs.

The ADLs—caring for yourself personally, cooking, cleaning, doing laundry, and so forth—are important activities. Unlike human breathing or heartbeat, the ADLs do not happen automatically, without intentional effort on the part of the patient, yet many clinicians tend to regard them as such unless the patient is completely bedridden. Few people regard cleaning an apartment or washing clothes as equal to conducting a shareholders' meeting, but cleaning or washing very likely requires more physical effort. Daily activities are not minor issues, but central to a patient's ability to survive and to that person's self-esteem as well.

Clinicians need to help their patients comprehend just exactly the kinds and amounts of activity they have been doing and then help establish realistic new boundaries. Together, they modify daily activities so that the patients are once again performing within the realm of the possible. Although a formal exercise program may represent a realistic and desirable amount of regulated activity in a clinician's mind, simply shopping for groceries and putting them away in cupboards may be all the exercise the patient can actually sustain. Clinicians need to help patients learn to trade off activities. On a day when patients shop for groceries, for example, they may not wash their hair, prepare any meals, or pick up the children from day care. For severely compromised patients, a day's activity may consist solely of getting out of bed, dressing in street clothes, and eating a meal with the family. For working patients, clinicians may recommend that patients change their shower time from the crowded morning schedule to the evening and then to limit hair washing to once or twice a week. They may suggest that patients set out their breakfast the night before. They may help patients to develop simple, nutritious menus that require little preparation and simplify food shopping.

In Phase 2, clinicians teach much more complex activity restructuring in all areas of action—not just ADLs—but during Phase 1, the clinician's primary effort is to contain the patient's urgency and help provide a structure for living that returns some small degree of control to the patient's life.

Most chronically ill individuals, especially in Phases 1 and 2, have little realistic sense of their physiological, cognitive, and psychological boundaries. Physically and psychologically, they frequently struggle to pass in the outside world as normal and healthy. They usually attempt to hide their cognitive difficulties completely, fearing that any cognitive slippage will indicate to others that they are crazy or have Alzheimer's. In all areas, patients usually attempt to do more than they can possibly sustain—that is, they usually try to do everything they did before they were ill—only to suffer even further erosion of self-esteem when they collapse from doing too much. Unfortunately, they rarely learn that they collapsed because they have done more than they can possibly do now that they are sick. First, they do not really want to believe that they are sick, and second, they believe they collapsed because they failed to try hard enough. Phase 1 patients blame their own character, not their illness. And in this misplaced self-judgment, they are, unfortunately, often abetted by their families, coworkers, and the society at large.

Physical Safety Plan

Early in treatment, clinicians need to establish a physical safety plan with their chronically ill patients. Clinician and patient work together to set realistic parameters for what patients can do without harming themselves or others. If patients are severely depressed, they may also require a psychiatric safety plan. They need to recognize when suicidal thoughts may be endangering them and know what specific steps they should take when they feel at risk. But a physical safety plan sets somewhat different boundaries. If patients suffer cognitive confusion when they are tired, for example, and cannot remember where they are when they are out driving, they need to learn to recognize occasions when they must not drive at all. Patients with CFS, for example, may have to give up jogging, even though they long to run, because it seriously exacerbates their physical exhaustion. The destructive effects of summertime heat and humidity for some patients may make it essential for them to acquire air conditioning.

Examples

Everett suffered a good deal of confusion following his stroke, and he had little understanding of his boundaries. He sometimes fell when he tried to get out of bed unassisted, and his body often failed to respond the way he thought it would. He was prone to attempting activities that were beyond his current capacity without asking for help. Because his stroke had left him with serious cognitive dysfunction, his understanding and judgment were not always reliable. He was in great need of a physical safety plan. He and I worked together to establish easy-to-follow safety rules that he could honestly agree to adhere to. Essentially, he learned to not "get brave" on his own, but to save his heroic efforts until people were around to help if necessary. We also worked on the concept of asking for help until he had developed the skills to perform an action solo. An example of a small practical action was the purchase of a small bell to keep beside his bed so that he could call for help easily. He even agreed to try wearing a bell when he was up and about so that his wife or other caregivers would know where he was.

   Everett also required education about the concept of activity itself. Having always understood activity to mean heavy or exhaustive physical effort, he needed to acquire a meaningful understanding that ADLs constituted significant actions. Despite being paralyzed on the dominant side of his body, **Everett** had learned to dress himself, could for the most part toilet himself, and fed himself if his food was cut for him. He needed to learn that his hard-won battle to perform these ADLs demonstrated effort that was just as real and meaningful as mowing the lawn, fixing the toilet, setting up tents, or hiking 20 miles.

There was a great deal of similarity in the physical treatment goals for **Christine** and **Sophia**. For both, it was necessary to collect detailed data on what ADLs they could or tried to accomplish. It was then necessary to establish specific physical boundaries to keep their activities from exhausting them and possibly precipitating relapses.

Sophia was very impaired physically and cognitively, and she lived alone, without any immediate family support network. She was supposed to follow numerous medical protocols, which included taking a variety of medications and supplements, preparing a complicated diet, and getting exercise. Not only were these all hard to keep straight, but also she was so exhausted from, for example, trying to shop for fresh vegetables and then prepare them that she clearly had no energy for a formal exercise program. However, when she was feeling more rested, **Sophia** was capable of driving a car.

Sophia needed a physical safety plan that included two main components. First, although she hated to "be a bother," she had to contact one of two neighbors who agreed to get necessities such as milk or other perishables when she was too sick to leave the house. Second, because **Sophia** was seeing a number of doctors, each of whom was trying different ways to treat her, she needed a medications safety plan. Occasionally, she had bad reactions to new medications, and she had had the experience of being unable to contact the doctor during one such reaction. I became the person whom she called as soon as she detected any adverse reactions, and I took the responsibility of contacting the necessary doctors.

Sophia also needed serious restructuring of her ADLs because she was constantly exacerbating her condition by doing too much. She was even further endangering herself by, for example, collapsing at the stove or driving when she was cognitively impaired. I worked with her to reduce ADLs to the minimum. She would make her bed and dress every day but bathe less frequently (three or four times a week) and journey outside her house only once every other day. She was encouraged to cook larger quantities of her favorite rice and lentil dishes on those days when she was feeling strong and alert.

Sophia's sister had come from abroad for one extended visit during the time that **Sophia** was trying to obtain a medical diagnosis, but thereafter the sister could come only briefly, about once a month at best. As a consequence, **Sophia** had to create grocery lists that would carry her through 30 days. She still had to buy perishables, but these she got at a nearby convenience store so she did not have to walk long distances or wait in line. When she couldn't go at all, she asked her neighbors for help and eventually contacted a local shopping service. I also suggested that **Sophia** buy enough cheap underwear, towels, and sheets to survive for about a month without doing laundry.

Sophia had the advantage of already practicing a very advanced spiritual life. She regularly devoted part of every day to prayer and meditation, so it was easy for me to show **Sophia** how this activity could also help moderate her difficulties.

Christine was very impaired physically, but she did not have as many cognitive difficulties as **Sophia**. Although she had many responsibilities—she was still a landlord with property even though she had stopped practicing as a nurse—she had the benefit of a husband living with her who could help with many things, and her husband's family was also willing to pitch in. The marriage was beginning to experience a good deal of strain because of **Christine**'s illness, but her husband was still willing to perform jobs such as grocery shopping. He would also carry the dirty clothes that **Christine** had sorted to the basement to put into the washing machine (and later into the dryer).

Christine always tried to do more than she should, but she came to see that she had to ration her efforts on those days when she could get out of bed. If she did not shower when she got up in the morning, for example, she would have enough energy to make breakfast. She might even be able to wash the dishes as well. On a day when she wanted to cook dinner, she made sure to take an afternoon rest. But **Christine** was often unable to get out of bed at all, so she had to change many aspects of her life. I helped her set realistic goals for housekeeping. For the most part, she would simply attempt to keep the house picked up. Every two or three weeks, if she was able, she would vacuum one or two rooms. But on that day, she must do nothing else—make no meals, wash no dishes, sort no laundry, and make no attempt to go outside. **Christine** learned to make up menus for a week at a time that were composed of simple, easy-to-prepare foods (pasta and sauce from a jar, frozen entrees, rice and sauce packets). These she and her husband supplemented with fresh fruit and vegetables they could eat raw (carrots, peppers, celery, beans). If she felt up to cooking, preparation was simple; if she did not, her husband did not face a daunting task.

Christine easily became dizzy and lost her balance, so, as part of her physical safety plan, she had to recognize that she must not drive at all. She also needed to agree to have someone watch her when she bathed to make sure she did not fall. Because she was losing necessary sleep and her husband often snored heavily, they had to arrange to sleep apart some of the time, but not always, because that would have been damaging to them both emotionally.

I insisted that **Christine** include as a necessary ADL—although strictly speaking, it was a personal enrichment activity—a daily period of time devoted to contemplation. **Christine** was not a reader or an intellectual. Never in her preillness life had she ever sat quietly listening to music, let alone meditating. I encouraged her to take up needlework, which would give her slight physical action that, at the same time, would not require much mental attention. **Christine** came to find real pleasure in needlepoint, and the time spent sewing allowed her mind and spirit to enter a quiet place.

Lewis needed to have a sleep plan. Tourette's syndrome exhausts patients, and **Lewis**'s overall neurology did not allow him to absorb the same level of physical stress as most people. Moreover, his sleep was disrupted by his trauma history. He had a very difficult time making any transition (such as that from waking to sleep or sleep to waking), which was made even worse by the agitation that tends to accompany Tourette's. **Lewis**'s sleep hygiene plan included when to sleep, when to get up, what to keep by the bed, what to do before sleep, and how to calm himself for sleep. He learned to eat a healthy dinner and then not to eat immediately before sleeping. A couple of hours before bedtime, **Lewis** was to turn off his computer and cease engaging in anything emotionally or physically stimulating. About an hour before sleeping, he was to make sure all the overhead lights were off so that his body could prepare for sleeping. He was to sit in the living room in a comfortable chair watching TV or reading something relaxing. About a half-hour before going to bed, he would take a warm bath. At his bedside, **Lewis** kept a variety of calming books, a tape recorder with soothing music tapes, and a radio. If he woke during the night and was unable to fall back asleep quickly, he could play music for a while or even read. **Lewis** woke fairly regularly at 7 A.M., but he learned to turn on the radio while in bed or to read a bit to ease the transition into the new day.

Kim needed to contain her anxiety and get rest, two closely interrelated goals. She had enormous difficulty focusing on any constructive activity, tending instead to dart from one thing to another without completing anything. Using an egg timer helped her train herself to stick to one action, initially for a short period of time. Eventually, she was able gradually to increase the time periods for specific activities. Because her restless legs interfered with getting to sleep, she learned to bicycle with her legs in the air while lying in bed until she had calmed sufficiently to rest. A weighted blanket then helped her body remain quiet. During the day if **Kim** found her restless legs causing her to engage in undirected, repetitive action, she used the egg timer to train herself to reduce this activity. I worked closely with **Kim**'s physician to determine an effective combination of medication and mild exercise to help relieve her persistent back pain.

TREATMENT: PSYCHOLOGICAL DOMAIN

Relationship Establishment

The most essential intervention in the psychological domain is the establishment of a warm, candid, egalitarian relationship between patient and clinician (S. L. Baumann, 1997; Rood, 1996). Clinicians need to continually convey to patients by statements and actions that the two are comrades in their activities together. Clinicians need to demonstrate that they and their patients are equally human, made of the same flesh and subject to the same ills and suffering. Clinicians have to believe this deeply and personally; it cannot be a stance merely assumed to deal with clients. Clinicians have to show that they are not simply interested in the patients clinically, but that their job is something they have consciously chosen—that it is a vocation that they feel called and privileged to do (Erlen, 2002). While acknowledging that they are experts in matters that patients may not understand, clinicians must clearly indicate that expertise does not make them better or otherwise superior human beings. That clinicians should acknowledge countertransference, assess it, and then use it to benefit the relationship with patients is a central pillar of the Four-Phase Model. Clinicians who have or seek out strong collegial support in the form of thoughtful mentors or attentive supervisors can usually overcome the difficulties that clinicians experience with relationship establishment.

Illness Affirmation

One of the first activities in the establishment of clinician-patient relationships is the clinician's sympathetic affirmation of the patient's illness (S. L. Baumann, 1997; Rood, 1996). Clinicians convey this through their words, their eye contact, their body language, their general affect. Clinicians must not only listen but also be willing to hear and process what patients tell them and react with empathy and feeling. Countertransference issues come into play here, too. Do clinicians need to like every patient? Should they treat patients they do not like? These issues are discussed in a subsequent chapter, but in practice, as clinicians examine themselves and learn to process honestly their reactions to what they experience with patients, they frequently find that their range of sympathetic understanding grows.

Trauma Affirmation

Immediately related to but extending well beyond the patient's illness is the patient's experience of trauma. It is essential that clinicians help patients to identify and then affirm the trauma that has occurred in their lives (Saigh & Bremner, 1999; van der Kolk et al., 1996). In Phase 1, the trauma of illness onset is particularly important. By teaching patients to recognize and grieve for the ways their illness has disrupted or even destroyed their old lives, clinicians can assist patients in the process of beginning to take control of their new reality. This reality includes, among many other things, an enormous change in the patient's sense of time.

Examples

Everett was both older than I and male. His children had all been sons, so he did not even have the experience of relating to daughters to help us build a relationship. Furthermore, it was contrary to every notion **Everett** had of himself as a man to complain or confess difficulties to anyone except occasionally his wife. Building a relationship, therefore, took time and care. I introduced myself by my first name but addressed **Everett** as Mr. Jones or as "Sir." Even when some relaxation and cordiality was established, I asked **Everett** whether I might call him by his first name before doing so. Finding that **Everett** was more comfortable with me when I behaved like a young man, I adopted an authentic stance, but one that was straight, frank, businesslike, with no frills. **Everett** had worked in plumbing supplies, but his real life occurred outside work when he cared for his house and yard or took weekend trips camping. He had never been interested in reading or intellectual activities through which I might have forged a bond. Discovering that **Everett** was a Giants football fan gave me a way to dissolve any awkwardness at the start of our sessions together.

Because it was so hard for **Everett** to acknowledge his sufferings, I began by affirming his illness and his traumas indirectly. While in the presence of both **Everett** and his wife, Joan, I would comment to Joan about how extremely difficult **Everett**'s experiences had been, but how bravely and consistently he was working to achieve as much functionality as he could. I made no bones about my admiration for him and the qualities he clearly demonstrated. At the same time, I expressed specifically some of the difficulties he faced and their ongoing nature.

Kim, on the other hand, was approximately the same age as I and working toward a graduate degree. Her urgency made her desperate to form a close relationship immediately. Later, I had to make sure that a kind of professional competition was not aroused, but at the start, it was most important to demonstrate to **Kim** that I recognized how disabled she was. **Kim** was, after all, attractive and well dressed. She did not appear to be in pain, even though she was and even though she brought a mat with her so she could lie on the floor. I articulated that it was a good thing for **Kim** to rest her back on the floor, and I sat in a low position near **Kim**'s head. I said that I was trying to position myself so that she could be comfortable talking, and I asked whether I had succeeded. The symbolic attempt here was to be on essentially the same level so as to emphasize the caring, egalitarian position I was trying to communicate. **Kim** was eager to enumerate her many physical problems and was openly gratified to have her numerous traumas acknowledged and affirmed.

Like **Kim**, neither **Christine** nor **Sophia** looked ill, especially on a good day. Both dressed attractively and understood how to behave to avoid public censure. Both related to me as a peer, **Sophia** because she related intellectually, and **Christine** because she regarded herself and me as fellow health care professionals.

Sophia had always been a smiling, bouncy, good-natured woman, and she continued to project that behavior even when it did not in the slightest reflect how she felt. In fact, it was often exhausting and depressing for her to do so. She had, however, been so iatrogenically and institutionally traumatized, first by the clinicians who worked for her company and then by a disability investigator who had expressed open resentment at her having attended a first-tier college, that she had become very distrustful. She was unfailingly gracious and polite, but it took a while for her to credit my sympathy and speak candidly about her condition. As a matter of fact, it was probably my presence at a scientific conference that **Sophia** also attended that finally established our rapport. From then on, the relationship resembled that of two decent, cordial colleagues.

Christine, although anything but intellectual, quickly related to me as a comrade-in-arms in the health profession. We had dozens of crazy clinical experiences that quickly established a bond between us. These stories also introduced a level of humor that in later sessions helped lighten **Christine**'s bleaker moments. Because **Christine**'s urgency related to her family and their increasingly intrusive and harmful behavior, I immediately helped her set protective boundaries. I also shared carefully edited personal material, which modeled the rare but sometimes vital necessity to take a leave from family altogether.

Lewis's obsessive-compulsive personality made him want to get right to the problem that was preoccupying him, namely, whether he was a monster. I listened attentively as he described his ideations. I acknowledged the possibility that a person, even **Lewis**, could be a monster, but said that nothing he had said so far indicated that he was one. Reassurance on this score did a great deal to form an initial bond. As **Lewis** became more comfortable, he began testing me with a kind of teasing behavior. Instead of being put off by such comments, I took advantage of them to begin teasing him back. In this fashion, we succeeded in establishing a kind of relaxed humor that became very useful later for defusing resurgences of anxiety.

Experience of Time

Patients experience time very differently over the four phases (Agnetti, 1997; Agnetti & Young, 1993; Young, 1994). During Phase 1, the most salient issue is the sharp divide in time that occurs after the illness begins. It is similar in significance to patients of B.C. and A.D. in the Western calendar. In Phase 1, most patients feel that time has stopped for them and that they are now imprisoned in a time warp while the rest of the world hurtles forward at what appears to be ever-accelerating speed. Part of the extreme urgency of Phase 1 patients is caused by their seeing life all around them racing on while they are held captive. Their intrusive ideations, their pain, and their fear keep them perpetually in the confines of their illness experience.

Examples

Obviously, **Everett** experienced the most dramatic instance of time dividing into B.C. and A.D. His stroke was like a knife that surgically divided his life into before and after. He also had the most immediate and persistent feelings of captivity, trapped inside a body (and, increasingly, a mind) that was nothing like the person he had been before the stroke. He remembered his former freedom with the utmost longing and felt doomed by what looked more and more like a life sentence in a ghastly prison.

Sophia and **Christine** also experienced the B.C./A.D. effect, although the line dividing the two was fuzzier. For them, also, the advent of their illnesses introduced a new form of time. In it, they slogged through events as though fighting their way through a swamp of thick mud while they watched other people, particularly their colleagues in **Sophia**'s case, move swiftly and effortlessly ahead in the career path they had once shared.

Lewis and **Kim** did not have a before/after effect, but they did experience periods when time was different for them. When **Kim** was in serious pain or beset by a new somatic problem, time would stop for her. Eventually, the condition would ameliorate, the clock would once again start ticking, and **Kim** would have to scramble to catch up developmentally with all her friends and later her colleagues. This disrupted chronology—the stopping and starting of time—was true for all five examples, and indeed for most patients I have seen. **Lewis**, for example, wanted to get married. He wanted to find a woman with whom to spend the rest of his life. With the upsurge of ideations, however, he retreated to square one, believing that he could not possibly be a fit partner for anyone. He consciously felt himself lagging behind everyone developmentally, particularly in forming a permanent relationship.

Emergence of Child Ego

At the same time that patients become swamped by their illness and trauma experience, and in part as a useful coping mechanism, their private, primitive, child-ego state wells up and takes over more and more of their lives (Bose, 1995; Klein & Schermer, 2000; Morse, 1997; Perrig & Grob, 2000). Clinicians may observe that patients speak in a small, young voice and comport themselves in a diffident, unsure, awkward manner as they try to express what they are feeling. Patients frequently report that they cannot maintain their public persona to others or even to themselves. Unbidden feelings erupt and sabotage the careful control and presentation of self that the patients have developed over the years.

This sudden emotional regression occurs with Phase 1 patients regardless of their emotional hardiness before the chronic illness. For some patients, it is a temporary method of handling a novel and devastating experience. As these patients begin to map out the dimensions of the problem and learn practical techniques for surviving in their new environment, they have less need of primitive ego protection and return more speedily to mature social behavior and functioning.

If, however, patients have significant personality disorders before their illness—if, for example, they are narcissist, borderline, or dependent—their Phase 1 experience can be much more extreme. It is not atypical for clinicians to take the ego collapse as proof that the chronic illness is psychogenic rather than physical, just as it is not atypical for clinicians to interpret the grieving of illness for clinical depression.

But, in fact, some degree of ego regression occurs even in patients who have previously been well-integrated personalities in response to the accumulating traumas of the illness. Moreover, because patients do not understand where their childlike feelings and responses come from or why, the very emergence of the child ego publicly shames them, privately horrifies them, and makes them increasingly fearful that they are going mad or deteriorating from some dreadful disease. Their ego loss can be substantial.

Examples

Everett's lack of control and his enormous physical changes caused the unexpected, unwanted emergence of his child ego in public. In church, which he forced himself to attend to please his wife, he was overwhelmed with the magnitude of all the changes that had occurred and tears began pouring down his cheeks. He was horrified and helpless before this manifestation of feeling that in the past he would not even have permitted himself in private.

Similarly, **Christine** and **Sophia** found tears simply oozing out of their eyes when they would be doing something so simple in the past, such as waiting in the checkout line or removing clothes from the dryer. **Sophia**, in particular, related an instance of this in a very small, high-pitched voice, then stopped and commented on the fact that she never spoke in such a voice ordinarily, which was true. She described how small she felt when she was weeping in public, how diminished, and especially how exposed.

Bernadette, another patient, suffered from CFS but also had a border-line personality. Although she appeared to understand the importance of restructuring her ADLs, she would not alter her activities at all. She would promise to do so, then lie to her caregivers about what she was doing. In-evitably, this would lead to a collapse, which she would furiously blame on her caregivers. They, in turn, became frustrated with her noncompliance. They also felt especially strong countertransferential issues because most of those trying to help **Bernadette** worked with other nonpsychiatric CFS patients, and they improved. The caregivers could see how **Bernadette** was being used as a bad example—a negative poster child, as it were—by those who had doubts about the reality of CFS or about the ability of clinicians to treat it as anything other than a psychiatric or malingering condition.

Emotional Passing

Despite all, patients in Phase 1 usually try to pass for normal emotionally, just as they do physically (Saylor, Yoder, & Mann, 2002). Many patients have very little sense of their emotional boundaries. Some sincerely deny that their illness has caused them any loss or diminution of functioning. They report emotional outbursts or cognitive confusion and impairment, yet simultaneously deny that they, as individuals of their educational or professional attainments, could have such difficulties. But other patients engage in their emotional passing quite consciously. They believe that their actual emotional life probably indicates that they are crazy or bad, and they are trying to hide this "fact" from everyone around them.

Emotional passing is a coping technique. In Phase 1, it is usually an uncon-scious response that arises from patients' shame. To behave in any way but their most familiar would, most patients feel, reveal to the world how inade-quate and flawed they really are. Hence, the goal of the clinician in Phase 1 is to help patients recognize when they are engaging in passing behavior, both physical and emotional. Later, beginning in Phase 2, patients learn how to use emotional passing behavior consciously and for rehabilitative purposes. But even in Phase 1, clinicians start teaching patients to recognize their losses and their suffering so that they will be able to grieve appropriately and move into new and more effective ways of coping. Clinicians also need to introduce patients to palliative techniques for dealing with the grief and loss that chronic illness produces in their lives. New understanding and better coping techniques allow patients to cease passing except for consciously chosen reasons.

Examples

All patients, indeed all people, try to pass when they are in social situations and feel less than normally confident or secure. **Christine** was actually using a wheelchair because she was unable to walk, but she would act as though being in a wheelchair was just some quirky thing she was doing and that actually she was just like all the people around her.

Everett would repeatedly say to all his clinicians, including me, that he was fine cognitively, even though he would just as regularly tell his wife that he just couldn't think normally and that she would have to do things such as write the checks and balance the checkbook. He could no longer pull people's names out of memory, so he called all his sons "honey" and "dear," even though those were the affectionate names he had previously used only with his wife. He would tell his wife he was too tired to watch TV, but actually he could not follow the plot line and simply did not want to have attention called to this. He wanted to pass for his old self.

Sophia wanted to pass not only because of who she was and how she was raised, but also because she was aware of the fact that class is a very important issue when approaching any authority, including a doctor. She perceived that if she acted "inappropriately" in a doctor's office, she would be considered of a lower social class, particularly in this country with its racial problems, and would very likely be given a psychiatric diagnosis. Moreover, she guessed that the diagnosis would be worse the more inappropriate her behavior was judged. Consequently, she dressed for the occasion and behaved with great cordiality, asking after the doctor's well-being. Nonetheless, she still managed to irritate one physician by bringing a ring binder containing various medical reports and a written list of questions. Both these items had actually been prepared for her by her sister, but the doctor interpreted them as her productions and diagnosed her, among other things, as a person with Axis II Obsessive-Compulsive Disorder.

Passing is actually a very important component of successful living. It is extremely important, however, for patients to conduct a kind of cost-benefit analysis of their passing activities. Some behaviors do not produce any or enough benefit to be worth the effort. I often engage patients in antipassing exercises in which they are told to come to my office in sweatpants, with hair uncombed, and all disheveled. Patients need to think about when it is worthwhile to engage in passing and when it is not. They need to develop a clear understanding of how much energy they use to pass, and they also need to become aware of how their passing behavior not only misleads others, but actually confuses them about themselves.

Christine, an experienced health care professional, always tried to put her best foot forward in the doctor's office. She emphasized any advances and improvements and simply suppressed any negative information, including the fact that she was feeling lousy at the very moment of being in the doctor's office. She was, in effect, trying to please the doctor, but telling the truth would also have reminded her of just how bad she really was. Her husband finally had to intervene to give a more accurate picture of her condition. One thing about passing that **Christine** came to learn with me was that *awareness* allows individuals to decide—to make a choice—about when they are going to expend the energy to pass.

Patient Education: The Phase Model

An essential and ongoing part of the clinician's function is educational. To initiate this teaching process and give patients a vision of where they can hope to go in their illness experience, clinicians should introduce the concept of the Four-Phase Model. Partial understanding of the phases will not only help patients comprehend where they are at the moment, but also show them a better future they may actually hope to attain. Education to the phase concept includes not simply the phases themselves, but all the cultural and sociocultural influences and factors mentioned in Chapter 2. It also includes the concept that family and work systems are deeply interconnected with the private lives of individuals.

Learning the sequence of phases introduces patients to the general illness narrative, which will eventually help them reconfigure their personal illness narrative in a sustaining and meaningful way. Patients have already begun this personal narrative process during assessment.

Process and Content

During Phase 1 treatment, clinicians involve patients in a number of insight-building activities. They introduce patients to the distinction that exists between the content and the process of their lives. The content may be said to include all the different things individuals do over time, whereas the process is the way they do these things. Content varies greatly, but processes tend to be consistent over time. Patients can be guided to recognize the themes that characterize how they act. How, for example, do patients behave when they meet new people? How do they relate? How do they handle conflict? How do they establish trust? One way clinicians and patients can gain understanding of these common themes is if patients report the events of the preceding week and then examine their behavior with the clinician to discover common threads.

Clinicians can selectively use their own feelings and behaviors to model the ways they want the patients to regard themselves (Chin, 2002; Mattoon, 1985; Stein, 1996). To work effectively, modeling requires great candor and equality on the clinician's part.

Observing Self

Inextricably interwoven with the examination of content and process is helping patients to develop an observing self (Kornfield, 1993; Levine, 1979; Morse, 1997; Stein, 1996). Clinicians introduce patients, often by modeling, to that self that can stand apart from the suffering, frantic, illness-driven self the patient is living with now. The observing self can look at the suffering self's experience dispassionately, yet at the same time regard it with compassion. Useful activities include exploring the following questions: How does the patient actually feel? What is it like for the patient to suffer? What anxieties drive the patient?

It might seem that such exercises in the building of insight would be difficult with a less educated clientele. It is my experience, however, that this is not the case. Character and personality appear more important than formal education, and many poorly educated individuals are nonetheless very intelligent. When less educated patients indicate they are uncomfortable completing written forms, clinicians can devise less stressful forms of data collection (checkmarks under pictured activities, for example) or can rely on oral questioning.

Examples

Patients' intellectual ability, their personalities, and their level of insight before their illness obviously play roles in how easily they comprehend the concept of the observing self and begin to distinguish content and process. **Lewis** grasped the notion instantly. He became an assiduous collector of data and soon was able to separate how he processed distressing ideations from their actual content. He also began to observe his repetitive behaviors "objectively" and relate them to other aspects of his life, such as how alert or tired he was, how stressed, and so forth.

Sophia also saw these activities as fitting into the objective scientific model that she knew and loved. She, too, cheerfully collected and sorted data and developed an objective observer stance about herself and what was happening to her that did wonders for reducing her growing self-loathing.

Kim could gather data and occasionally stand apart to observe herself, but she was very easily confused and so regularly distracted and unfocused that it took longer for her to develop these skills.

Christine found the exercises much more difficult. Because she did not like to read, I introduced her to selected meditation and breathing techniques so that she could begin to understand the notion of the observing self. Eventually, **Christine** was persuaded to begin journaling, something she found acceptable because she recognized it as a technique now used in the training of some nurses.

Everett found it very hard to grasp the difference between process and content. I worked with him initially to count and track data. The number of times he got up at night—for which he needed assistance but did not want to request it—was a source of contention at home. **Everett** was asked to count how many times he got up each night for a week. In my office, his numbers for times getting up, times trying to do it on his own, and times when he requested help conflicted with those of his wife. I made no comment on the discrepancy, but asked **Everett** to count again the following week. I also asked him what he thought about doing all this counting business. Gradually, **Everett** was able to begin talking about his "style" of behavior, which was not to say he was having a tough time, and to see that this style was increasing the difficulty of his life (and those around him) rather than reducing it.

Isabella, another patient, worried all the time that her husband would become fed up with what she had become and leave her. I asked **Isabella** to observe herself during the next week every time she felt this particular anxiety. She was not supposed to try to change her thoughts, but simply to pay attention to them and to the circumstances in which they occurred. She was to collect data. Using such terminology in itself started to normalize this highly charged and emotional material, moving it into a more neutral and "scientific" world where **Isabella** was able to reflect on it more objectively.

Identification and Differentiation

Clinicians also teach patients how to identify, differentiate, and affirm their fears, losses, and suffering, as well as their functional and dysfunctional adaptations (Jung, 1990; Mattoon, 1985; Stein, 1996). It takes time and patience to tease specific fears and losses out of the welter of emotions that patients are experiencing, especially because many patients are strongly in denial. Denial is, after all, a potent coping technique, and it requires some coaxing for patients to give it up to move forward.

Clinicians begin by helping patients to differentiate their chaotic experiences (Gershuny & Thayer, 1999; Klein & Schermer, 2000; Parson, 1999). How does the patient feel? What is changing in the patient's life? How diminished do patients feel before the world at large and privately before themselves, compared with the person they used to be? To start the process, clinicians may suggest kinds of fears or typical losses. For some patients, the sheer naming of possible fears and losses proves that such fears and losses are real.

To help patients differentiate their fears and losses from past events in their lives, clinicians need to be very observant of patients' physical cues and body language, as well as their speech. Frequently, an occasion of fear or loss in the immediate context has raised issues from the past, which act as emotional accelerants, fueling the current fears or enlarging the sense of loss. Clinicians need to work very attentively with patients, carefully making sure to retain their attention and involvement during this process that can cause great anxiety and distraction, to separate past from present, and to identify the process that the old emotional context generates.

When past and present are differentiated, it may then be possible to see that the process occasioned by past emotions does not necessarily apply to the current situation. Differentiation also breaks patient experience into manageable parts that more easily offer opportunities to engage problem-solving techniques and other interventions. Affirming with patients the reality of their fears and losses helps free them from their additional fear that they are crazy or bad. Eventually, it also comes as a vast relief to patients, even if it simultaneously fills them with apprehension because they also learn that the clinician cannot immediately and magically remove them.

Example

For **Christine**, it was particularly useful to develop dichotomous techniques for comparing the past and the present. She began by comparing her current social abandonment by her family with what had happened two years earlier when she had contracted hepatitis. She had been rescued from her family's failure to support her or care for her then by a fellow nurse, whom she later married. **Christine** needed to differentiate her new from her old losses, but she also needed to reflect on her real as opposed to her perceived responsibilities to her birth family. She needed to distinguish her legitimate responsibilities to herself and her marriage as opposed to her responsibilities to her birth family. In the process of differentiation, she was also able to begin grieving for her losses, both past and present.

Fear of the Future

Most patients are terribly scared about what is going to happen to them in the future (S. L. Baumann, 1997; Henderson, 1997; Kahn, 1995; Morse, 1997). They often ask how much worse things can get or how long they will suffer. Obviously, clinicians cannot answer these questions with any certainty, but at this point, it is better to meet the patient's terrified experience of ambiguity with something more supportive than scientific accuracy. Clinicians can stress the truth that, over time, patients' situations will change and change again. As clinicians see more and more chronic patients, they will also be able to assert with conviction that although they do not know precisely what will happen with that particular patient, most patients they have seen experience an improvement in how they feel and in the quality of their lives. Just as important, especially for patients in Phase 1, clinicians can assure patients that they are committed to continuing in a supportive relationship and that it is possible for patients to arrive at a place where life will once again be meaningful.

It is very important for clinicians to assure patients that they can be in a diminished state and still identify, and then articulate clearly and cogently, what they need and want. It is possible for individuals to cry like children and, at the same time, be competent. Clinicians need to affirm that suffering does not obliterate the ability to think, and they can help patients script the information the patients need to convey even when patients' emotions seem to be swamping them.

Loss and Dissociation

Clinicians also need to begin educating their patients about ego loss and about dissociation (Bose, 1995; Drench, 1994). Patients in Phase 1 have suffered terrible, yet often unrecognized, ego losses. Following the traumatic experience of illness onset itself, patients may be said to bump into loss walls constantly. They have lost the ability to perform their roles at home and on the job the way they used to. They cannot participate in relationships with family or friends as they have in the past. They feel they are barely hanging on even though they are making a superhuman effort, yet they are frequently criticized for failing to perform as they used to. No one knows how hard they are working, most especially those who have always been closest to them.

The external losses patients suffer are more than matched by inner losses. Patients have usually become so different from what they once were that they no longer even have a sense of who they are (Kahn, 1995). Often, they fear they are crazy or that they are dying.

The enormous grief such losses cause needs to find expression and processing, but almost everything in the day-to-day lives of patients makes expressions of grief unwise or unworkable (Bose, 1995; J. W. Brown, 1999; Tallandini, 1999). Deep processing of illness-related grief occurs most significantly in Phase 3, but even in the early days of Phase 1, clinicians can begin to teach patients that loss produces grief and that grief needs to be continually engaged, felt, and understood if patients wish to move toward a more meaningful, positive life (Bose, 1995; Cutcliffe, 1998; Prigerson et al., 1997). In other words, patients need to learn the connection among loss, trauma, and grief, and to understand that acknowledging and processing their grief is a powerful move toward a better life. In Phase 1, clinicians permit unstructured grieving (tears or expressions of suffering that occur during sessions together or reported by the patients as happening away from the clinical setting). But they also seek to create structured times for grieving within the basic ADLs they establish with Phase 1 patients. They encourage patients to set aside a certain amount of time each day to listen to music or read or write in a journal or meditate or pray. They teach patients that such opening of themselves to feeling, and especially to their feelings of grief, is as necessary an activity as bathing or dressing or eating. This activity not only begins to acquaint patients with their true feelings of loss, but also helps reduce the number of uncontrolled spontaneous expressions of grief at times that may be inappropriate or embarrassing to patients. Such activities actually fall into the personal enrichment group, but it is important for patients, and clinicians as well, to treat them as being as essential and life-supportive as those more mundane activities usually associated with physical ADLs.

When Phase 1 patients are not awash in confused suffering, they have often dissociated. Indeed, dissociation is a curiously healthy coping tool for patients who have no one to help guide them through their experience. They split themselves off from their diminished selves and try to live as though the suffering self does not exist. When does dissociation become a clinical problem? Those patients who consciously dissociate to alleviate their experience of suffering are performing a healthy action. As they come to have a better understanding of where they are and what they can do about it, the dissociated self can transform into the observing self. Clinical dissociation is uncontrolled dissociation. It happens completely without the patient's acquiescence or desire.

In Phase 1, most of the clinicians' efforts are concentrated on the physical and social/interactive domains. In the psychological realm, they work principally to achieve damage control and containment. They begin teaching patients the techniques of self-awareness and self-examination because in the process of learning about the illness phases, clarifying the differences between content and process, and engaging the observing self, patients can begin to demystify some of the terrors and fears associated with suffering (Chuengsatiansup, 1999; Neimeyer, 2000; Witztum, Dasberg, & Bleich, 1986). The self-examination encouraged in Phase 1 acts to help quiet and contain the patient. The emotionally neutral, "scientific" process of information-gathering is calming and therapeutic in and of itself. Clinicians do not attempt to achieve serious insight-building until Phase 2 when patients have achieved a stability that makes it possible. At that time, however, the patients will continue to use and refine the techniques they have learned in Phase 1.

During the initial efforts in Phase 1, clinicians will find that metaphor can play an important role, especially images of captivity and imprisonment. Patients can be helped to see that although they have experienced profound personal loss and often great restriction in their lives, they need not lose dignity or human value, any more than Nelson Mandela did during his many years in prison (King, 1986; Mandela, 1994). The experiences that patients are undergoing are certainly not ones they would have chosen, but they can still be safe and have value as human beings.

Value of Child Ego

Eventually, clinicians lead their patients into an understanding that even the suffering, diminished self, and the parts of the self that the patients despise have purpose and positive value (Bose, 1995; Klein & Schermer, 2000; Morse, 1997; Perrig & Grob, 2000). These elements have served to protect the patient; to communicate much that the patient cannot otherwise articulate; and to gain attention, help, or other benefits for the patient. The difficulty with the primitive child ego is that it develops when people are young; hence, it does not have the discrimination and differentiation that come with developmental advance. It finds practically every event or change huge and scary and reacts to every change equally powerfully and primitively (Bose, 1995; Klein & Schermer, 2000; Perrig & Grob, 2000). Contrary as it seems, for patients to advance, they must make an ally of their child-ego self. If they do not, therapy is nearly always useless because the primitive self is strongly entrenched and, if attacked, will not give up without a fight.

Patients go through this ego-regression process regardless of whether they have had well-integrated personalities up to this point or whether their personalities have long been more fragile or traumatized. Nearly all people automatically bring such primitive defense systems into play when they are assaulted as they are in chronic illness. The better-integrated person tends to engage in defensive activities that are not illegal or dangerous, but more disturbed individuals may well seek to meet their needs through alcohol, drugs, or antisocial behavior. Whatever the defensive modes, however, clinicians still need to help patients ally with the ends sought by the diminished self. Clinicians adopt an apparently neutral stance, pointing out what the child-ego self is trying to achieve and, when these are inappropriate, helping the patient to arrive at better methods of fulfilling these needs. The important point here is that patients should come into alliance with the protective self, even when they intend to move beyond it as soon as possible.

Some patients decide to name this primitive self, giving it a separate identity. But another approach is for clinicians and patients to observe and understand how the child ego functions in general and how it has served in this particular illness crisis. Rather than discarding the primitive self, patients and clinicians try to grow it up a bit. Eventually, it will be reintegrated with the patient's new self, the self who will have learned how to live with the illness. Although reincorporation of the primitive self hardly seems a pressing concern to patients in Phase 1, the concept will later help them to deal more expeditiously with relapses, when they initially feel shot right back to their former childlike sick self again. By that time, however, patients have learned that the suffering, diminished self serves important functions and that they will eventually reintegrate it because they have done so before.

Patients often express with anguish or anger that clinicians cannot possibly know how they feel. If clinicians have had personal experiences of illness or trauma like the patient's, this is an excellent time for them to share aspects of it. Countertransferential material can build bridges across what appears to be a gulf of experience. As with all countertransferential sharing, discretion is paramount. Clinicians need to be sure that patients are at a point where they can process the information appropriately and benefit from it. If clinicians have never had comparable experiences, they should frankly admit the fact, saying that they nonetheless wish to understand patients' experiences and journey together with them as they continue trying to move toward integration of the illness into a meaningful life. They should then sincerely ascertain whether patients wish to continue working with them.

Examples

Both **Lewis** and **Sophia** had highly constructed public selves, which required enormous effort to maintain. **Lewis**'s career as a high school teacher would certainly be endangered if he let down his guard, yet he was not getting what he needed emotionally. He needed to share his ideations selectively, in a safe place, so that he could maintain his public persona on the job. Checking regularly with me to determine whether his thoughts were monstrous or not was a childlike dependence on outside assurance that allowed **Lewis** to continue living his adult life while he worked on the issues behind his problems. **Sophia**'s child self, who emerged in public tears, was an excellent barometer of **Sophia**'s emotional weather. Her public bubbly graciousness had sternly held her seething anger and desperation in check, but when **Sophia** was sufficiently traumatized, her child self simply broke through unbidden. Gradually, **Sophia** learned that if she let what her child self had to say come through at certain times, it did not appear when she did not want it to. She began to process the real issues behind her tears and respond to them directly.

Asserting Positive Values

During the often painful process of sorting out and then affirming fears and losses, clinicians constantly assert positive values—the worth of the patient, the value of the suffering and the experience, and the ongoing willingness of the clinician to work with the patient (Nouwen, 1972). Clinicians model an attitude of calm and tolerance in the face of all the suffering, ambiguity, and chaos of the patient's situation. They assert that there is a bottom to the pit into which patients feel they have fallen and that there is a process through which patients can come to understanding and a meaningful life. Because clinicians know that patients are unlikely to accept this possibility at this point, they ask that, for now, patients borrow the clinicians' lack of fear about the patients' situation, their affirmation of the patients' losses, and their allowance of the patients' suffering. In other words, the clinicians ask patients to borrow the clinicians' faith until the patients have built faith of their own.

Humor

If possible, clinicians should allow the emergence of some humor or at least an occasional lightness of tone. If patients perpetually regard their situation solemnly and seriously, life can sometimes seem even grimmer than it actually is. Humor helps patients acquire or maintain a sense of balance about their relative difficulties and miseries. Laughing can lighten their burden both psychologically and physically. Humor also demonstrates that patients can, at least temporarily, achieve a certain objectivity about their situation. Humor is, however, a very delicate matter, and clinicians must be particularly sensitive and observant about its use and its effects.

Examples

As mentioned previously, early on in treatment, **Lewis** and I developed a lighthearted teasing. This subsequently proved very helpful in the therapeutic process. We got to the point where I could ask him jokingly how his self-loathing had been going the previous week, and he could respond with equal humor. It served the observation process particularly well because it allowed **Lewis** to stand back from his desperation and look at it with different eyes. **Christine** and I were constantly able to joke about the absurdity of how damned sick a person had to be to get any attention. This both acknowledged **Christine**'s serious difficulties and assured her that I was her committed advocate, who would stick with her through the hard process ahead.

Clinician as Witness

As patients engage in all of these educational activities, the clinician's role is largely one of witnessing (S. L. Baumann, 1997; Bose, 1995). Witnessing as a principal activity can often frustrate clinicians, whose culture and training have led them to measure their effectiveness and value by achieving a cure. But clinicians can learn to transform even this countertransferential response into a positive treatment tool. Witnessing eases the deep loneliness that patients feel and builds a sense of community or esprit de corps. It brings dignity to the experiences of patients, elevating them again in their own eyes to a level of human respectability. Through witnessing, clinicians focus patients' learning process and make it clear. Witnessing is a way of sharing patients' experiences and affirming them. Witnessing, finally, begins the building of a critical spiritual mass, which is indispensable for patients when they arrive at Phase 3 and begin to work through the difficult process of meaning development.

Psychological Behavioral/Structural Goals

Behavioral and structural goals in the psychological domain in Phase 1 deal with emotional and attitudinal issues rather than physical ones. They are, or one might say they make possible, the implementation of the physical plan— both the safety plan and the revised physical activities plan. Just as in the physical realm, it is important for clinicians to establish what patients' psychological and emotional lives were like before their illness. Were patients emotionally "hardy," able to experience difficulties and surprises with calmness and measured response, or did stressful events and situations make them nervous, confused, or upset? As in the physical realm, clinicians need to understand what kind of emotional constitution patients had before they became ill.

Contemporary Therapies

Clinicians may use many traditional therapies to alleviate the presenting problems of Phase 1 patients—the intrusive/numbing trauma ideation cycle, the concurrent problems of anxiety and depression, and the ideations typical of this phase, such as those about death. These include, but are not limited to, Freudian and Jungian therapy, narrative therapy, problem solving, grief/strategic, interpersonal/transpersonal, cognitive-behavioral, rational-emotive, Rogerian, Gestalt, neurolinguistic programming (NLP), eye movement desensitization (EMDR), and family systems therapy. Whatever techniques are employed, the goal is to develop patients' sense of containment and control. Gradually, as patients move out of Phase 1, they cease to feel completely at the mercy of outside threats, whether physical or emotional. They discover that a small degree of control has returned to them.

TREATMENT: SOCIAL/INTERACTIVE DOMAIN

Social systems issues are essential in the treatment of chronically ill patients, yet they are often ignored (Agnetti, 1997; Axtell, 1999; Lubkin & Larsen, 2002; Nicassio & Smith, 1995; Rolland, 1984). Patients do not live in a universe uninhabited by others and free from obligations except to themselves. Clinicians need to keep cognizant of both the practical issues relating to family and work systems and the trauma these systems can be inflicting on patients.

In Phase 1, the participants in the patients' social systems have some of the same reactions that the patients have. What is happening to the patient imposes an unwanted change on the social worlds of the patient as well as an unwanted change on the patient. Unlike the patient, however, the social system does not suffer the symptoms the patient does, which constantly force the patient to recognize that something is wrong. Social system actors can more easily deny it. When the social system actors are forced to acknowledge the illness, they usually respond as if the patient were suffering an acute illness. How they behave usually depends on their response to illness in general. Many social system actors at this point will tend either to attempt to control the situation or to flee. Their reactions resemble those they would have toward acute illness. It is in Phase 2 that truly distinctive changes occur in the social/interactive world of chronic illness patients.

Family Systems Issues

Early in meetings with patients, clinicians should also start to work on patients' family systems issues (McCahon & Larsen, 2002). Clinicians need to help patients identify hostile or judgmental attitudes that emanate from family members and teach them appropriate methods for responding to such attitudes. This includes guiding patients about choosing battles to fight and minor stupidities to ignore. Illness usually brings changes to roles and responsibilities in the family, and these need examination.

Sexual relations are often a crucial concern. Pain or exhaustion markedly reduces sexual functioning, but, in addition, the emotional traumas associated with Phase 1 and the regression to a childlike ego state often make sex of no interest to patients. This indifference on the part of an otherwise mature-seeming partner can generate other tensions that increase patient difficulties.

The reduced child state of the patient can elicit or demand an inappropriate parental state in the partner. Although it is important for clinicians to help patients and their partners recognize and allow the temporary reduction in the patients' ego age, it is also desirable to encourage both partners to enter temporarily into a more equal, brother-sister relationship than to establish what is often a destructively controlling parent-child dynamic.

Chronic illness in a parent can have a decided impact on children, and children with chronic illnesses generate profound reactions in their parents (Falicov, 1988). Each family presents a different constellation of issues, and it is the clinician's responsibility to sort out what particular needs each particular family has. Clinicians need to monitor how the children of sick patients are handling the situation and give them opportunities to ask questions, express fears, feel grief, and the like. Conversely, when the patient is a child or young person, the parents have complex needs and reactions, and their problems need the clinician's careful consideration and attention.

Family Trauma Care

Clinicians need to work with family members to identify their traumas as these relate to the patient and the chronic illness. It is essential that both patients and families understand that families, too, suffer because of the chronic illness and that their sufferings need to be affirmed. They, too, need to grieve for their very real losses.

Example

Everett's wife, Joan, had suffered a succession of traumas to which almost no one paid any attention because the focus was understandably on **Everett**. First, she had been terrified that **Everett** would die, and her hopes and prayers aimed entirely at seeing him come out of his stroke-induced coma. With this desire granted, she now had **Everett** alive, but he was a totally different individual. She lost the husband she had known their entire marriage and in his place had a strange person who was suffering tremendous losses of his own and who needed constant care. He not only could not do all the things he used to, but also thought and behaved differently. Moreover, they no longer had the friends they used to, not because people intentionally dropped them (although some did), but because Joan and **Everett** could no longer participate in most of their friends' activities. Moreover, **Everett**'s appearance made some people uncomfortable, so even when friends were well-intentioned, they tended to avoid seeing **Everett** and Joan or to cut their visits very short. No one really considered what life was like now for Joan. Knowing her, they were sure that she would take care of **Everett**. They mistakenly believed that she would know what to do and would do it well. It never really occurred to anyone that Joan had not the slightest notion of how to care for a stoke recovery patient. Joan needed not only open recognition from me of her traumas and encouragement and support for her own grieving, but also guidance about her new role.

Family Case Management

In addition to the emotional aspects of the family trauma situation, there are also practical family issues that clinicians should help address. These relate to coordinating care, carrying out household activities, financial issues, long-term care, and so forth.

Example _____

Everett's wife, Joan, needed a great deal of practical advice and assistance. For the first time in her marriage, she became responsible for paying bills and keeping the checkbook. She had to arrange for lawn mowing and call the plumber when the toilet backed up. She had to file their federal income tax returns. In every practical sense, she became the head of the house. Although she had grown sons and helpful friends, she still had to learn skills she had never expected she would have to develop. In addition, she had to learn how to care for **Everett** and what services were available to support and supplement her. She needed to learn and reassess the family's overall financial picture so that she and **Everett** could budget for their new circumstances.

Family and Couples Intervention

Phase 1 patients frequently want to bring their partner or other family members to see the clinician because interaction with the partner or these family members is so central to the patient's life and has often been severely impacted by the illness. When family members do come, clinicians should carry out some of the same actions that they have with the patient; that is, they should establish a relationship and affirm both the patient's illness and trauma and the family member's loss and trauma as well.

Frequently in chronic illness situations, one family member or one partner can become very controlling (Agnetti, 1997; Doherty & Colangelo, 1984; Doherty, Colangelo, & Hovander, 1991). Clinicians may be able to initiate self-observing processes that will help the family or couple work on this, and clinicians can also model for family members both what the patient needs and what the family members need. It is probably not desirable for a patient's clinician to attempt couples or family therapy as well as individual therapy, but periodic family visits can keep everyone abreast of what is happening and how the patient's understanding is evolving.

In a very important acknowledgment of vicarious traumatization, clinicians affirm to the family members that they have suffered losses that are as real as, although different from, those of the patient. Clinicians model for the patient how to respond to their family's needs, and conversely, clinicians model for the family what the patient requires. It is always possible that a partner or family member will be unwilling or unable to act in the way that is necessary for the patient, and the clinician has to affirm this as a valid stance. But the clinician also has to affirm that the patient must receive the understanding that the clinician is modeling from someone, even if it is not the spouse or the particular family member.

It is necessary for both patient and family members to understand that it is acceptable to be upset with the illness, but not with the patient. In cooperative situations, family members can learn to grieve with the patient over their mutual losses. Clinicians can help to dismantle cultural myths about being strong and not acknowledging suffering. They can also guide family members in how to listen to and support each other.

Example

Christine was becoming very fearful when she first came to me because her birth family not only was violently angry and disbelieving of her, but also aggressively sought her out, in large part to browbeat her for failing to maintain her former responsibilities. At this stage, **Christine** could not imagine cutting off from her family altogether, but she also could not sustain this kind of abuse. Ordinarily with such salient family issues, I would talk with family members to clarify the patient's condition and limitations, but also to hear and affirm the family's losses and difficulties. But **Christine**'s family were adamantly opposed to meeting with me because they regarded me as symptomatic of **Christine**'s refusal to get control of herself and also as enabling **Christine** to continue along what they regarded as a willful and irresponsible path.

As a consequence, I had to approach the family issues with **Christine** alone. I had to help **Christine** establish safe contact rules with her family. Because family members had already let themselves into **Christine**'s house one time when **Christine** was in bed and had asked to be left undisturbed, I suggested that **Christine** change the locks and have keys only for herself and her husband. I also recommended that **Christine** get a phone answering machine so she could screen her calls. Both actions allowed **Christine** to determine when she would engage with her family. The family took to writing cards and letters, the contents of which distressed **Christine**, but she now had time to consider her responses to all forms of contact.

As a longer term effort, I began working with **Christine** about not allowing abuse or verbal battery. On a practical level, if her family demanded that she appear at a family gathering and bring certain foods as her contribution, **Christine** had to set parameters. She had to explain that she could not prepare any food and that she could stay only a short time. If family members began berating her when she was visiting, she was to leave immediately. This was not as easy because **Christine** was usually confined to a wheelchair on these occasions and her husband was rarely at her side when such things happened. **Christine** learned that if she had explained her limitations to a family member three or four times already and if they still ignored what she had said, she should stop excusing herself and simply say no.

I also encouraged **Christine** to examine the individual occurrences she would relate and to compare them to see if anything had changed in the process or whether she was simply enacting the same, harmful cycle.

Couples Management

All of the issues pertaining to families apply to couples, but, in addition, chronic illness almost always raises issues of sexuality (Agnetti, 1997; Doherty & Colangelo, 1984; Doherty et al., 1991; Flodberg & Kahn, 1995; Reiss, Gonzalez, & Kramer, 1986). Both partners need to learn that although the illness may severely restrict the sexual activities they have known in the past, there are many ways to express closeness and physical engagement. Often in Phase 1, the urgency and pain of the patient are so great that they more or less preclude much active sexual life. Here clinicians can educate both patient and partner to the likelihood that this will change in time and can help them learn ways to be with each other in the meantime. Issues of socializing and companionability also become important, as do roles and responsibilities. Clinicians should also help arrange couples therapy for patients and partners who are having a difficult time adjusting to the new situation created by the illness.

Examples

Christine's husband, Michael, unlike her family, wanted very much to talk with me, and those talks proved very productive. Not only was he **Christine**'s primary caregiver and the buffer between her and her family, but also he had been forced to take over many of her former activities around their house and other property that **Christine** owned. Because

Michael was also a nurse, he believed in the reality of her condition and was not ashamed of her. But his very knowledge meant that he was often second-guessing **Christine** as to how she managed her condition, and this created friction.

In addition, **Christine** wanted him to do all the things she had done before, and she wanted him to do them her way. But Michael did not like to mow lawns, fix plumbing, paint walls, or glaze windows, all jobs **Christine** had happily performed when she was healthy. She knew she was asking a lot of him, so she tried to do things on her own, but this almost inevitably caused her symptoms to flare up. Michael was getting frantic. He did not want **Christine** overextending, but he also did not want to do much of the work himself.

I helped **Christine** and Michael work out reasonable rules of engagement. But, more importantly, I gave both parties opportunity to express to me and to each other the impact that **Christine**'s disability was having on both of them. **Christine** felt guilty and, at the same time, struggled against her dependence on Michael. Michael, too, felt guilty, particularly because he sometimes felt angry and resentful at what he was forced to do. Both needed to talk about their grief and anger and to become conscious allies rather than secret enemies. They needed to learn to be angry at the disease, not the person.

I also suggested that they review their budget carefully. Although their income had gone down when **Christine** went on disability, so had some of their expenses—they no longer went out to dinner and the movies. This meant some funds were available for Michael to hire people for some jobs. For her part, **Christine** had to accept that the lawn would not get mowed as regularly and only necessary repairs would be made.

Lewis was dating a young woman regularly at the time he came to me. Indeed, part of his urgency in seeking treatment arose from the increasing incidence of disturbing ideations, which seemed related to his increased sexual life. When he tentatively shared some of their content with his friend, she decided to end the relationship. This decision further contributed to **Lewis**'s notion that he was monstrous. I offered to meet with the woman and speak with her about **Lewis**'s condition, but she did not agree. In time, it became clear that the woman had ended the relationship for reasons other than the fantasy information **Lewis** had confided to her.

Everett had never conceived of sexual life as comprising anything other than intercourse and, at the time he came to me, he was functionally impotent. Among the many other issues related to male and female role considerations in **Everett**'s and Joan's marriage, I needed to introduce them to the concept of being sexually intimate in ways other than intercourse. In larger ways, however, **Everett** felt emasculated. The couple had always had a traditional relationship, and now it was necessary for Joan to assume a more assertive, commanding role. The fact that she felt uncomfortable doing this and inadequate to the task did not reduce the tension that was growing between them. **Everett** felt that Joan was bossing him around, and Joan resented the fact that she was no longer being cared for and at the same time was annoying **Everett** for doing jobs he couldn't do and she didn't want to. I worked with both partners, individually and together, to help Joan take charge without ceasing to have feminine characteristics that **Everett** appreciated. And **Everett** learned that he was still a man, even in his condition, and that he could still contribute advice and support in the management of the household.

Health Care System Management

Clinicians need to educate patients and their families about how to behave concerning the health care system in general, especially doctors and HMOs (Landro, 2000; Newcomer, 2000; Weber, 1997). They can aid the family in finding and selecting the clinicians that the patient needs (Burton, 1995). The clinician acting as case manager for the patient takes responsibility for seeing that all the clinicians involved in the patient's care share assessments and protocols with one another and work collaboratively as a team.

Examples _____

Sophia learned that she did not need to accept the traumatic treatment she had been receiving up to the time she met with me. I helped her locate an attorney to help with her disability claim and gave her a list of primary physicians who were familiar with the complexities in conditions like hers. I also helped **Sophia** develop a collection of experts whose assessment of **Sophia** would help build an appropriate medical record for her.

   Lewis and I became fellow coordinators in his health care management. He needed the combined services of a primary care doctor, a psychiatrist, a sleep specialist, and occasional consultations with a neurologist and a specialist in Tourette's syndrome. I helped guide him to appropriate clinicians and made sure that all parties shared their findings with one another.

Work System Issues

When chronic illness patients are still functioning well and continuing to work, they often face difficulties at work similar to those at home (Gulick, 1991; Houser & Chace, 1993; Roessler & Rumrill, 1998). They may not have been able to work at their usual pace and may have frequently taken sick leave. Their coworkers may have become judgmental and stigmatizing. In addition, patients may face practical problems in a workplace not geared to their level of disability.

Patients often ask clinicians to help them educate their employers about their illness and what they need to make the workplace functional for them. Many employers are willing, even eager, to cooperate. Clinicians may arrange for a specialist to analyze the work environment so that it can be made ergonomically appropriate for the patient. They may recommend alterations in work-rest patterns to make best use of the patient's energy patterns. They may speak to the employer or coworkers about the nature of the patient's disease to provide accurate information and to relieve fears about contagion.

Examples

A patient named **Fan** had a disfiguring facial cancer. Her coworkers were becoming very uncomfortable in her presence, so **Fan** asked me to conduct a consultation at her place of work. I spoke with **Fan**'s boss and fellow workers, both separately and together. I urged them all to speak out about their concerns, which not only let them vent their feelings, but also gave the concerns legitimacy. It turned out that **Fan**'s office had some interface with the public, although **Fan**'s particular job did not. Some of her office mates thought that her appearance would distress clients, but they also didn't know what her medical problem was or what effect it might have on them. I explained that **Fan**'s condition was not contagious and that she was not going to die. **Fan**'s appearance, however, would not improve. I noted that **Fan** did not, in fact, come into contact with the public except accidentally. I also helped guide **Fan**'s coworkers about behavior. They were upset because they did not know what to say to **Fan**. I told them that they need not talk about her condition at all unless **Fan** brought it up, when they would respond compassionately. I advised the group not to talk among themselves about **Fan** because this isolated her and made her feel very uncomfortable. If they needed to talk together, they should do so somewhere other than the office. Essentially, I recommended that they talk out their feelings now and then try to behave with **Fan** as they would with anyone else. I also made myself available for future consultations if the office members wanted it. In time, as **Fan** demonstrated that she could continue to perform her job adequately, the other members of her office became used to her appearance and it ceased to distract or disturb them.

Carmen, a young woman with CFS who was working in a large business organization, was having trouble with her employer because she became exhausted about halfway through the day and her work was suffering. I consulted with the company and suggested that they put a sofa in the ladies lounge. As soon as **Carmen** was able to take a 20-minute rest once or twice a day, her work performance returned to normal. Other employees, incidentally, also appreciated having a place to lie down for a few minutes, and office morale as a whole improved.

In some cases, employers may ask clinicians to speak with a disability specialist hired by the employer. Clinicians should remember that they can be both objective and dispassionate and still remain the patient's advocate (K. M. Boyer, 1999; Hummel, 2002; Stephens, 1989). In many cases, patients will eventually apply for disability benefits. To do so successfully requires forethought in all aspects of patients' relationship with their health care providers. Unnecessary mistakes made out of ignorance can cost patients desperately needed financial assistance. Clinicians may not be able to keep up with the intricacies of disability insurance personally, but they should make sure that the patient has assistance from someone who does and who works as a team member with the clinician and the patient.

Clinician Advocacy

Clinicians have an obligation to advocate for their patients. They need to speak for them vis-a-vis other health care providers, the patients' HMOs, the disability companies, and the federal and state governments (K. M. Boyer,

PHASE 1
Checklist for Treatment

Physical/Behavioral Domain

_____ 1. Who are the members of the multidisciplinary team that are addressing the patient's needs? Are you able to keep members of the team informed about the findings/protocols of the others?

_____ 2. What medical protocols have been established for the patient? What medications have been ordered? Have you asked the medical team about potential interactions between these medications or between ordered medications and others the patient is already taking?

_____ 3. Have you worked with the patient to ensure that the patient structures his or her life to incorporate recommended physical protocols? How will the patient accomplish what has been recommended?

_____ 4. Using the patient's activity data, have you helped restructure the patient's activities of daily living? What is that plan?

_____ 5. If the patient needs one, have you developed a physical safety plan? What is that plan?

Psychological Domain

_____ 1. Have you begun establishing a warm, egalitarian relationship with the patient? What indicators seem to show this to be so?

_____ 2. Have you affirmed to the patient both the difficult fact of the patient's condition and the hurts and difficulties that the patient has experienced as a consequence?

_____ 3. Have you begun educating the patient in the phase process so that the patient has some roadmap for what lies ahead?

_____ 4. Have you begun teaching the patient about content and process and the distinction between the two?

_____ 5. Have you introduced the patient to the observing self (in particular, in relation to the collection of activity data)?

_____ 6. Have you begun teaching the patient about identification and differentiation (of fears, losses, suffering, functional and dysfunctional adaptations)?

_____ 7. Have you begun teaching the patient about ego loss and dissociation?

_____ 8. Have you helped to provide comfort and containment, asserting positive values and perhaps even humor?

_____ 9. What form of therapy have you employed to help the patient work toward psychological behavioral/structural goals?

_____ 10. Is a psychological safety plan necessary? If so, what is that plan?

(continued)

Social/Interactive Domain

_____ 1. Have you worked with the family/partner to identify their traumas as they relate to the patient's condition?

_____ 2. Have you worked with the family/partner to help make necessary practical adjustments?

_____ 3. Have you worked with the family/partner on changed interpersonal relations?

_____ 4. Have you helped educate the patient and family on interaction with the health care system?

_____ 5. If the patient is still working or is on sick leave, do you need to intervene with the employer, coworkers, or the physical work situation? What actions have been carried out?

_____ 6. If the patient cannot work, have you provided assistance or helped find expert assistance as to disability?

1999; Hummel, 2002; Stephens, 1989). Disability companies, for example, often sell policies to other companies, which ostensibly reinvestigate claims to see whether the patient is ready to return to the workforce. Although the investigation has all the trappings of objectivity, the company may actually intend to move as many people off the disability rolls as possible. Clinicians need to teach their patients to act as consumers in the health care system, to insist on their rights, and to accept their responsibilities. They need to teach patients to become their own advocates (Anderton et al., 1989; S. L. Baumann, 1997).

COUNTERTRANSFERENCE

Countertransference is the name given to the responses stirred in clinicians by patients or by patients' illnesses and experiences. In traditional analytic circles, countertransference was thought to occur only rarely and to be completely undesirable when it did. It was an untoward occasion when the subjective/nonscientific erupted unbidden into the objective/scientific arena. Because the clinician's feelings were not objective, countertransference was thought to distort observation and, therefore, needed to be suppressed or eliminated. What the health care profession deemed desirable was "clinician neutrality" (Alexandris & Vaslamatzis, 1993).

Today, most clinicians acknowledge the concept that illness of every sort includes physiological elements, which may be measurable and quantifiable, but also elements of psyche, which are rarely measurable and distinctly qualitative. Many also agree that health care providers cannot conceivably work as totally objective scientific machines. They know that in their professional activities, clinicians, like everyone else, are affected both by their personal emotional lives and by their experiences with patients (Pearlman & Saakvitne, 1995; Rood, 1996; J. P. Wilson & Lindy, 1994).

It is a basic assumption of this book that countertransference happens to all clinicians all the time. If these ubiquitous countertransferential responses are acknowledged and processed properly, they can actually produce greater understanding, closer patient-clinician relationships, and creative treatment possibilities. Ignored or repressed, the responses can negatively impact the patient-clinician relationship and make effective treatment unlikely.

Some countertransferential responses may be called "objective" because nearly everyone experiencing the same stimulus reacts the same way (Pearlman & Saakvitne, 1995). Most people exposed to bodies mutilated in massacres or children dying of starvation, for example, feel revolted and horrified. They are angered, fearful, and sometimes roused to action. Not to feel this way may be taken as a sign of trauma in the observer, which indicates that the affected observer should be removed from the scene and helped to recover human perspective.

Other responses may be called "subjective" because they are triggered in individuals by associations particular to that individual (Pearlman & Saakvitne, 1995). A clinician whose mother was alcoholic will almost certainly react more powerfully to patients suffering or inflicting abuse because of alcohol. A clinician whose sister died of MS may feel tremendous stress and frustration if unable to effect improvement in an MS patient.

The words *objective* and *subjective* are neither and both objective and subjective. In this society's quantitative scientific culture, feelings and responses are burdened with negative connotations because they are qualitative and lack obvious measures. But no matter how they are regarded, they are real, they happen all the time, and they can either enhance or destroy a therapeutic relationship.

It is a central principle of the Four-Phase Model that clinicians as well as patients go through the four phases in response to the clinical situation at hand and in terms of their own life trajectories. Although their experiences differ greatly and clinicians usually develop skills for proceeding through the phases more swiftly on subsequent journeys, clinicians as well as patients personally experience responses to crisis, stabilization, resolution, and integration.

Phase theory sees countertransferential responses not as negative intrusions that need to be suppressed, but as experiences that help clinicians to achieve more creative, effective work. It is not simply an act of self-preservation for clinicians to understand their countertransferential responses-though it is that as well. Understanding and transforming them produces better treatment.

TRANSFORMATIVE STEPS OVER THE FOUR PHASES

Over the course of the four phases, as patients create and rewrite their illness narrative, clinicians also take a series of transformative steps, which help them to process and then use their countertransferential responses. These are not simple actions, quickly accomplished, but are deep attitudinal changes that require time. By coming to meaningful terms with their own feelings, however, clinicians are then able to model these understandings for their patients as the patients try to come to grips with and develop meaningful responses to their illness experiences (Chin, 2002). The countertransferential transformation steps follow this progression.

Allowance of Suffering

In Phase 1, clinicians develop an allowance of suffering. This is not the same as accepting suffering, in the sense of considering suffering a desirable phenomenon, but rather it is the development of a stance that recognizes that the suffering is there with the patient, it is there in the world at large, and it is also here, in the clinician and here in the clinical relationship. Suffering happens, and the clinician needs to learn to allow its existence. The clinician's attitude needs to evolve from one of resistance or denial to an acknowledgment that suffering can be present regardless of what people prefer or desire and that it is wise to pay attention to its existence.

To allow suffering, clinicians must learn to tolerate both their own affect and that of their patients. They must come to acknowledge, examine, and accept that ambiguity pervades the situation. They need to gain insight into the concept that people need not fear feeling bad in and of itself. Feeling bad, feeling pain, and so on—suffering—simply is, and they can let it happen without stress or resistance once actual threat, physical or psychic, has been ascertained and treated to the extent possible. Clinicians allow themselves to experience surrender; that is, they let go of trying to manage those things in life that are not, in fact, accessible to human control. When they feel attuned to this in themselves, clinicians can begin to model it for their patients.

Meet Suffering with Compassion

In Phase 2, clinicians learn to meet the suffering with compassion. This is the very slow, but important process of beginning to learn to regard the suffering in oneself and others from a loving place. Individuals get to compassion by actively engaging the grief reaction to suffering and by feeling the emotions that trauma and losses justifiably evoke. Consciously identifying and grieving for their suffering also defuses the danger of neurotic suffering because neurotic suffering cannot survive exposure to clear examination and understanding.

Meet Suffering with Respect

As clinicians move into Phase 3, they work to meet suffering with respect. This represents a complete 180-degree turnaround from the situation that existed at the start of Phase 1, when both clinician and patient were dealing with society's and their own intolerance of suffering and their perception of its inadmissibility. Coming to an attitude of respect does not occur as a major "conversion" experience, but in many little breakthroughs or insights. Although there are no big epiphanies, a sense accumulates that the most despised thing, the suffering, has become almost holy or sacred in its importance.

In Phase 3, the suffering, rejected self becomes the bedrock on which patients begin to construct their new selves. They can do this now because they and the clinician have together discovered that respect for suffering can help patients create and find meaning for their present lives. This is a very exciting process for both clinicians and patients because development of meaning occurs most successfully when the creative processes are engaged. During the course of achieving this new stance, clinicians model and witness for patients the concept of standing with the self, of being an advocate for the people they actually are.

Integration of Suffering

In Phase 4, clinicians and patients carry out an integration of suffering into their lives. Most practically, and yet most profoundly, this occurs by freely making the daily commitment to small acts of bravery. Clinicians and patients both choose to meet the hard, difficult moments the patient's condition presents with courage and even grace. For many people, taking advocacy action in society about the condition helps to give substance to the integration of suffering in their lives. This is not a matter of speaking out one day a year, though it could be, but of daily witnessing the experience of chronic illness in themselves and for the world. This may take the form of speaking up when someone at work makes an inappropriate remark, rather than simply letting it pass. Or perhaps patients choose to use their handicapped stickers for parking even though they use neither crutches nor give other obvious indications that they are eligible for these places. Other people find that creative actions or activities make the integration evident or real and hence purposeful for them. They write journals or poetry, they paint or play music, they build models or work in wood, they tie fishing flies. In Phase 4, clinicians and patients have incorporated conscious suffering into their lives. They comprehend deeply that all humans, chronically ill or not, live with paradox, but that paradox does not destroy meaning or purpose in life. They treat themselves with honor and integrity, meeting the issues of living, which include suffering and the inevitability of dying, with all the resources available to the human spirit.

COUNTERTRANSFERENCE IN PHASE 1

Revulsion, Fear, and Anger

At the same time that clinicians are assessing their chronic illness patients, they need to maintain a running review of their own countertransferential responses. Crisis characterizes Phase 1 for both patients and clinicians. Clinicians can find that patients' stories or sometimes simply the situations they know the patients are in stimulate feelings of revulsion, fear, and anger (Figley, 1995; Schwartz-Salant & Stein, 1995). These emotions may arise in reaction to the patient's problem or method of dealing with the problem, but clinicians may just as easily feel them in reaction to what has happened to the patient or what other people have done to the patient. Emotions can also accumulate in clinicians as they see a number of different chronically ill patients, so that at some

---

PHASE 1
Countertransference

Revulsion, fear, anger
Ambiguity and chronicity
Forbidden impulses
Distraction
Disbelief
Traumas
Patient avoidance
Rejection/overidentification
Medical school syndrome

Clinical Stance
Allowance of suffering
Empathetic relationship
Equal, open exchange
Affirmation and compassion
Modeling toleration for ambiguity

---

point the sheer fact of meeting the next new patient stimulates revulsion, fear, or anger that has accumulated over time.

Ambiguity and Chronicity

All three emotions relate directly to the sociocultural factors discussed earlier, especially the nearly universal intolerance of suffering, ambiguity, and chronicity (Figley, 1995; Schwartz-Salant & Stein, 1995). Exposure to the patient's situation stimulates the clinician's cultural fears of contagion and frequently animates an atavistic "just world" rationalization for negative characterological judgments. Negative feelings are also magnified by clinicians' concerns with professional status and hierarchy, by fears of stigmatization for treating a marginalized patient population, and by the sense of failure or inadequacy that the ambiguity of treating chronic patients induces.

All three emotions exist on continua of strength. Revulsion ranges from mild aversion and distaste to true revulsion. Fear stretches from mild twinges of awareness that the clinician could suffer similar symptoms to full-blown terror of illness and death. Anger may manifest as annoyance that a patient must be exaggerating or overdramatizing, but it can also arise from clinicians' feelings that no one could possibly pay them enough to absorb this sort of pain. Anger at the patient may even spring from a general fury over the health care system's inability to cope adequately with chronic patients or society's unwillingness to support its poor and disabled.

Forbidden Impulses

Listening to the possibly violent, often compelling, needy outpourings of a Phase 1 patient, clinicians may suddenly find themselves having "forbidden impulses," such as sexual or sadistic thoughts or passing notions of humiliating the patient (Alexandris & Vaslamatzis, 1993; Pearlman & Saakvitne, 1995; J. P. Wilson & Lindy, 1994). Even these feelings can be turned to useful effect if the clinician examines them carefully. Sometimes they may actually point to important aspects of the patient's experience, which are unaccountably missing from the patient's account.

Distraction from the Patient

Whatever the intruding emotion, however, in all instances it distracts the clinician (Alexandris & Vaslamatzis, 1993; Olkin, 1999; Pearlman & Saakvitne, 1995; J. P. Wilson & Lindy, 1994). The clinician stops listening to the patient's story and begins instead to pay attention to and think about his or her own story as it unfolds in relation to the patient. Obviously, when clinicians stop listening to patients, they are not performing adequately and will ultimately not treat effectively. Learning to listen both to patients and to their own countertransferential responses is a skill that takes practice and guidance for clinicians to learn and maintain. As a consequence, those who work intensively with the chronic illness population need to share their issues periodically with a valued colleague or group of colleagues to maintain balance and insight. The establishment of such mentoring or supervisory relationships is discussed later in the book.

Disbelief

In addition, Phase 1 patients often stimulate disbelief in clinicians (Pearlman & Saakvitne, 1995; Rood, 1996; J. P. Wilson & Lindy, 1994). This response involves a combination of cognitive and emotional elements. Most clinicians have not, as a matter of fact, seen so many chronic patients that they have become aware of all the manifestations that chronic illness has in even one patient. As a consequence, they may not credit patient narrations as authentic descriptions of reality. They may feel that they cannot be hearing the truth, especially because they cannot recall ever hearing of such things happening to people like themselves (B. A. Boyer et al., 1996; Kwoh et al., 1992; Starfield et al., 1981).

Professionally, clinicians, like all people, tend to prefer situations with clear and relatively direct explanations and solutions. It requires a rare and dedicated person who takes the time to listen to patients, establish rapport, and slowly tease out consistent patterns. Individuals may go into the field of social work, psychology, or psychiatry without a complete understanding of the level of vocational services required. But even those with true desire to help and serve may, nevertheless, find that their personalities and skills are ill-suited to the challenge presented by chronic patients.

Clinicians' Traumas

The problems or situations of Phase 1 patients may trigger old traumas in a clinician's life (Figley, 1995; Nouwen, 1972). Recalling the profound misery and hopelessness that a clinician's father felt when he became bedridden with prostate cancer may stir up powerful emotions when dealing with a chronic fatigue patient at wit's end because he cannot move his limbs properly. And in the experience of most clinicians, there is also the patient "who gets to you," the patient whose problems and experiences arouse the clinician's most potently upsetting and disabling anxieties.

Patient Avoidance

Countertransferential responses to Phase 1 patients may lead clinicians to avoid the patient by missing or habitually rescheduling appointments or by trying to pass the patient along to some other clinician. Or clinicians may distance themselves emotionally, creating such a chill that the patient quickly learns to report only selectively (Rood, 1996; J. P. Wilson & Lindy, 1994).

Overidentification and Failure to Set Boundaries

Clinicians may just as easily overidentify with the patient and become careless about setting appropriate internal or external boundaries (Figley, 1995; Pearlman & Saakvitne, 1995; J. P. Wilson & Lindy, 1994). In this context, it is important to remember that countertransference responses may be positive as well as negative. Patients may arouse strong feelings of admiration. Clinicians may idealize any people who suffer as having some deep connection to truth or meaning. Clinicians may be fascinated by their patients, engaged with their personalities and minds, or personally enriched by contact with them. But even if the countertransferential responses are positive, they can distort assessment and treatment and complicate successful evolution through the phases unless they are consciously recognized and processed.

Medical School Syndrome

Finally, some clinicians may see their patients' symptoms in themselves and fear that they may be suffering the same illnesses. This phenomenon resembles "medical school student syndrome," where fledging doctors are convinced they have each new disease they study. Chronically ill patients in Phase 1 often struggle to maintain the activities and behaviors of normal life even though they have enormous difficulty and even though their attempts to live as they did before are increasing those difficulties. Seeing patients who in so many ways appear "normal" can make clinicians wonder whether they, too, are fooling themselves and trying to pass. It is easy to believe that they, too, may be ignoring levels of exhaustion and confusion that signal something pathological.

This brief list of countertransferential responses to Phase 1 patients is merely suggestive of the most important reactions, ones that require particular attention on the clinicians' part. But whatever the responses, the essential issue is for clinicians to recognize and process them so that their personal reactions can enhance rather than hinder patient assessment and treatment.

Examples ─────────────────────────

My distinctly different reactions to **Everett** and **Kim** are illustrative of these instantaneous, gut responses. **Everett** was disturbing to look at. His stroke had left him slumped on one side, and he moved clumsily. He had difficulty making eye contact, slurred his speech, and because of his uneven control, he tended to drool. In other words, he presented a frightening vision of the horrible things that can happen to a human body, even one's own. I had had extensive experience with patients who looked as bad or worse than **Everett**, but, nonetheless, my immediate, instinctive reaction was one of revulsion and fear. Furthermore, **Everett**'s whole conception of himself as a man and his relationship with his wife was one that had little appeal for me because I believe in feminist ideals of equality between the sexes. But it was going to be essential, if I was to help **Everett** at all, to enter into his mind-set in some way that would allow me to understand his pain and loss. In addition to **Everett**'s multiple traumas, his wife, Joan, was also severely traumatized. **Everett**'s care depended almost entirely on her, so the return of Joan to some state of well-being was vital to **Everett**'s treatment.

Kim, on the other hand, appeared to be completely healthy. She was well dressed, quick of movement, bright, and alert. As I listened to **Kim** itemize her extensive list of diagnoses and describe her unremitting pain, I felt as though she were being buried under the avalanche of disparate information, which was increasingly hard to credit the longer the catalog became. Despite my knowledge of the invisibility of pain in most people, when I looked at **Kim**, it was hard to believe in her pain. A glance at **Kim**'s X-rays demonstrated that she must be telling the truth, but my gut reaction was that no one could suffer as much pain as she claimed without its showing on her face or in her stance. **Kim** was also so demanding and had so many problems and traumas that it was hard to relate to them all. **Kim**'s agitation made her unable to focus well, so she tended to skitter from one subject to another in a fashion that irritated me enormously even though I understood why it was happening.

Without doubt, **Lewis**'s ideations would have bothered many clinicians. It is hard to say why I was not disturbed. Perhaps I had the good fortune to notice his subtle physical tics while he was talking and was processing this information more attentively than the ideational content. Perhaps my past work with an incarcerated population had familiarized me with the kinds of ideations typical of actual sexual criminals. **Lewis**'s enormous accomplishments during his life, his overcoming of poverty and racial barriers, produced strong positive countertransferential feelings in me. I wanted **Lewis** to continue to succeed, so I actively wanted to support and assist him.

Neither **Sophia** nor **Christine** looked ill when they first saw me. Although **Christine** frequently used a wheelchair before this time and did so afterwards, past experience with other clinicians made her carefully arrange her first visit to occur when she could navigate under her own steam. **Sophia**'s presentation was so gracious and charming that it would have been hard not to like her. Both women had conditions in which diagnosis involved subjective information, but this was such familiar territory for me that it did not inspire the kind of distrust that self-reported information has for some clinicians. Both women, although different from each other, resonated with me for many reasons. **Christine** and I had similar professional experiences, whereas I enjoyed **Sophia**'s brilliant mind and was moved by her deep and meaningful spirituality.

CLINICAL STANCE IN PHASE 1

Allowance of Suffering

As mentioned previously, clinicians transform their Phase 1 countertransferential responses by learning to *allow* suffering and to tolerate affect and ambiguity. They examine their reactions until they can honestly experience a surrender to a clear and specific knowledge that suffering does exist in their lives and the lives of their patients. It is not possible to exclude suffering from life. Nor, in the last analysis, is suffering such a negative thing that we cannot learn from it and grow because of it.

Empathetic Relationship

In the crisis and urgency that characterize Phase 1, the most important activity for clinicians is to establish a warm, empathetic relationship with their patients. This relationship is often a fragile thing, easily ruptured by missteps that clinicians make out of ignorance or unwillingness to confront the issues that arise for them when they are in the presence of their chronic patients.

Equal Exchange

Equal exchange is the cornerstone for building a solid relationship that can withstand the occasional buffeting that may occur. *Equal,* here, refers to the shared humanity of clinician and patient. The clinician presumably has greater specific expertise—which is why the patient comes to the clinician in the first place—but expertise is the only way the clinician differs from the patient.

Expertise does not permit the clinician to become a listener who from a height of assumed superiority affects to hear impartially the pains and inadequacies of a patient and then to pronounce treatments that will improve the patient's situation. When clinicians are convinced that they alone can promote patients' best interests, they project—and patients quickly internalize—a sense of patients' incompetence and dependency, which simply exacerbates patients' Phase 1 sense that their illness is totally outside their control.

Honor of Work

It is important for clinicians to recognize that patients entrust them with important confidences, about which the patients are often deeply ashamed. Often, the most significant discussions include substance that seriously distresses the clinician as well. Clinicians should be humble in the face of such risk-taking on the patient's part and openly demonstrate gratitude that the patient sufficiently trusts the clinician to talk about matters that the patient knows are regarded by most people with aversion, possibly anger, or sometimes even fear. If clinicians honor the work in this way, even when the work includes distressing material, they make it possible for the patient to begin honoring the work also. And honoring the work is a first step for most patients toward developing a new attitude toward their whole illness experience.

Affirmation and Compassion

Clinicians have to affirm the illness and trauma experiences of their patients and convey genuine compassion for their patients from the beginning of the relationship. They have to exude a sense that they will act toward their patients in a loving way. It is important that clinicians also act, and show that they act, in a loving way toward themselves. This is best accomplished by clinicians' acknowledging and examining their countertransferential responses and speaking of these openly with their patients when discretion indicates this will benefit the patient. Clinicians should preface any sharing by considering the emotional state of the patient, the context of the situation, what the clinician feels the patient can handle, and whether such sharing will enhance or detract from the clinician-patient relationship. By sharing carefully chosen and modulated responses, clinicians can help to model concretely that the work the clinician and patient do together is an exchange between human equals.

Open Communication

Clinicians must also take care not to direct all conversations with patients or to set limits on language and expression that exclude important aspects of the patient's experience. The isolation created by suffering can create experiences for patients, which feel beyond the possibility of communication. Words may fail altogether, yet the patient wants someone to understand that has happened. As a consequence, all patient utterances are approaches to the truth of their experience and clinicians should consider them in that light.

Seeking Advice

When clinicians are baffled by patient information, they need to acknowledge this openly and seek advice from others. They need to demonstrate that they, too, must learn all the time. By being willing to exhibit fallibility and humility, yet with dignity, authority, and self-respect, clinicians increase their ability to engage with their patients.

Modeling Toleration for Ambiguity

Clinicians importantly model toleration for the broad range of patient (and clinician) affect and for the ambiguity that suffuses the chronic illness experience. The calm witnessing of what patients consider the horrors of their world helps bring patients' experiences back to the realm of the normal. The events and experiences may be unpleasant and not ones patients would willingly choose to undergo, but they are not extraordinary, bizarre, or even unusual. Normalization of patient experience, occurring in the context of a warm, supportive patient-clinician relationship, helps prepare the patient to move into Phase 2.

Example

As I began to find ways to bond with **Everett**, I was able to model for him and Joan how to allow and discuss his traumas and suffering in a style that would be comfortable for **Everett**. Initially, I would, more or less, sneak it in. In what would sound like a side comment to Joan, I would say how impressed I was with what **Everett** was able to do and how he had really taken on a lot of extremely difficult stuff. I would also say how impressed I was with Joan, who was assuming so many responsibilities and learning to do so many new things. Time and again in conversations, both when Joan was present and when she was not, I would comment, essentially to myself, on the severity of the situation, on how

Everett had survived it and was battling to extend his functionality as much as he could.

This running commentary helped label the experiences that **Everett** and Joan were having. Putting the discourse into heroic language—saying that such work was not for the faint of heart—continuously impressed on **Everett** how brave, how manly, he was because of what he was making an effort to do every day. Gradually, **Everett** was learning to be proud of what he was doing.

In these conversations, I kept reiterating that **Everett** and Joan were not alone and that I would stick with them and do this difficult work with

PHASE 1
Checklist for Countertransference

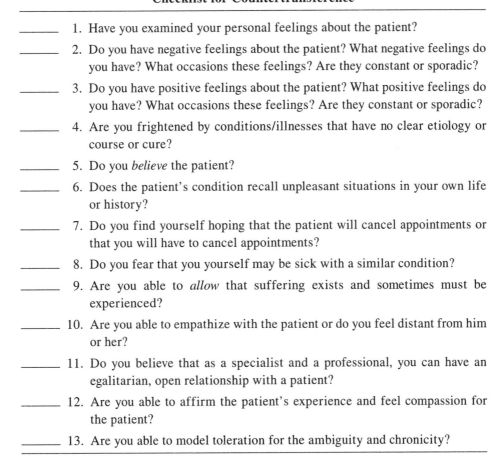

_____ 1. Have you examined your personal feelings about the patient?

_____ 2. Do you have negative feelings about the patient? What negative feelings do you have? What occasions these feelings? Are they constant or sporadic?

_____ 3. Do you have positive feelings about the patient? What positive feelings do you have? What occasions these feelings? Are they constant or sporadic?

_____ 4. Are you frightened by conditions/illnesses that have no clear etiology or course or cure?

_____ 5. Do you *believe* the patient?

_____ 6. Does the patient's condition recall unpleasant situations in your own life or history?

_____ 7. Do you find yourself hoping that the patient will cancel appointments or that you will have to cancel appointments?

_____ 8. Do you fear that you yourself may be sick with a similar condition?

_____ 9. Are you able to *allow* that suffering exists and sometimes must be experienced?

_____ 10. Are you able to empathize with the patient or do you feel distant from him or her?

_____ 11. Do you believe that as a specialist and a professional, you can have an egalitarian, open relationship with a patient?

_____ 12. Are you able to affirm the patient's experience and feel compassion for the patient?

_____ 13. Are you able to model toleration for the ambiguity and chronicity?

them. I emphasized that I was not surprised by their situation, beginning the process of normalizing it. I also worked to normalize the concept that **Everett**'s disability would continue, although it was dynamic and might not always have the same characteristics.

Everett had always thought of himself as a fighter, so I used battle imagery. I got **Everett** to look at the strategy and tactics needed to fight different battles. I helped him to conceptualize their new activities as clever tactics to outwit a powerful opponent. I also employed many football analogies.

Throughout, I would regularly express gratitude for **Everett**'s sharing confidence with me. I would also thank him for the time that he spent working with me. I would articulate that I both cared about **Everett** and about the work. Having established myself in **Everett**'s eyes as a kind of guy's girl, I would emphasize that I didn't ever waste my time on useless efforts. Our work together was definitely not a waste of time.

When **Everett** got really comfortable with me, we sometimes joked about his situation, usually using football metaphors. He was a quarterback who constantly got sacked, but who kept getting up and working to improve his team's strategy and, especially, to improve their defense of their quarterback. But humor was never allowed to become disrespectful, and I stopped it dead if it threatened to go in that direction.

SPIRITUAL/PHILOSOPHICAL PERSPECTIVE IN PHASE 1

One element of the phase process that has increasing importance as patients move forward through the phases is the spiritual or philosophical perspective. This aspect of both the patient's and the clinician's mind-set deals deeply with meaning and cosmology. During Phase 3 especially, patients accomplish some of their most intense work in this area.

Primitive Punishment or Abandonment

In Phase 1, the urgency and lack of control that patients feel in their somatic and psychological life may manifest in very primitive spiritual or philosophical ways. Because they believe they are bad for being ill and yet cannot in any fashion change the facts of their situation or fix themselves, they tend to

---

PHASE 1
Spiritual/Philosophical Perspective

Experience
   "Godlessness"
   Primitive punishment or abandonment
   Highly structured beliefs
   Spiritual/philosophical perspective externalized

Clinical Action
   Generalized comfort and containment

---

believe either that God has abandoned them, that there is no God at all, or that God is punishing them (Dyson, Cobb, & Forman, 1997; Rehm, 1999; Sugarek, Dyo, & Holmes, 1988; C. H. Sumner, 1998). They frequently feel this way even if they have not been involved at all in regular religious practice before their illness. Culturally, most people in Western society carry deep fears that an angry, avenging deity may exist and that bad fortune, particularly in the form of illness, is a sign of deserved punishment. Those who believe there is no God often express deep existential despair, asserting that they have no reason to continue to live because there is no point to living. The ambiguity of their spiritual situation mirrors the ambiguity of their clinical and social situation and causes them equal, if not greater, grief.

Clinicians may have similar feelings or worries, especially if they have not meditated on these issues in the past. Their clinical practice itself may also lead them to question how God, if they believe in God, can permit the suffering they see in their offices every day. Many clinicians are in a constant evolution of personal meaning themselves, and they may find themselves shaken by patients' specific issues, especially because patients' arguments can be very compelling. Clinicians may also experience countertransference in response to the philosophical role that patients often thrust on them. Patients may come to regard them, at least temporarily, as the ultimate arbiter of philosophical or spiritual meaning, and such responsibility is more than most clinicians can shoulder easily (Allport & Ross, 1967; Fowler, 1982; Kelly, 1995; Kohlberg, 1981; Krippner & Welsh, 1992; Payne,

Bergin, Bielema, & Jenkins, 1991; Peck, 1987; Richards & Bergin, 1997; Scotton, Chinen, & Battista, 1996; Shafranske & Gorsuch, 1984).

Parallel Development of Meaning

As clinicians and patients move through the phase process, both work on the development of meaning. Patients are focused on their individual lives, but clinicians carry out a parallel process. Concurrently, they examine and revise their personal beliefs while helping their patients construct meaning that is individually significant to the patients. Patients' ultimate beliefs and understandings may very well not coincide with clinicians', but that is as it should be. Conceptions about the meaning of life are highly individual, even if there are many shared elements.

Generalized Spiritual Comfort and Containment

In Phase 1, patients, for the most part, express spiritual or cosmological issues in terms of being punished, damned to hell, and other such statements. Because they are beset by the immediate problems of their illness, they are incapable of doing any deep or meaningful work now. In Phase 1, clinicians should seek only to provide a generalized sense of philosophical and spiritual comfort. They need to receive their patients' fearful and self-condemnatory statements compassionately and with understanding but then suggest that there are other ways to view the situation and affirm that the patient is not going to hell. If patients express total existential despair, especially if suicide seems a possibility, clinicians need to work with them to get them to hold open a space in their minds for eventual meaning. Although the patient cannot imagine meaning now, the clinician needs to argue persuasively that it will exist in the future. Until patients arrive at a later phase and engage in more sophisticated philosophical development of meaning, clinicians mostly act as comforting, empathetic, witnessing presences to this aspect of the patient's experience.

Examples _____

As mentioned earlier, **Sophia** came into treatment with an unusually high level of spirituality. Daily prayer and meditation were part of her life. The community of her childhood had a highly structured, intense level of religious belief, and **Sophia** was sustained by this. She had a profound sense of the God without and the God within. As with many people, however, **Sophia** had been so attentive to her education and her career that although she went through the forms of her religious practice, she was often doing so automatically. I worked with **Sophia** to tap back into the deep meaning that her practice had had for her. For a Phase 1 patient, however, **Sophia** was extraordinary in the supportive meaningfulness of her spiritual practice.

Everett was far more typical of Phase 1. He had never had much use for religion and rarely attended church after he got married. He could not conceive of why his suffering was happening to him and wanted to blame something or someone. Because he had no cosmology and no God that he believed in, he didn't even have God to blame. He felt both trashed and abandoned.

Church was, however, important to Joan, who had taken her children to Sunday school and later to church and participated in church activities. This is the way she had grown up, and she felt it was the right way to live. Religion had meaning for her in the sense that it seemed to make the social world she lived in three-dimensional. When her parents died, she found the services and prayers comforting. They made the deaths, which occurred at what seemed like reasonable times and without great pain or distress, fit into an orderly progression of a sensible universe. But the situation she found herself in now was horrible, and she was desperately trying to do what God wanted of her so that God would relieve **Everett** and her of this terrible circumstance. She felt that **Everett** must come to church now as well, so **Everett** faced the ironic situation of embarrassing himself weekly trying to get to church to pray to a God he didn't think existed to provide some comfort to his wife.

The farming community **Lewis** had grown up in was deeply religious, and **Lewis** had attended church from the time he was a little boy. He had found solace there from the secret difficulties he had at home, and the pastor had taken an interest in this bright little boy. The pastor had intervened to make sure that **Lewis** was allowed to complete his high school education, and the church had even managed to find money to help finance his college education. **Lewis** was convinced that even if he was not a monster, he was being punished for some colossal failure, and he feared that the failure was his overweening pride in putting himself so far above his family. Fortunately, his old pastor was still alive. I urged **Lewis** to

PHASE 1
Checklist for Spiritual/Philosophical Perspective

_____ 1. What spiritual/philosophical attitudes has the patient expressed to you?

_____ 2. Have you been able to offer general comfort, particularly as to any fears of the patient of "going to hell" or being "forsaken by God" or being "punished for sins"?

It is important to note that spiritual/philosophical issues come most actively into play in Phase 3. During Phase 1 and 2, the clinician attempts largely to provide comfort and containment, passively assenting to the patient's actions as long as they are not harmful to the patient.

---

contact him to talk about these issues, and the pastor helped reassure **Lewis** that God did not act that way. Whatever evil was befalling **Lewis**, God would help and support him through his trials. **Lewis** did not feel God working with him at this point, but he did, gradually, become convinced that he was not an object of punishment.

Table 4.1 provides a summary of Phase 1 of the Four-Phase Model.

Table 4.1   Phase 1: Crisis

1. Course of Illness

Physical/behavioral domain
    Coping period—symptoms interpreted as normal
    Onset period—symptoms recognized as beyond the normal but bearable
    Acute/emergency period—symptom severity demands assistance
Psychological domain
    Loss of psychological control
    Ego loss
    Intrusive shame, self-hatred, despair
    Shock, disorientation
    Disassociation, fear of others, isolation, mood swings
Social/interactive domain
    Others experience shock, disbelief, revulsion
    Vicarious traumatization
    Responses dependent on family/organization maturation
    Suspicion-support continuum

2. Identifying Characteristics

Urgency
Locus of treatment outside self
Self-pathologizing

Table 4.1 *Continued*

Intrusive ideations and denial
Ego loss
Low tolerance for ambiguity

Clinical Goal

Trauma and crisis management

Clinical Summary

Bond
Affirm
Teach
Observe
Safety plan

3. *Assessment*

Physical/behavioral domain
Medical review
Activity level review
Physical benchmark
Neuropsychological review
Sleep assessment
Other assessments
Psychological domain
Phase placement
Psychosocial assessment
Initial trauma assessment
Psychiatric evaluation
Personal narrative (combined assessment and treatment)
Social/interractive domain
Family and couples evaluation
Work evaluation

4. *Treatment*

Physical/behavioral domain
Multidisciplinary team
Medical protocols
Physical structural/behavioral goals
Restructure activities of daily living
Physical safety plan
Psychological domain
Relationship establishment
Illness/trauma affirmation
Education to illness phases
Introduction to process and content

(continued)

Table 4.1 *Continued*

Introduction to the observing self
Introduction to identification and differentiation
Education about ego loss and dissociation
Assertion of positive values, humor
Establishment of psychological behavioral/structural goals
Social/interactive domain
Family trauma care
Family case management
Health-care system management
Workplace/employer intervention
Clinician advocacy

5. *Countertransference*

Revulsion, fear, anger
Ambiguity and chronicity
Forbidden impulses
Distraction
Disbelief
Traumas
Patient avoidance
Rejection/overidentification
Medical school syndrome

Clinical Stance

Allowance of suffering
Empathetic relationship
Equal, open exchange
Affirmation and compassion
Modeling toleration for ambiguity

6. *Spiritual/Philosophical Perspective*
Experience
"Godlessness"
Primitive punishment or abandonment
Highly structured beliefs
Spiritual/philosophical perspective externalized
Clinical action
Generalized comfort and containment

Chapter 5

PHASE 2: STABILIZATION

PERSONAL ENERGY PROCESS AND ACTIVITY CATEGORIES

How the personal energy process of patients functions and the necessity for patients to understand this process and to adapt their lives to it are salient aspects of Phase 2. It is vital to recognize that this process encompasses both the physical and the psychological manifestations of an individual's energy. It is significant in all phases, but in Phase 2 most patients first become capable

PHASE 2 Course of Illness
Physical/Behavioral Domain
Plateau
Stabilization
Psychological Domain
Increased caution/secondary wounding
Social withdrawal/social searching
Service confusion/service searching
Boundary confusion
Social/Interactive Domain
Interactive conflict/cooperation
Vicarious secondary wounding
Vicarious traumatization manifestation
Normalization failure

of recognizing and then attempting to adjust to the changed energy process that their chronic illness has generated (Bedell, 2000; Hinojosa & Kramer, 1997; Polatajko, 2000; Rebeiro & Polgar, 1999).

Four Activity Categories

The personal energy process is the pattern that an individual's actions follows, but it is also the number of actions that an individual can perform successfully in a specified time, typically daily. The actions fall into four general categories:

1. All the personal activities of daily living (ADLs)—all self-care—beginning with rising out of bed, washing, dressing, feeding, caring for clothes and surroundings, and so forth.

2. All the activities that enrich the individual's being and inner world. These range from physical activities such as exercise programs and sports to intellectual, artistic, and spiritual activities, such as reading, attending plays, growing a garden, playing a guitar, attending church, meditating, and so forth.

3. All of the individual's social activities, including sexual life and family and friend relationships.

4. All activities related to work or employment (Bedell, 2000; Hinojosa & Kramer, 1997; Primeau, 1996).

Accomplishment of an Action

Typically, the accomplishment of any action follows a simple curve. Individuals decide to perform an action. When they actually begin, however, they must almost always overcome an initial resistance, as though they were starting to roll a large stone. This is true for healthy people as well as sick ones, and even if the activity is a simple one such as washing the dishes. Once into the activity, the work proceeds more smoothly and easily, rather the way a car can shift into higher gear once it has overcome the initial inertia of moving from a stationary position. Ordinarily, individuals continue an activity to completion, at which point they feel a pleased sense of accomplishment and enjoy a brief period of rest or relaxation as a reward. The ability to have, let alone enjoy, this somatic or physical sense of accomplishment and deserved break depends, however, on individuals having some energy remaining after they finish the task (Bedell, 2000; Hinojosa & Kramer, 1997; Primeau, 1996; Rebeiro & Polgar, 1999).

Exhaustion

If the activity has totally absorbed all their energy, leaving them completely exhausted, not even the knowledge of a job completed permits true relaxation. In most healthy people, working to exhaustion tends to produce only irritation and a sense of overwork. But even among the healthy in today's society, many people have unreal expectations of being able to accomplish far more than they reasonably can; and over time, they suffer repeated frustration as well as physical exhaustion. In the sick, working to exhaustion has even more serious consequences physically and emotionally (Bedell, 2000; Hinojosa & Kramer, 1997; Primeau, 1996; Rebeiro & Polgar, 1999).

In addition, people who are ill are far more likely to have to stop an activity midcycle. This may be due to exhaustion, but it can also be due to cognitive failure or the physical inability to complete an action because it requires lost capabilities. Among the cases mentioned in this book, **Christine** sometimes was unable to carry out a task because she would became confused and unable to figure out what to do next. **Everett**, on the other hand, could not complete certain tasks, such as buttoning a shirt completely, because he could not manage the small muscle coordination required. When people are forced to abort a job midcycle, they have no pleasing sensation or satisfaction of a job done, but instead experience a sense of failure and inadequacy.

Normal Multitasking Needs

Normal healthy people accomplish many tasks, often doing several at the same time, over the course of a day. It is somatically and psychologically necessary for a person's well-being to complete a number of tasks each day. Although not quite on a par with the human need for food, shelter, and water, the physical need to complete multiple tasks—to work—is arguably as important as the need for sex, socialization, and recreation. It is the accomplishment of tasks that creates in individuals the sense that they have a high quality of life (Christiansen, 1999; Hinojosa & Kramer, 1997; Rebeiro & Polgar, 1999).

Culture's Activity Demands

In addition, the nation's culture dictates that hard work and doggedness will, in the end, produce success or the results that individuals desire. Yet even with healthy, normal individuals, repeated attempts to execute tasks that are either beyond their current abilities or performed in a manner not geared to their capabilities will lead only to failure. When people fail in an activity, they often try even harder to do what they have already been doing, rather than standing back and reconsidering whether they are pursuing a wise course to begin with. Even in healthy people, this leads to repeated failure and the diminished sense of self such failures produce (Burckhardt et al., 1989; Ware & Kleinman, 1992).

Activity Elimination

When normal people have personal goals and expectations that exceed what can be accomplished in their actual life schedules, they, like sick people, start to eliminate activities from the four general activity categories because they simply cannot accomplish all that they set out to do. Activities related to an individual's inner life are usually the first to go. People cut down on their exercise classes, read fewer books, or cease attending church. In the social sphere, sexual life diminishes, as does time playing with children or visiting with friends and relatives. Then ADLs begin to suffer—the laundry accumulates, no one cleans the apartment, people buy takeout meals rather than cook. For most adults, employment-related activities are the last to suffer erosion because most adults depend on their jobs for survival (Gignac, Cott, & Badley, 2000).

Personal Energy Process in Phase 1

The chronically ill suffer lowered, often severely diminished, personal energy processes. If the onset in Phase 1 is gradual, patients gradually cannot perform all the activities they used to, although they are often unaware of this consciously. They simply begin to cut out activities or fail to complete activities they attempt. They first cease to perform activities related to their inner well-being, then cut back on most social activities, and often cease to keep up with the ADLs. Most struggle to accomplish work activities to their employers' satisfaction, but the toll that chronic illness extracts from the personal energy process usually reduces activity levels in all areas of the patient's life. If the chronic illness comes on severely and abruptly in Phase 1, however, patients may find themselves bedridden, unable to do anything at all. They cannot even carry out the basic activities of personal care (Bedell, 2000; Hinojosa & Kramer, 1997; Polatajko, 2000; Rebeiro & Polgar, 1999).

The failure to complete activities with satisfaction, with a feeling of energy to spare and a sense of deserved rest, badly erodes an individual's physical and psychological well-being. Many chronically ill individuals complete tasks, but only at the cost of complete, debilitating exhaustion. Others constantly attempt to carry out activities, which they fail to complete at all. In either case, these individuals experience repeated frustration, loss of competence, and erosion of personal and social worth. Some patients, unable to carry out such commonplace actions as walking to the bathroom unassisted, washing their hair, or making their beds, suffer profound humiliation and distress. Higher level activities are frequently impossible to accomplish or only if all lower level activities are eliminated. Moreover, the attempt to perform activities as in the past frequently exacerbates the patient's chronic illness and may cause a relapse or severe symptom episode.

Changes in Phase 2

In Phase 1, fear and urgency often distract patients from reflecting consciously on how restricted and truncated their activities have become. They may enumerate to their clinician a list of actions they can no longer perform or have difficulty carrying out, but they do not perceive an overall, persistent pattern. In Phase 2, however, as patients' symptoms plateau and they regain some degree of personal control, their ability to examine their activities objectively—to gain data and insight about what they can reasonably accomplish—becomes a significant element in treatment.

Because Phase 2 patients are more contained and controlled, they are now capable of doing intentional work. Most clinicians want to engage patients in taking action from the beginning, but Phase 1 patients are often incapable of doing so. As a consequence, they frequently ignore or give up on activities they are urged to perform at that time and may cease to believe that such activities could help them at any time. In Phase 2, however, patients can take action. They are capable of being compliant, although they may not be for other reasons. Other stage models have noted that health-change clinicians and programs tend to be action-oriented, but that because patients are not prepared to take action in the early stages, these programs fail to achieve change or do so only temporarily (Prochaska, DiClemente, & Norcross, 1992; Prochaska & Velicer, 1997b; Prochaska et al., 1994). The argument is pertinent even though this model is one that addresses imposed change and does so in all three systems of a patient's life.

IDENTIFYING PHASE 2 PATIENTS

Some Control and Ego Strength Regained

In Phase 2, patients begin to gain a tiny modicum of control over their experience. The locus of control is very slowly returning to the self, and patients exhibit a bit more ego strength than they were capable of in Phase 1.

PHASE 2
Identifying Characteristics

Some control and ego strength regained
Seeking behavior: others of like kind, other treatments or clinicians
Low tolerance of chronicity
Reduced self-pathologizing
Fewer ideations
Normalization failure

Clinical Goal
Stabilization and basic activities restructuring

Clinical Summary
Collect data
Differentiate
Develop insight
Develop norms and goals

Seeking Others of Like Kind

Given the small, but growing sense of self, patients begin to engage in seeking behavior. They start to search for others like themselves—those with their particular illness if the condition has been identified. They also seek new sources of support and identification, as well as treatment. In part, this searching results from the rejection and secondary wounding that patients experience because they upset those around them by continuing to remain sick, by failing to return to preillness normal. Stabilization and order return in part because they find others who will not discriminate against them (Gilden, Hendryx, Clar, Casia, & Singh, 1992; Hinrichsen, Revenson, & Shinn, 1985; Humphreys, 1997; Nash & Kramer, 1993).

Locating others of like kind or people who will exhibit nonjudgmental empathy can have positive and negative outcomes. On the one hand, illness support organizations can provide patients with acquaintances who understand how they are feeling and with information that is helpful to them. But not all the information has been subjected to critical scrutiny and some may be of poor quality. Moreover, patients in different phases have markedly different experiences with support organizations. Phase 1 patients, for example, are often frustrated by such groups because the organization does not instantly provide decisive remedies and doctors who can produce cures. Young patients in less privileged socioeconomic groups may seek acceptance and sympathy in gangs, further compounding their health problems with social maladaptations. On the other hand, some patients who have abused alcohol or drugs in an attempt to palliate their suffering may experience significant support and encouragement from 12-step recovery programs or religious commitments. By Phase 2, the lowered sense of urgency allows patients to make better use of support organizations because Phase 2 individuals do not have the same insistent need or expectation of immediate remedial help from such groups.

Seeking Other Treatments or Clinicians

Seeking different treatments or different clinicians frequently results when patients perceive that their current provider is not the best-informed clinician for their problem. They then begin to look for experts on their illness with the hope of finding better information, more successful treatment, and perhaps a cure. Some patients also leave clinicians who stigmatize or reject them, that is, when the patients experience iatrogenic traumatization. So-called "doctor hopping" can actually be a healthy choice either when patients are seeking expert advice or when they have been harmed by prior clinicians, even if unintentionally. It is certainly an appropriate response to incompetent treatment. Clinicians are trained to be suspicious of this possibly clinically borderline behavior, but it may sometimes be a sign of growing mental health and smart consumerism.

Low Tolerance of Chronicity

During Phase 2, most patients first become deeply aware of chronicity, and they find it intolerable. In Phase 1, they firmly believed that someone would eventually identify and cure their problem even when they actually knew there was no hope of a cure. But in Phase 2, they slowly begin to realize that their condition may well last a long time, if not forever. Coming to understand the issues associated with chronicity is central to treatment in Phase 2.

Less Self-Pathologizing, Fewer Ideations

By contrast with the increased difficulty caused by chronicity, self-pathologizing starts very slowly to decrease in Phase 2 patients, partly as a result of chaos stabilization and partly because the patients have located new sources of support with others of like kind. Their language changes; they are less apt to present themselves as bad people, but rather as people who are having difficulty finding help for their condition. At the same time, troubling ideations begin to diminish in frequency and intensity or, at the very least, become housebroken by familiarity.

Normalization Failure and Its Consequences

Phase 2 patients and those around them become acutely conscious of patients' failure to return to normal. When patients reach a plateau of symptoms, they generally believe that they are on the way to a cure and that they shortly, if not immediately, should be able to resume their former life and activities. Their family, friends, and coworkers share these expectations. Because Phase 2 patients are not in the crisis mode of Phase 1, where they were totally preoccupied with immediate pain or life problems, they can actually come to recognize that they are still not able, as a matter of fact, to do many of the things they used to do. At best, they can accomplish activities by trading off other activities. This failure to normalize and the ambiguity of their condition generate a new kind of suffering in Phase 2 patients (Agnetti, 1997; Axtell, 1999; Rolland, 1994).

New Examples

Most patients come to clinicians either in Phase 1 or Phase 2. One patient who entered my practice while he was in Phase 2 was **Joshua**, a Black man in his early 60s. He had been suffering heart disease and high blood pressure for several years. Standard medication, although it reduced the blood pressure somewhat, did not bring it down to safe levels. He was now suffering from severe headaches as well, which he claimed had developed only after he began taking the blood pressure medicine. His doctor tried other medications, but none reduced the blood pressure adequately and all apparently caused **Joshua**'s debilitating headaches. In an attempt to address the pain management issue, which the physician believed to be a psychological problem, and also in the hope that my phase approach would reduce **Joshua**'s blood pressure to reasonable levels, the doctor referred **Joshua** to me.

Joshua did not have the intense urgency that characterizes Phase 1 patients. He did hold himself responsible for his condition when he experienced symptoms—in his case, either the headaches or a very flushed face, which he believed indicated that his blood pressure was soaring. **Joshua** refused to accept the notion of a chronic condition at all. He demanded a cure and declared an interest only in those activities or medications that would make him symptom-free forever. **Joshua**'s work and home life had not been seriously affected by his condition, so he had not experienced the normalization failures typical of Phase 2. Nor had he considered finding others with his problem, even though he was conscious of the fact that many older men he knew suffered from it and that his father and his uncles were all dead by the time they were his age.

Gina, a White woman in her early 40s, also came to my practice when she was in Phase 2. She was a middle school teacher, married, with two children, both of whom suffered from severe attention deficit disorder. She herself had been diagnosed about a year earlier with fibromyalgia (FM) and chronic fatigue syndrome (CFS). **Gina** sought me out on her own. She was not in crisis. For more than a year, she had held things together, but it was becoming increasingly difficult, and she wanted to learn better ways to cope.

Gina suffered pain and fatigue. The latter caused some cognitive dysfunction. Exhaustion and fatigue caused her to become confused and temporarily experience a sense of being overwhelmed. **Gina** had a good deal of ego strength and an internalized sense of control. After her first diagnosis (CFS), she had sought out others of like kind, but she now wanted to go beyond the anecdotal recommendations of her fellow sufferers to seek expert help. She faithfully followed her doctor's protocols, but she was clearly seeking other clinical help to improve her life.

Gina's experience with her children had developed in her a fairly high level of tolerance for certain chronic conditions. But she did keep trying to behave as though she and her children were normal healthy people, and she kept failing. As a consequence, her self-pathologizing was still relatively high. She believed that she should be able to do everything she had done before, especially in relation to her children. Every time she failed, she felt unhappy and inadequate. At these times, she became preoccupied with thoughts of her failure, her unfulfilled life, and the prospect of being unhappy for the rest of her life.

Gina was also entering menopause, and age-related issues were beginning to slow her down. During the summer break, she had been able to manage, but with her return to teaching in the fall, she was suffering more pain and less ability to cope. Her husband was becoming angry because he had to do more and more of her jobs. It also turned out that his younger brother, now dead, had suffered from cystic fibrosis, and he felt the unhappy and demanding experiences of his childhood beginning to repeat themselves.

Previous Examples

All five cases discussed in Phase 1 moved into Phase 2 as they increasingly contained their crises and their symptoms stabilized. This became apparent, however, in different ways. Here are a few examples.

Lewis showed he was regaining ego strength when he began turning less to me to determine whether the content of his decreasing ideations was crazy or evil. He gradually became more tolerant of his symptoms, which bothered him less when they occurred. He learned not to try stopping them midthought, and when they were over, he interpreted them less drastically. As a consequence, his self-pathologizing began to reduce. Along with coming to believe that his behavior was not heinous, he was becoming less upset about his other tics. He was slowly coming to comprehend that he was not failing because he was not being cured. This sense came and went. He would become upset about not sleeping and still became uncomfortable when I gave him a five-minute warning before the end of a visit, but he was developing good insight and was maintaining it with some consistency.

Everett also showed greater ego strength as he began to contain the crisis of his situation. He began to feel a more internalized sense of control, which took the form of seeking other treatment, particularly related to rehabilitation. Although he had reached what the rehabilitation hospital regarded as a plateau, he felt that he was continuing to improve and wanted to locate additional physical therapy. Although **Everett** still had a very low level of tolerance for the chronicity of his situation, he was starting to grasp that it was permanent, even though it might be improved somewhat. His self-pathologizing that he was not a man any more was beginning to recede a bit as he felt the strength and bravery required to retrain the left side of his body and to accomplish what he had once considered simple tasks. He was still struggling with the more or less static nature of his disability, however. Complicating his adjustment was the pressure he was receiving from his attentive, but uncomprehending, sons. Because they lived relatively nearby, they and their wives tried to help Joan with **Everett**'s care. Inevitably, as it became clear that **Everett** would not return to his prestroke level of functioning, they felt this imposition on their lives and that of their mother. As a consequence, they tended to urge **Everett** to do things he was not ready to do and perhaps would never be ready to do. They assured their mother that he could go to the mailbox by himself, when actually he still required spotting. They incorrectly believed that Joan could leave **Everett** alone in the house for extended periods of time. Because **Everett** shared many of his sons' notions about what he should be able to do, he continued to overextend and suffer setbacks that then greatly depressed him.

Christine moved into Phase 2 as she comprehended that she could put limits on her family's behavior. It continued to be extremely difficult for her, but she learned to say no to some demands and to protect her own home space. When she had first become sick, **Christine** lost her two best friends. She didn't understand why and could never get them to explain what was wrong. As she entered Phase 2, she began to want to find new friends who, like her, had to deal with chronic syndromes. Her difficulty here was that her serious physical limitations truly did isolate her socially. **Christine**'s profession had prepared her to tolerate chronicity as to her illness in itself, but not its chronicity as to her family and work. In Phase 2, **Christine** also began seeking other treatments, even though she continued to follow all her medical protocols. She found an alternative practitioner, who succeeded in changing her diet in a more whole-grain, natural-produce direction. This probably benefited **Christine**. Her self-pathologizing was still strong. She felt that if she were a good person, she would be able to do what both she and her family wanted, and a new level of anxiety was added in that she was often afraid I would be disappointed with her if she acceded to family demands. Despite the fact that she did try to protect herself from her family, she still lived in hope that her family would change their ways, bring her back into their midst, support her in her illness, and treat her with sustaining affection.

ASSESSMENT: PHYSICAL/BEHAVIORAL DOMAIN

Typically, clinicians first meet new patients when they are in Phase 1 or Phase 2. If patients are presenting in Phase 2, the clinician ultimately needs to consider all the assessments discussed for Phase 1 patients to obtain a full clinical picture. After determining that a new patient is, in fact, in Phase 2, the clinician still needs to decide whether, for example, a neuropsych review or sleep studies evaluation is necessary in addition to the Phase 2 assessment measures. If, however, the patient has been assessed for phase placement previously, the clinician will rely primarily on Phase 2 assessment measures. All patients receiving phase method care will require ongoing reevaluation as they move through the phases.

Medical Review

Whether patients are new to the clinician or under ongoing phase method treatment, the clinician needs to obtain an updated medical review. This record review should include the entire medical-psychological-rehabilitation team involved in a patient's care so that all team members keep abreast of any

---

PHASE 2
Assessment

Physical/Behavioral Domain
    Medical and medications review
    Activity threshold review
    Medical and rehabilitation coordination

Psychological Domain
    Phase placement
    Personal narrative
    Trauma assessment: premorbid, comorbid,
        iatrogenic, disease/syndrome, cultural

Social/Interactive Domain
    Effect of normalization failure on family
    Review of family roles and responsibilities
    Family narrative
    Vicarious trauma evaluation
    Couples evaluation
    Work evaluation

---

changes in patient symptoms and coordinate their different treatment protocols. For example, a chronically ill patient who had a medical review in Phase 1 may have since undergone thyroid treatment. The treatment may have had a significant impact on the patient not only physically in terms of enhanced energy levels, but also psychologically in terms of improved cognition, socially in terms of increased ability to interact with others, and perhaps heightened self-esteem because of weight loss and greater functioning. Any such changes need to be shared among the team members and their interventions altered accordingly. It is also important to determine how well the various protocols that different team members established are working together to see whether they need to be readjusted.

Medications Review

A medications review is a very important component of the overall Phase 2 medical review. The medical team needs to be aware of all the medications and supplements the patient is taking—prescribed, over-the-counter, and alternative. They need to be sure that all of the medications work together positively rather than exaggerate or neutralize one another. The team also needs to discuss whether the various medications are still necessary or still necessary at the same dosages.

Activity Threshold

As with Phase 1 patients, clinicians may find activity sheets and body charts useful to determining how Phase 2 patients feel and what their current activity threshold is (Fennell, 2001). Because Phase 2 patients have usually attained a degree of stability and their symptoms exhibit a certain predictability, the body and activity assessment offers clinicians several different sorts of useful intervention options, from potential rehabilitation programs to psychological self-awareness activities. If the Phase 2 patient is new to the clinician, the clinician should try to determine how the patient felt and what level of activity he or she performed before the chronic illness occurred and during the first, crisis phase of the illness.

An activity threshold reassessment is key for determining appropriate rehabilitation measures. As in Phase 1, the review considers the ADLs, work activities, and personal and social activities. Equally important is a reevaluation of the patient's general physical constitution and psychological hardiness. Even when patients have undergone a Phase 1 evaluation, their condition may have changed importantly by Phase 2.

Coordination of Rehabilitation

In Phase 2, medical, physical, and psychological rehabilitation coordination may become pertinent for the first time. Once patients have passed through the initial crisis phase and carved some order from the chaos they originally experienced, they may be able to benefit from rehabilitation efforts. They may now have enough actual physical strength and sufficiently stabilized symptoms to carry out a physical rehabilitation program. In addition, the gradual return of psychological control to the patients may permit them to tolerate the structure of the rehabilitation routine.

Examples _____

The new patients who entered in Phase 2, **Joshua** and **Gina**, required a full Phase 1-type workup. I worked particularly closely with **Joshua**'s doctor to learn about the course of **Joshua**'s response to different medications, the onset of his headaches, and what additional treatments had been tried. With **Gina**, it was important to follow the history that led to her diagnoses and to learn the full extent of protocols that **Gina**'s various doctors had prescribed. In addition, it was important that I collect information on the health histories of **Gina**'s children and of her husband and his family.

With **Everett**, I conducted a medical and medications review between six months and a year after I began seeing him. I consulted with both his primary physician and his neurologist. **Everett** was showing some progress, particularly in his speech and with use of his hand. He was, however, still having trouble sleeping. I was particularly concerned to know which antidepressants he was taking. I also learned that he had briefly been placed on an antiseizure medication, although he was no longer taking it.

After reviewing with the doctors, I then worked with **Everett** and his wife together to reevaluate his activity levels. In general, Joan would assess his function as better than **Everett** would assess it—which in part showed her still in the cheerleading role whereas he was still suffering from his sense of not being a man—but neither was too far off base in their evaluations. **Everett** no longer slept as much of the day as he had at first. He was more alert and able to participate more. He could now walk their long driveway twice, and he would sometimes do the dishes—not well, Joan said, but then that was nothing new. For the most part, **Everett** could toilet and dress himself.

Everett strongly wanted to increase the amount of rehabilitation he was receiving. Although it was important for me to monitor his activities to see that he didn't exceed his limits, I also began working with his primary care physician to locate additional rehabilitation services that **Everett**'s HMO would cover.

Christine needed a medications review. She had been given a sleep medication that seemed to make her sleep worse and a medication for depression that did not seem to improve her spirits but made her more fatigued. This in turn affected her sleep pattern, making her both desperate for sleep and unable to achieve it. **Christine** had, of her own accord, stopped taking both medications, so it was crucial for me to coordinate with her doctor about other potential medications. **Christine** also wanted to try some alternative treatments. She believed from anecdotal evidence gathered at an MS support group meeting that acupuncture could help improve her gait. I discussed this option and whether it would be covered by **Christine**'s insurance with the primary care physician. Given the great difficulty that **Christine** had getting around, the physical therapist in my practice, who made home visits, seemed to present a great opportunity, especially because she had excellent techniques for working on balance—help that **Christine** sorely needed.

Christine and I reassessed her activity threshold to discover what she was capable of managing. With some MS patients, and this was true for **Christine**, over time they unfortunately tend to get worse. **Christine** was having greater difficulty with mobility, as evidenced by her more frequent use of aids such as a cane and a wheelchair. She complained of some dizziness, but her fatigue level was the same once she went off the depression medication.

Although **Christine** was physically worse, she was coping better because she was selecting ADLs carefully. She no longer washed her hair every day, and on days when she did, she didn't wash the dishes. When she washed the dishes, she successfully tried the technique of leaving two dishes in the sink to prove to herself that she could.

ASSESSMENT: PSYCHOLOGICAL DOMAIN

Phase Placement

The first aspect of the psychological evaluation of chronic illness patients is always phase placement because the phase dictates many of the subsequent treatment interventions. The identifying characteristics of Phase 2 have been discussed previously.

As mentioned earlier, patients in Phase 2 are now capable of making intentional behavioral changes and of learning new coping techniques. In certain aspects, therefore, clinicians may find the literature on stage behavioral models useful (Brownell et al., 1986; DiClemente, 1991; Prochaska, DiClemente, & Norcross, 1992; Prochaska & Velicer, 1997a; Prochaska et al., 1994). It is essential to remember, however, that most of the changes chronic illness patients face are imposed changes, and intentional efforts on their part may make no difference in whether many aspects of their lives get better or worse.

Revisiting the Personal Narrative

If the patient originally came to the clinician during Phase 1 and has already constructed a personal narrative, it is desirable as the patient enters Phase 2 for clinician and patient to reexamine that document. They begin teasing out issues that may act as hindrances to integration of the chronic illness as well as those that may help the patient come to new understandings. If the Phase 2 patient is new to the clinician, the clinician should ask the patient to construct the same sort of personal narrative as described in the Phase 1 assessment section.

Trauma Assessment

The new or revised personal narrative offers patients and clinicians a useful tool for a deeper assessment of trauma than was possible with Phase 1 patients. During Phase 1, patients experience so much chaos and crisis that they can usually at best identify only the most salient aspects of the trauma issues in their lives. Within the relative stability of Phase 2 and the patient's growing containment, however, clinicians have the opportunity to explore trauma issues in greater detail. Patients examining their personal narratives may be reminded of premorbid traumas they put aside or of traumas specifically related to their chronic illness that they had not recalled before.

Iatrogenic Trauma

Chronic illness patients who have reached Phase 2 have almost always experienced some iatrogenic trauma. Their often-nebulous, hard-to-establish symptoms, in combination with the predispositions and cultural expectations of the health care establishment, can sometimes generate dismissive attitudes in the professionals they have approached for help. By the time they have reached the relative stability of Phase 2, the patients may recognize by themselves that they have been hurt by the medical care system.

Cultural Trauma

It is far less common, however, for patients to recognize the ways in which they have suffered from cultural trauma and stigmatization. This is particularly true for patients who had always been part of the mainstream culture.

People from poor and minority backgrounds are far more likely to recognize cultural stigmatization when they see it. For mainstream patients, however, their illness is usually their first experience of minority status.

Eliciting information on stigmatization is often a matter of doing a bit of cultural consciousness-raising. Patients need to think about how their families, friends, and coworkers react to illness. They need to reflect on the open and hidden content of stories in the popular press or TV shows for them to recognize and identify specific forms of stigmatization that they have suffered. Details become important because it is often minor, unrecognized issues that fester in patients' minds and prevent them from attaining a clear vision of their situation.

Examples

Joshua was thoroughly conscious of cultural stigmatization, and he believed strongly that he had suffered iatrogenic trauma. When his blood pressure did not go down with medication, his primary care physician assumed that **Joshua** had simply failed to take the medication. But when asked, **Joshua** insisted that he was taking it regularly, and the doctor believed him. However, the neurologist whom **Joshua** had been referred to did not. **Joshua** believed that racial issues were at work here. The neurologist was an East Indian, and **Joshua** was convinced that the doctor suffered from bigoted notions about behavior and compliance among African Americans. Moreover, as **Joshua** did not improve, and then when he began complaining about headaches, which the doctors could also not relieve, they began to wonder whether the problems were not essentially psychological. If they were truly somatic, they would have responded to treatment.

Gina, by contrast, had always been firmly located in the cultural mainstream, so she had great difficulty identifying cultural stigmatization. Before her illness, as she freely admitted, she had believed that CFS and FM were mythological diseases invented by lazy yuppie fakes so they could live off other people's efforts. Even with all the reality of her painful, debilitating symptoms, **Gina** felt guilty for failing to perform up to her culture's standard. In addition, for her entire lifetime, **Gina** had wanted to be, and had succeeded in being, a superwoman. She took care of her husband, children, and relatives; volunteered at school; and held a job as well. The brick wall of her illness stopped her from accomplishing even half of what she had done before, and her grief and self-condemnation at this failure were palpable.

Everett made an enormous advance psychologically as he entered Phase 2. He had never created a personal narrative—didn't "believe in that bullshit"—but in Phase 2, I introduced him to a small tape recorder. **Everett**'s delight with mechanical equipment of any sort made him enjoy investigating what he could do with it. Eventually, the pleasure of talking, recording, and listening gave way to an interest in what he was actually saying. He began to think about his childhood and youth, he recalled his days in the military, and he talked about what he had liked at work and what he had hated. Before I returned the tapes to him, I sometimes recorded questions or comments that stimulated him to think and talk about issues he hadn't considered.

Everett even found himself talking about issues such as the reactions people in the street had to him now. He had always been a good-looking man who continued to receive admiring glances from women even as he got older. Now, however, he was clumsy and misshapen, and people either studiously avoided looking at him or examined him with a kind of fear and loathing. By recording on tape, **Everett** had a certain distance from the emotional content of his material, and he was more able to comment on the shock of his stroke and how he felt about his loss of control. I could call attention to many elements of ego loss and to the isolation this formerly social man was now suffering.

ASSESSMENT: SOCIAL/INTERACTIVE DOMAIN

Effect of Normalization Failure on Families

In Phase 2, it is desirable to conduct a more extensive family review than probably occurred during Phase 1. In Phase 1, all family members usually understand that the patient is in crisis and, to some extent, are willing to adjust to what they understand to be a temporary situation. In Phase 2, however, the family as well as the patient expect that the patient will or should return to normal. They can be very disappointed or angry that patients, having reached a plateau of symptoms, are not taking up their prior responsibilities or not doing so successfully. It is hard to overestimate the level of impact that chronic illness can have on a family. True recognition of chronicity occurs in Phase 3, as it does with the patient, but in Phase 2 the sheer persistence of the changed family situation brings changes in the family response. It is not uncommon for families or partners to become tired and discouraged during Phase 2. They can give up on the patient and either divorce or cease to offer any meaningful support, aid, or assistance.

Review of Family Roles and Responsibilities

Clinicians need to clarify with patients and their families what roles and responsibilities each family member has. It is essential to determine what everyone's assumptions and expectations are before attempting any interventions that take the new realities into consideration.

Family Narrative

It is sometimes helpful to work with the family to develop a family narrative relative to the chronic illness patient's experience. The very creation of this story often helps family members by bringing contradictory understandings and unarticulated assumptions to light. If a narrative can be agreed on among all the family members, the family has a way, if they are so disposed, to move forward together.

Vicarious Trauma

Discussion of the family narrative allows for investigation of vicarious trauma suffered by family members. In one highly conventional Mormon family, for example, the wife and her family experienced extraordinary psychological and social disruption when the husband's illness made it impossible for him to continue his role as breadwinner. The wife had been prepared while growing up to act as housekeeper, wife, and mother but not as the financial provider, and her family reacted as though her husband's failure to support his family showed the wife's poor judgment in selecting her spouse. The wife, too, was ashamed of her husband's failure, but she loved her husband and they already had children, so the wife did not feel she could terminate the marriage. She also assumed that her husband's illness and the effects it produced in their marriage demonstrated that both her husband and she were insufficient and deserving of punishment in God's eyes.

Once again, it may take the clinician to draw out instances of vicarious trauma, especially culturally induced traumas. It is important for clinicians to acknowledge and validate these traumas and for the patients to recognize that their family members have suffered also.

Couples Evaluation

Phase 2 patients and their partners need to have couples evaluations, even if the patient has been with the clinician since Phase 1 and has already had a couples evaluation during that time. Because Phase 2 brings the reality of chronicity starkly home into the patient's life, it is very important to assess how the couple is adapting to what is going to be the long-term situation. The evaluation should include issues of sexuality and socializing.

Exhaustion in the sick partner may make sexual connection something the couple has to plan for. It is important for both members of the couple to recognize that chronic illness need not end sexual life altogether but that the couple may need to change their habitual sexual practices to accommodate each other's needs. Some patients, for example, suffer a sharp drop in blood pressure and faintness when they are too long in a supine position. As a consequence, the couple may want to experiment with sitting positions. Clinicians can help teach their patients and the patients' partners about different modes of sexual stimulation and satisfaction.

When chronic illness patients must restrict their social life, it may be desirable for the couple to change their usual patterns of socialization so that the healthy partner is not restricted to the limited contacts sustainable by the sick partner. The couple can consciously choose particular occasions when they wish to see friends together, but the healthy partner should be encouraged to see friends independently, even if in the past the couple always went out together.

Just as important as sexuality and socializing are the issues of friendship and companionability. Does the couple enjoy each other's company, share stories about their daily lives, and look to each other for advice and comfort? If there are children in the family, do the partners have a personal relationship with each other apart from their roles as parent or provider? Levels of companionability vary in any marriage, but friendship in marriage often forges the strongest bonds between partners. When one partner is chronically ill, companionability is put to a severe test. The illness can become like another person in the household, another "child" to be accommodated. The ill partner often has far more limited experiences to share in conversation with the healthy partner, and the preoccupations of the sick partner can often become irritating or boring to the healthy partner. On the other hand, the healthy partner's ability to function freely in the world constantly calls attention to the limitations and constrictions of the sick partner's new existence.

In Phase 2, both partners come consciously to comprehend the true meaning of chronic illness—the sick partner's condition is going to persist indefinitely, and the couple's life will never return to its preillness state. Because chronic illness changes the persons and conditions of the partnership so completely, many marriages have difficulty weathering the passage through Phase 2. Not only do patients need eventually to integrate their illnesses, but also their partners actually need to achieve integration of the sick partner's condition into their lives.

Work Evaluation

Phase 2 brings the same problems of normalization failure into the workplace. Although employers and coworkers may have accepted what they believed was a temporary disruption in a worker's productivity, they are not at all pleased with the prospect of a worker's performing at a lower capacity long term. Even more than in Phase 1, it may be desirable for the clinician or the physical or occupational therapist to conduct a workplace evaluation. The clinician is often the person best suited to teaching the employer or immediate superior about the chronic illness, how it may impact the sick person's work performance, and what general modifications in work arrangements will produce the best results. A physical or occupational therapist can often best assess what adjustments need to be made in the patient's actual workspace or work process to minimize physical stress. A lowered computer keyboard or raised monitor, for example, may minimize wrist or back and neck strain, whereas a headset phone can reduce hand/arm motion strain. Chairs on wheels and immediately accessible drawers for active files can help to keep taxing physical movement to a minimum. Such changes can make important differences for workers whose chronic illnesses require them to budget their energy very carefully.

Examples _____

Christine's failure to return to normal affected her marriage not so much in a physical way as emotionally. She and Michael had adjusted to her revised ADLs very well, and Michael was able to absorb many of the necessary tasks that **Christine** had to give up. **Christine**'s frustration at being so limited, however, took the form of wanting Michael to do everything she had done before, in the way she had done it, and Michael was getting angry. **Christine** was also discomforted by the change of roles. She had been the dominant figure in their marriage before her illness, and now she was playing a greatly reduced role in everything, including decision making. Michael, although he had a good understanding of MS intellectually, did not yet have a solid emotional grasp of what it meant in his wife's case. Just as **Christine** did, Michael knew some MS patients who had entered long periods of remission. The couple understandably wanted to believe that the same would happen with **Christine**. Neither wanted to acknowledge the slow but constant deterioration of **Christine**'s physical condition.

Christine's and Michael's family narratives had been severely impacted by her illness. They both came from large families and desperately wanted to have children. Despite her questionable health, **Christine** had succeeded in getting pregnant once, only to have a miscarriage a couple of months later. The couple had had dreams of using the profits from the rental properties **Christine** owned to start a health care business that would provide home-based medical support services.

Their sex life had been impacted by **Christine**'s physical pain and fatigue, but also more subtly by the changing family roles and by their current arguments. Their very high level of companionability was stressed by the fact that they no longer had special "dates" together. Although both had worked—Michael at two jobs and **Christine** managing her properties as well as working as a nurse—they had always made sure to make time for themselves when they would go out for a special dinner and a movie or some other entertainment. They had not done this for months, and both were feeling the strain.

Although **Christine**'s family was a distinct problem in her life, Michael's family members were becoming increasingly involved in a positive way. This was further exacerbating relations with **Christine**'s family, but their help was invaluable at times when **Christine** was forced to stay in bed. It was also providing **Christine** with some solace for the loss of her friends and family.

Gina's husband, Vince, did not understand her illness at all and was dealing badly with any increased responsibilities or role changes. Like

Gina, although he was willing to credit the reality of his children's conditions, he had never believed in the authenticity of CFS. Unlike **Gina**, however, he was not now experiencing the reality of CFS symptoms, so he still felt that it was a psychological condition at best. He thought she just needed to get her act together. When invited to come to speak with me about the illness, Vince refused. **Gina**'s children accepted the way she was, but they had no understanding of her condition and continued to make high demands on her time and energy. **Gina**'s parents were dead, but she had a good relationship with her younger twin sisters, who lived in New York City. Because of the distance, they could talk only by phone.

Gina's condition produced some difficulties in the couple's sexual life because her exhaustion tended to defeat any desire. But more problematic was the reduction in the couple's companionability. Not only did Vince not sympathize with **Gina**'s condition, but also he was having some worries at work. Rumor had it that layoffs were likely. Vince was convinced that he could find a new job if he lost this one, but he wanted the security of knowing that **Gina** would continue to teach full time while he searched. For her part, she could barely manage her work schedule in addition to the child-care demands in her own family.

Joshua had always gotten along with his wife, Maybelle, and their three adult children were a pride and joy to them both. Moreover, she had a very good job with the state, so their income supported them handsomely.

As **Joshua**'s headaches came on, he began to reject any changes in his life that he would have welcomed in the past. In particular, one of his firm's clients was opening a branch in South Africa, and they had asked whether **Joshua** would be interested in helping to set up their accounting department. Once, **Joshua** would have jumped at the chance, and he knew that Maybelle would have been equally thrilled. They had followed political events in that country with great interest and had always talked about someday going to visit Africa.

In addition, **Joshua**'s continuing high blood pressure made him secretly fear that he might die while having intercourse. He did not talk with Maybelle about this, but simply avoided having sex. Not realizing his fears, Maybelle thought that he was losing interest in her now that the children had left home. She thought she looked old compared with the girls in **Joshua**'s office, and she wondered whether he was involved with someone else.

The couple had always been very active in their church, and when **Joshua** first began having difficulties, they asked the church members to pray for him. Now **Joshua** was becoming reluctant to go to church. Maybelle didn't know that **Joshua** felt people were treating him strangely. He felt that they didn't believe he was sick. Moreover, he was angry with God for giving him this terrible invisible trial when he had always lived his life ethically, morally, and responsibly. As far as **Joshua** was concerned, no one believed he was a victim—not his doctor, his friends, or his God. So it hardly seemed likely that his wife would, and he did not confide in her.

Everett and Joan found they were developing an entirely new family narrative. Whereas once they had employed a hierarchical structure to run the family, with **Everett** in charge and Joan his faithful lieutenant, they now found that Joan had to take over more and more of **Everett**'s old functions. Joan attempted to take over as unobtrusively as possible, and at first she solicited his advice and approval constantly. As time went by, however, although she found her new responsibilities scary, she also found she could do most of them pretty well. She felt a distinct sense of personal enlargement and competence.

Joan's actions surprised her sons, who had expected that they would have to fill any roles their father could not handle. This relieved them somewhat, but nonetheless they still suddenly realized that they now had elderly parents who needed their help and care for the long term. None of the families were prepared for this eventuality. One of the daughters-in-law became very interested in and fond of the new Joan because she could relate to her better. But another was angry because **Everett**'s and Joan's problems distracted her husband from issues relating to her own parents and made him less willing to help her with them. **Everett** and Joan's sons did jobs they felt they should—cleaned out the gutters, changed the screens for storm windows, turned over the vegetable garden—but having put in caretaking time, they were less eager to go for the purely social visits that had been their custom in the past. Joan saw her grandchildren less and missed them terribly.

Their nonfamily social life was also somewhat complicated. Joan and **Everett** got along well with each other, and they enjoyed the families of the men **Everett** worked with. But **Everett** had always been the one to initiate social activities, and Joan was completely at a loss as to how to do

PHASE 2
Checklist for Assessment

Physical/Behavioral Domain

_____ 1. Has the patient received a medical review? Have the patient's medications been reviewed?

_____ 2. Have you reviewed the patient's activities with him or her?

_____ 3. Have you coordinated possible new medical or rehabilitation efforts?

Psychological Domain

_____ 1. What indicators place this patient in Phase 2?

_____ 2. Have you asked the patient to provide/update his or her personal narrative?

_____ 3. Have you made a trauma assessment? What traumas are particularly salient now?

Social/Interactive Domain

_____ 1. Have you evaluated the effect of normalization failure on the family/partner? What were the results?

_____ 2. Have you reviewed family roles and responsibilities?

_____ 3. Have you begun helping the family to construct their own narratives of this illness experience?

_____ 4. Have you evaluated for family trauma?

_____ 5. Have you evaluated vicarious trauma that members of the medical team may be experiencing?

_____ 6. Where appropriate, have you carried out a couples evaluation?

_____ 7. Have you conducted a work evaluation? Are there issues with the patient's employer or fellow workers?

---

this and with whom, especially because **Everett** was embarrassed to be seen by his old companions.

CLINICAL GOAL AND TREATMENT ISSUES IN PHASE 2

The overarching clinical goal of Phase 2 is to help patients stabilize and begin restructuring their activities to fit with the limitations imposed by their chronic illness.

The major treatment issues of Phase 2 are to help patients develop self-observation and analytic skills and then to teach them about the personal energy process and the desirability of maintaining a balance of activities among the four major activity areas—personal maintenance, personal fulfillment, social and familial, and work-related activities. During Phase 2, clinicians also work most intensely with the partners and families of their patients as these individuals learn to develop the new roles and responsibilities required by the patient's illness. Workplace interventions are also often useful during Phase 2 if the patient is able to continuing working.

TREATMENT: PHYSICAL/BEHAVIORAL DOMAIN

Medical Protocols

The medical and medications review may lead the clinician to recommend a number of changes in a patient's medical protocols. Once patients have reached a plateau of symptoms and have slowly begun to reacquire a small degree of control over their lives, it may be possible to stop interventions, particularly medications, aimed at dealing with the crisis situation. If medical protocols have stabilized various physical symptoms, the medical team needs to determine whether present interventions will maintain the status quo and perhaps lead to better functioning or whether a change will produce better results.

Activity Threshold Modification

In Phase 1, the clinician endeavored to determine what activity level patients could sustain without harming themselves and how that level compared with what patients had been able to do when they were healthy. At best, the clinician sought to discourage Phase 1 patients from so consistently exceeding their boundaries that they remained in a constant state of crisis. The relative stability of Phase 2 allows the clinician to begin real educational work with patients on their activity levels. Many patients in Phase 2 are not only physically more capable of action, but also, more importantly, they are psychologically capable of engaging in intentional change. By waiting until Phase 2 to carry out more extensive interventions, clinicians can achieve greater success.

PHASE 2
Treatment

Physical/Behavioral Domain
    Medical protocols
    Activity threshold modification
    Education on personal energy process, four activity groups
    Data collection
    Education on activity adjustment

Psychological Domain
    Self-observation refinement
    Insight maintenance
    Overcoming of psychological defenses
    Characterological interventions
    Expression of feelings, grieving
    Clarification of values/development of norms

Social/Interactive Domain
    Education of family about normalization failure
    Revision of family roles and responsibilities
    Family narrative/traumas
    Clarification of values/development of norms
    Education to illness etiquette
    Couples interventions
    Workplace interventions/strategy development/disability

The Personal Energy Process (PEP)

In the greater containment of Phase 2, clinicians can begin to teach patients about the personal energy process as it exists in all people, healthy and sick. They call particular attention to the curve of an action, how a person first decides to perform an action, then overcomes an initial resistance, then finds the job moving forward with greater ease, until finally the individual completes the action and experiences a deserved sense of relaxation. This relaxation comes, however, only if the person still has energy left over after completing the activity. If a person has worked to exhaustion, completion of the job does not bring the physical and psychological benefit that is necessary for a sense of well-being. It is important for clinicians to point out to patients that all people must perform many actions or tasks each day to experience a high quality of life.

Four Activity Categories

Patients need to learn that all life activities fall roughly into four categories: the ADLs and self-care, the activities that enrich an individual's inner being, the activities that relate to an individual's social and family world, and the activities that relate to an individual's work or employment world. To enjoy a meaningful life, people usually need to engage in activities from all four categories regularly. When people are overextended for any reason—they may be healthy but have taken on too much, or they may be ill and unable to do what they believe they must do—they usually begin to eliminate activities, starting most frequently with the activities that enrich their inner being. Social activities and ADLs tend to be the next to go, with work activities persisting the longest because they provide necessary financial support for the individual.

Education and Data Collection

Clinicians then need to teach their patients the very difficult concept that sheer doggedness and hard work will not, despite cultural assurances, necessarily produce the results individuals desire. If individuals, even healthy individuals, persist in tasks beyond their current capabilities, they will repeatedly fail. Patients need to comprehend deeply that the same is true for them. If they persist in attempting what is beyond their capacity, they will very likely fail and possibly precipitate a relapse in their illness.

A great deal of the education about the personal energy process occurs when clinicians and patients discuss the daily activity data that patients collect for clinicians (Fennell, 2001). In Phase 2, patients have attained sufficient containment to keep detailed activity sheets on their daily lives. On these sheets, they record exactly how much time they spend carrying out the activities they attempt throughout the day. In addition to recording what they do and for how long they do it, they also record how they feel and what their symptoms are during each activity. The sheets also include time spent eating, resting, and sleeping, with comments on the effects of the food and the quality of the rest or sleep. If the patient is a woman, it is advisable to include daily information about where in the menstrual cycle the patient is and how she is feeling.

Initially with the help of the clinician, patients place each of the activities they log onto their data collection sheets into one of the four activity categories, but in time they can usually carry out this sorting process by themselves. Eventually, this will become part of an intervention technique, but at first it is important simply to recognize what activities serve what purposes.

Listing Wants, Shoulds, and Responsibilities

On a separate page, or even on the back of the data collection sheet, clinicians ask patients to list things they want to do, things they think they should do, and activities they regard as part of their responsibilities (Fennell, 2001). This ultimately provides the measure of how well patients' actual activities match their desires and expectations.

Neutrality and Normalizing Effect of Data Collection

Throughout the data collection process, clinicians emphasize the scientific, emotionally neutral nature of the task. There is no moral or ethical evaluation. Patients simply keep track of what they do and how their body and/or mind feel during the activity. Clinicians tell patients not to attempt to change anything but simply to keep as accurate a record as possible. When patients and clinicians examine the data together with patients' statements of desires, expectations, and responsibilities, patients' normalization failure usually becomes dramatically apparent. Expectations and desires far exceed activities. Often for the first time, patients can see in black and white that their physical condition no longer permits them to live up to their expectations.

This often comes as a shock to Phase 2 patients. Usually, their symptoms have stabilized sufficiently so that they are beginning to test the waters of "normal life" again. They have not yet accepted the chronicity of their condition and believe that the plateau represents a slowly approaching cure. In this mistaken attitude, they are often strongly encouraged by family, friends, coworkers, and the society at large. Because they believe that a return to their former normal activities will demonstrate they are cured, many chronically ill Phase 2 patients push themselves to do more and more, and at first their slightly elevated energy levels permit this. Without guidance from a clinician, Phase 2 patients may well push themselves into a relapse and a return to Phase 1, setting up a vicious cycling between Phase 2 and Phase 1 that can continue indefinitely, but with deep emotional losses each time around.

Learning to Adjust Activities

Using the data collection sheets, however, clinicians can encourage patients to see how slight improvements in personal energy often cause patients to engage in more activities than they actually can sustain. The data sheets also permit patients to make better allocations of their energies. A patient can, for example, go with her daughter to pick out a wedding dress, but she cannot also make the catering arrangements. And even to accomplish the shopping trip, she may have to eliminate some activity of personal care, such as washing her hair or cleaning the house.

Clinicians carry out an important function when they help to make sure that patients select activities from each of the four activity categories. For some chronically ill patients, the work category consumes a large portion of their energy bank account. Clinicians need to encourage such patients, however, that there are alternatives to leading a totally disbalanced life. Part-time employment or going on disability are preferable to suffering a relapse because of overwork. For other patients, the work category ends altogether because they can no longer work at all. Their severely compromised energy status makes it all the more important to select activities carefully from the other three categories to enhance the quality of their lives as much as possible.

It is especially important for clinicians to urge patients to select some activities daily that nourish their inner life. If in the past the patients were totally involved in physical activities—they used to play racquetball, for example, or go mountain climbing—the clinician needs to help them find new modes of inner fulfillment. It may begin with physically oriented, but manageable, activities such as yoga or meditation, but ultimately the clinician usually encourages patients to write in some fashion, which allows them to reflect on what is happening to them and how they are responding to it. Expressive activities such as writing offer patients ways to confront their losses and grieve, and prepare them to move forward with the work of integration.

Data Collection as Activity Modification

Readers will have recognized that the data collection is a treatment intervention, not simply a source of information for the clinician, although it is that as well. If writing presents an obstacle to patients, clinicians may be able to make picture charts that they can check, which the clinician then supplements with oral information from the patient. Sometimes it may be necessary for the clinician to rely almost wholly on conversation with the patient. Objective examination of their lives not only allows patients to see what is actually happening to them and how, to a degree, they can manage it, but also helps to remove unreasoning fear and terror. The patients' conditions may not be what they would wish for themselves, but they can still examine their situation matter-of-factly and perhaps even alter it to their benefit.

Examples

As a new patient, even though she was in Phase 2, **Gina** received a total physical review. She was taking a large number of medications for pain, headaches, congestion, allergies, and sleep. She wore an A-TENS unit for pain but had anti-inflammatories to take in pill form as she needed supplementary pain control. In general, **Gina** felt the medications were working, at least if she didn't exert herself, but she described how long it had taken to locate an anti-inflammatory and a decongestant that didn't cause troublesome side effects. When **Gina** was taking all of her medications, she sometimes felt woozy, and she had a certain amount of gastrointestinal distress. She felt that these effects, however, were acceptable trade-offs for the pain relief.

The doctors suggested that the pains in her neck and back might stem in part from osteopenia. Because **Gina** was also entering menopause, they had suggested she go on hormone therapy. **Gina** wanted to hold off on that until she could do without some of the medications. She was very anxious to investigate any methods, other than pharmacology, for alleviating her symptoms. She had been given stretching exercises to do in the morning, particularly when she awoke in pain. These did ease the pain, but they also took a significant amount of time during a hectic part of her day.

Gina also had some sleep difficulties. She tended to wake several times during the night and often had trouble getting back to sleep. As a consequence, she did not get the rest she needed, and she often woke without feeling refreshed.

I felt that **Gina**'s sleep difficulties could probably be improved with some simple techniques. I recommended that **Gina** start layering nightclothes and coverings so that if she awoke because of night sweats, she could adjust her temperature easily, without becoming fully conscious. I taught **Gina** that she could even stick one bare foot out from under the covers to reduce her temperature. If **Gina** was overly uncomfortable in her sweaty nightclothes, she could put clean ones right beside the bed where she could change quickly, again without fully awakening. Because **Gina** was often hungry or thirsty when she woke, I suggested that she keep water right beside the bed, as well as either plain crackers or grapes. I suggested presetting the radio clock to a soothing talk station so that she could turn it on very low as background noise to help her slide back into sleep.

I agreed with **Gina**'s desire to explore other methods of coping and spoke with **Gina**'s physician about activity interventions that might help reduce the number or frequency of **Gina**'s medications. The doctor enthusiastically endorsed the proposed program and requested reports on its progress.

Gina was an excellent candidate for activities analysis and intervention because she was motivated and orderly in carrying out recommended data collection. Because all patients in Phase 2 need to engage in activity analysis, **Gina** can stand as an ideal example. The following psychological treatment section discusses **Gina**'s psychological difficulties with the analysis work and the difficulties experienced by some of the other patients as well.

When I first introduced **Gina** to the concept of the personal energy process, we discussed **Gina**'s individual experience with task initiation, process, and completion. I emphasized the notion that, contrary to popular thought, sheer persistence at an activity does not necessarily produce the desired result, including the psychological satisfaction of a job done. **Gina**, it turned out, was able to start, carry out, and complete tasks most of the time. Only when she was very depleted physically did she suffer any cognitive or physical difficulties in finishing tasks. **Gina** was dynamically disabled. That is, if she was reasonably rested, she could carry out almost any activity without difficulty. If, however, she was tired, she became disabled in her ability to perform even ordinary, habitual actions.

In this, **Gina** contrasted sharply with **Christine** or **Everett**, who had much more static disabilities. **Christine**'s MS interfered with her ability to carry out simple tasks all of the time. She easily became confused part way through and had to go very slowly and concentrate to finish. She was also losing her ability to fine tune certain motor skills. Her cursive handwriting was becoming progressively unclear, although she herself could still usually interpret it. I worked with her to print in block capitals, particularly on forms.

After his stroke, **Everett** relearned many basic care and other activities, but he, too, still became confused very quickly. He had to consciously think about actions such as putting on his shirt and buttoning most of the buttons. If he stopped concentrating, he became confused and couldn't think what he was supposed to do next. Fatigue had a severe impact on him. **Everett** had always enjoyed police shows on TV, but he now had trouble keeping track of the plot, particularly of any quick-cutting program. At my suggestion, he started to keep a pad beside him and write notes about what had just happened at each commercial break.

I also taught **Gina** about the four general categories of activity—ADLs, personal fulfillment, social, and work—and about the importance in everyone's life of carrying out some activities in each category. I told **Gina** to write down all the things she did each day for a week. The following week, we examined the list together. Each day began with getting up and doing stretching exercises. **Gina** then listed getting ready for school, school, appointments after school, making dinner, and doing homework. I showed **Gina** that she had not itemized most of her activities. **Gina** had not simply "gotten ready for school," but had dressed, made breakfast, overseen her children getting ready for school, and made lunches for everyone. "School" encompassed contact hours in the classroom, meeting time with other teachers, conferences with individual students, and so on. "Appointments" consisted of driving her children to their psychologists' appointments. Because the children were tired and irritable afterward, she treated them to a snack at a crowded fast food restaurant before going home. Once home, she spent nearly an hour sorting through the mail before starting to get dinner ready. "Doing homework" meant more than helping oversee her children's homework. It included doing her own preparations for the next day's classes, grading papers, and completing forms she'd received from the school administration.

Gina got the point. The following week, she began to keep more detailed notes about her activities. After a couple of weeks, she and I examined the lists and inserted each activity into one of the four categories. I reminded her that ADLs for someone else (her children, her husband) did not constitute ADLs for herself, but actually belonged in her work category. It quickly became obvious that **Gina**'s life consisted almost entirely of ADLs and work. She no longer had the time or energy for social life apart from some activities with her family, and she engaged in no personal fulfillment activities at all. **Gina** had a large imbalance among categories, but her personal energy cycle was more or less in tact.

Next, I had **Gina** begin keeping a daily symptom journal (Fennell, 2001). She kept daily track of her sleep, the number of times she awakened, and whether she had symptoms at rest. She noted what day she was in her menstrual cycle. Then for each day, she assigned a pain evaluation number for morning, afternoon, and evening for a number of symptoms: fatigue, headache, cognitive, body ache, sore throat, GI problems, and food. In addition, she now listed her activities on the same sheet so that she could track symptoms and activities simultaneously.

I asked **Gina** to create one final list detailing what she wanted to do, what she felt she should do, and what her responsibilities were during the same time periods as the previous list. With the data she had amassed, **Gina** was finally able to begin examining her life objectively. Moreover, because she had been collecting information for more than a month, she could look at longer term as well as daily patterns.

She and I together identified cycles of increasingly frantic, exhausting, painful effort, followed by collapse and enforced rest. The collapse would produce guilt in **Gina** and mild to strong recriminations from her husband and the school. Consequently, as soon as **Gina** was feeling better, she tried even harder to make up for her past deficiencies and thus set herself up for even more painful and humiliating failure.

Gina responded ideally to the neutrality of the data collection process. She believed that she was indeed seeing objective proof that she could not continue to lead her life the same way. This was not a personal opinion, but a clear "fact." However, it took some time for her emotional acceptance to catch up to her intellectual understanding.

Gina was also beginning to learn that the skewing of her activities around work and ADLs was bad for her physically and psychologically.

She realized that she needed to reduce or eliminate some activities altogether and replace others with social contacts. She needed to begin nourishing an inner life. By the sheer business of collecting the data, **Gina** was also beginning to examine her life in a serious, conscious way.

Given direction, **Christine** also scrupulously made lists of everything she should do, everything she wanted to do, and everything that she did do. At first, on reviewing the list of what she had actually done, she would discover in conversation with me that she had left off many activities because she didn't think of them as activities. These would include items such as talking for an hour to a friend or going out to pick up the mail. Although there was still a great disparity between what **Christine** thought she should do and wanted to do and what she could do, she was learning from the list-making activity and was beginning to make more thoughtful decisions about where to put her energy.

In contrast to **Gina**, **Christine** learned to rebalance her activity categories so effectively that she actually accomplished more than she had in the past, besides feeling less stressed. But she still suffered from an impaired personal energy cycle. **Gina**, when rested, had no symptoms, but **Christine** had symptoms even when resting. For a time, however, **Christine** had a better quality of life than **Gina**, despite being in worse shape, because she distributed what energy she had more meaningfully and effectively.

TREATMENT: PSYCHOLOGICAL DOMAIN

Relationship Establishment

If the Phase 2 patient is new to the clinician, the clinician must first establish a warm, equal relationship with the patient and affirm the patient's illness and trauma. All of the issues discussed in Phase 1 on this topic are relevant here. It will then be necessary for the clinician to teach the patient about the phase process and to begin introducing the patient to the observing self and to the distinction between content and process. Because Phase 2 patients are more contained and less desperate than Phase 1 patients, it is sometimes possible to move through the initial steps more quickly.

Ignorance of Boundaries

Unaided, the principal problem Phase 2 patients face is their inability to recognize appropriate boundaries for themselves, whether these boundaries relate to physical activities, psychological stamina, cognitive abilities, or social activities. Patients lost their old activity governors when they contracted their chronic illness, and they have not yet replaced them with new measures of what they can do without harming themselves. The slightly increased energy levels of Phase 2 encourage patients to do all sorts of things they have missed, which initially often makes them feel wonderful. The old life beckons most seductively. For aggressive, achieving personalities, this is a particularly attractive lure, but the same happens with patients who were generally easygoing before their illness. Because Phase 2 patients still expect a cure, they are doubly betrayed when increased activity not only makes them much worse but also causes a relapse.

Refining Self-Observation

The absence of appropriate boundaries makes it essential for patients in Phase 2 to refine their capacities for self-observation and deepen their ability to analyze process. The collection of activity and symptom data, plus reflection about desires and expectations, gives patients and clinicians the actual individual substance of patients' lives to work with. Patients can learn to see that they habitually spend more energy than they have and that when they do, they suffer disproportionately. They learn to compare how much energy different activities require, and over time, they can learn to choose lower energy-consuming activities that they also enjoy. They come to know their own parameters objectively.

Throughout the four-phase process, patients need to accomplish a number of psychological tasks. Individual tasks pose greater or lesser difficulty depending on each patient's personality and history. To work effectively with the clinician, patients need to form a strong, trusting bond with the clinician. They need to learn to observe and to collect data and then to differentiate experiences or analyze them. They need to develop insight, almost always with help from the clinician, and then they must struggle to maintain these insights over time. Throughout this lengthy process, they must endure because that is much of what they are learning—the daily experience of what they cannot do and of what they have lost (Bedell, 2000; Gignac & Cott, 1998; Gignac et al., 2000; Small & Lamb, 1999).

Maintaining Insight

It is very difficult for patients to maintain insight over time. What is perfectly clear in the clinician's office when examining the activities chart and discussing symptom levels disappears from patients' consciousness before a week is out. Insight usually has painful components. It forces the patients to look at what they are now as opposed to what they were. It causes grief as patients keep being forced to look at their losses. People tend, after all, to feel bad about themselves when they do not live up to their expectations, even if they know their expectations are unrealistic and they think they have altered them. The insights they gain are almost never things they want to acknowledge as so. Outside the clinician's office, patients are once again swamped with social attitudes, many of which they still covertly share. Away from the reassuring acceptance of the clinician, patients once again feel like losers, like the disabled kids they studiously ignored in school. Living with their chronic illness requires daily surrenders, which exacerbate their sense of worthlessness (Hatcher, 1973; M. H. Horowitz, 1987; Pulver, 1992; Silbermann, 1967).

Psychological Defenses

All individuals have erected psychological defenses against what they perceive as potentially harmful attacks, but it is necessary to overcome these defenses, to become vulnerable to pain and loss, if patients are to acknowledge their new situation, grieve for their suffering and losses, and then attempt to develop new coping skills. All people have protective psychological defenses, but patients with certain characterological traits or even full-blown personality disorders will have greater difficulty allowing themselves to gain insight into their situations. This adds additional challenges to the work of Phase 2.

Team with Psychologist, Psychiatric Social Worker, or Psychiatrist

When clinicians have chronic illness patients with any pronounced personality disorder, it is advisable to have another specialist see the patients for that aspect of their health care needs. A clinician attempting to bring patients through the phases of the chronic illness experience needs to focus on a different set of issues. A psychologist or psychiatric social worker should be involved to focus on the personality disorder itself. As with all professionals involved in the patient's health care, it is absolutely essential for the chronic illness clinician and the mental health specialist to work collaboratively and to keep each other informed of pertinent issues. The impact of characterological difficulties on treatment within the phase paradigm differs depending on the specific disorder.

Characterological Difficulties: Narcissists

Narcissists may find it difficult to acknowledge that they suffer the personal diminution of a chronic disease. They persist in preillness behaviors because to do so meets their expectations for themselves. When this overextension stimulates a relapse or increased symptomatology, narcissists regard the phenomena as totally unrelated to any action of theirs, regardless of charts and data sheets, because the only essential truth for them resides in their unrealistically high estimation of themselves.

Clinicians will find it difficult to establish an effective working bond with narcissists. Initially, narcissists doubt that anyone can perform up to the standards they require. If clinicians have an extremely high reputation or work in a prestigious institution, they may be acceptable until they present analysis contrary to the understanding that most narcissists have of themselves. When clinicians attempt to guide narcissists to greater insight, these patients tend to believe that the clinicians' "criticisms," as they perceive them, merely confirm an assessment that the clinician is inadequate. They do not perceive that they are trying to live up to unrealistic, and often unjustified, expectations they have for themselves.

By emphasizing how experienced and well credentialed they are, clinicians can sometimes persuade narcissists that they are taking them on because the narcissists are so clinically interesting that they are worthy of an expert's attention. The clinician must show concern for the patient, but not too much because that may stimulate the narcissist's rejection of any personal inadequacy. The concern should be expressed almost as scientific curiosity, as the intriguing special aspects that make the narcissist of interest to this very busy professional. Narcissists can also be challenged by the notion that learning to live with chronic illness is Darwinism in action—that only the smart and the clever survive. Among the psychological tasks, narcissists find bonding and insight the biggest stumbling blocks (Coderch, 1991; Goldberg, 1974).

Characterological Difficulties: Compulsives

Compulsive personalities may find it difficult to tune down their expectations for order and perfection. Even when it is essential, they often cannot select any activities to eliminate because they consider all of them necessary. Their need to maintain control via rules, lists, and schedules, as well as their inability to delegate activities, makes it difficult to shift their priorities.

Compulsives can, however, bond with clinicians. And if they regard the clinician as a higher authority, they may begin by taking directions for rearranging and substituting less strenuous activities until they can be brought to recognize the value of these things in themselves and can henceforward make some of these changes on their own. Their biggest hurdle is relinquishing control of every sort. Control for them usually means being able to take on any task and do it better than others (DeVeaugh-Geiss, 1993; Foster & Eisler, 2001; Gournay, 1998).

Characterological Difficulties: Dependents

Some argue that dependent personalities appear frequently among chronic illness patients. Phase 2 patients or those who have been struggling with their condition for some time are particularly likely to exhibit dependent traits because they have, in fact, been forced to solicit help from others. They, therefore, often seek to appease or placate those who care for them in an attempt to forestall potential or imagined abandonment. Dependent patients may bond quickly with their clinicians, but they can often assume a posture of pleasing the clinician rather than actually engaging in the insight development or the kind of behavioral change that might help improve their situation. To please other significant people in their lives, dependent personalities often engage in excessive passing behavior, which worsens their condition. In many cases, dependent patients use their clinician as the person to stand up for them against significant others in their lives, rather than trying to make the necessary changes in themselves or their relationships. In terms of the four kinds of activities, they often carry out excessive work and social activities at the expense of any personally rewarding activities or even of self-maintenance activities. This, again, expresses their fear of displeasing others in their lives. As dependent personalities develop a bond with their clinician, however, and as they find others of like kind, they become more willing to rearrange their activities because they have others who care about them.

Characterological Difficulties: Avoidants

Avoidant personalities can, with effort on the clinician's part, be gradually coaxed away from their unsubstantiated fears of inadequacy toward genuine insight into the actual deficits created by their chronic illness experience. Their hypersensitivity may make the phase journey a rocky one for clinicians, but with special care and attention to the countertransferential issues these patients arouse, progress can be made (Perugi, Nassini, Socci, Lenzi, & Toni, 1999; Rettew, 2000).

Characterological Difficulties: Histrionics

Patients with histrionic personality traits find interaction with clinicians highly satisfactory because they are, in fact, guaranteed to be the center of attention. Clinicians tend to find their greatest difficulties proceeding from the difficulty these patients have in achieving deep insight or maintaining it over a significant period of time. Histrionic personalities are easily influenced by others and tend to engage in whatever behaviors draw the attention of those who happen to be around them at any given time. Because most chronic illness patients need to take a stance against certain attitudes in the popular culture if they want to integrate their illness experience, the playing to the crowd characteristic of histrionics is not usually conducive to improvement (Chodoff, 1982; M. J. Horowitz, 1997; Morrison, 1989).

Characterological Difficulties: Nonbonding Personalities

Those personality traits and disorders that militate against intimate, honest interpersonal connections—paranoid traits, schizoid, schizotypal, and antisocial ones—make effective therapeutic connections difficult to establish. In many cases, chronically ill people with these traits do not seek clinical aid at all, but handle their problems themselves, using whatever anodynes they have always relied on. Of this group, schizoid personalities are the type most frequently seen by clinicians. They are usually brought in by family members, and although they do not bond easily with the clinician, the clinician can often encourage schizoids to introduce a bit more social content into their lives. When this works, it usually increases their quality of life and makes them more amenable to similar kinds of therapeutic intervention (Akhtar, 1987; Fossati et al., 2001; Harvard Mental Health Letter, 2000, 2001; Quality Assurance Project, 1990; Siever & Gunderson, 1983; P. J. Taylor, 1986).

Characterological Difficulties: Borderlines

One of the most frustrating groups for clinicians is that of patients with borderline traits. Although they more typically present in abuse and traumatic stress syndromes, it is not uncommon to find them among chronic illness sufferers as well, particularly when the patient comes from a deprived or marginalized background. Borderline personalities frequently idealize the clinician at first and make assiduous shows of cooperation concerning interventions. They then suddenly reverse themselves to show intense contempt and fury that the clinician has not solved their problems. Although borderlines long for connection, they cannot bear intimacy. When a relationship appears to be developing—often the clinician is finally feeling that progress is being made—borderlines tend to sabotage it. They often try to manipulate their clinicians and are perfectly willing to lie and misrepresent what is happening in their lives.

People with borderline personality traits often prefer crisis to calm and swing violently back and forth between endless dichotomous poles of black and white. Their instability and self-destructive tendencies often force clinicians to engage in perpetual Phase 1 crisis intervention rather than permitting the quieter, more stable work that clinicians hope to accomplish with patients in Phase 2. Borderline patients are usually ill equipped to observe themselves dispassionately or to collect data. They can rarely develop the necessary insight, let alone maintain it for any significant period of time. They do not achieve much balance among the activities in the four areas. In addition, patients with borderline traits often have substance abuse problems, which further complicate work relating to the chronic illness itself (Gunderson & Zanarini, 1987; Yen & Shea, 2001).

It is often desirable to see patients with borderline traits in small groups rather than individually. The group defuses the focus on patient and clinician and diffuses intimacy over the entire group. The group members tend to keep one another honest because they will not credit many of the misrepresentations others may present. The clinician can also actively encourage the group to talk about how they use hyperbole and exaggeration as a safety mechanism to make sure they are seen and heard. After developing confidence among the group members that everyone is listening to one another, the clinician can then teach that hyperbole and exaggeration actually cloud and obfuscate their experience. This in turn leads to their erroneous sorting of experience into unshaded black and white. The clinician can model qualified responses by helping the group attach degrees of difficulty to situations. Group members can bring to the weekly group meeting examples of hyperbole and exaggeration that they used the prior week. With the group, they then discuss whether acting this way produced the ends that the patients wanted. This exercise helps patients develop conscious knowledge of how they function and introduces them to observation and analysis or differentiation.

Encouraging Patients to Express Feelings

Most patients, however, do not have full-blown personality disorders. Clinicians can and should encourage most patients to express their rage, grief, and frustration in ways that allow the patients to overcome their personal defenses and process their pent-up feelings about their illness. Some patients with strong religious faith can pray and tell God how awful their experiences have been and how miserable they feel. Others, especially patients in Phase 2, find that people like themselves are a source of mutual complaint and empathy. Whereas their acquaintances in the general population, and even their family and old friends, may be getting tired of being understanding, illness support groups usually provide patients with unfailing sympathy. In addition, members of such groups have a real understanding of the patient's situation (Johnson-Taylor, Jones, & Burns, 1995; Schirm, 2002).

Encouraging Grieving

Clinicians can inform patients—can predict for them—that they will feel an overwhelming sense of loss and grief, but can assure them that such feelings are completely normal. Clinicians encourage patients to express what they feel, whether to sympathetic others, in prayer, in writing, or whatever works for them. Clinicians particularly encourage patients to seek out others because this accomplishes two things at once: It allows patients to grieve as they must, and it introduces them to a new social life in which they are accepted (Johnson-Taylor et al., 1995; Schirm, 2002).

Soothing Activities

Clinicians can also recommend regular soothing personal self-care activities. These may range from curling up in an old quilt with a steamy romance novel to stretching out on the couch to watch a stack of football videos. With very poor clients, whose housing may be crowded and whose resources are slim to nonexistent, it is still important for the clinician to work with the patient to find soothing activities that are possible. Clinicians impress on their patients that self-care can be substantially more important at certain times than, say, cleaning the refrigerator or mowing the lawn.

Tracking Trauma

In Phase 2, clinicians also teach patients to use their increasingly refined insight to observe and track their traumas and their moments or periods of dissociation. Often, the losses that patients must come to acknowledge as part of their chronic condition trigger memories of old traumas and old griefs. Clinicians encourage patients to consider these old experiences in light of their new situation, to reflect on how their original responses to the old trauma may be reflected in their responses to the illness, but also to differentiate their current illness experience from their prior experiences. Similarly, when patients find themselves experiencing intrusive ideations—or conversely, when they sink into periods of numbness—clinicians urge them to track these experiences as closely and attentively as they have learned to track their daily activities and symptoms.

Values Clarification and Norm Development

Throughout activity restructuring, new norms are, perforce, developed. At first, this is often not articulated between patients and clinicians, but as work proceeds, clinicians help their patients to engage consciously in value clarification and norm development. Patients are also encouraged to share their revised values with their families and negotiate new norms for behavior in the setting in which they live (Fennell, 2001).

Phase 1-Phase 2 Loop

The work of Phase 2 is very difficult for patients to accomplish and even harder and more painful to maintain. Building insight is never easy, but it is especially difficult when it involves recognizing the permanent loss of their former life. The work of insight exposes patients repeatedly to grief. It is equally difficult to change values and norms, especially when patients did not choose to do so, but were forced to by their illness. The internal personal pressures to reject what has happened is enough to make patients ignore what they have learned and attempt a return to the old life. This may cause relapse, or relapses may happen totally apart from patient behavior, in either case throwing the patient back into Phase 1. Sometimes patients are able to move again into Phase 2 on their own because they learned how to reduce their activities and contain the crisis the first time around. But some patients simply seek solace in easily accessible anodynes such as alcohol. Some move from crisis to crisis in a perpetual experience of Phase 1. Social pressures tend to encourage the Phase 1-Phase 2 loop. The social actors in a patient's world usually want a return to the old life. Because this pressure conforms so completely with the patient's own wish to return to the precrisis life, it is hard to maintain insight or a commitment to new values and norms.

Examples

Gina was quickly capable of collecting accurate, informative data, and she was equally quick to make insightful evaluations. She could see that when she did too much, she had increased pains in her neck, back, thighs, and hip and that frequently her glands began to swell. With growing fatigue, she could chart that her cognitive difficulties increased. It was extremely difficult, however, to overcome **Gina**'s deeply entrenched notions of how to be the perfect mother, wife, and teacher. Her internalized guilt at failing to maintain her high standards was reinforced by her family and the administration of her school, both of whom benefited greatly when she performed well. Her psychology was constructed around the belief that she should be able do all these jobs, and her self-worth was entirely bound up in her doing them well.

At first, **Gina** and I set some daily boundaries on activities. For instance, when **Gina** came home in the afternoon, she did not even look at the mail but instead went to her room and rested or slept for at least 45 minutes. The children were gradually trained to help dry the dishes after dinner, set up the breakfast things, and make lunches before they began their homework.

But daily boundaries were only part of the problem. **Gina** would try to do everything she needed to do each day and would feel progressively worse until the weekend arrived, when she would attempt to sleep a little later in the morning and get a bit of rest during the day. If the weekend had nothing scheduled, this break sometimes provided the respite **Gina** needed. But frequently the children had games scheduled, or Vince wanted the whole family to go on an excursion together. On those occasions, **Gina** not only failed to get rest but also was unable to accomplish the tasks she usually completed on the weekend. Instead, she would begin the workweek exhausted, in pain, and with a backlog of jobs waiting for her when she came home in the evening.

Sometimes **Gina** felt so bad toward the end of the workweek that she would take a sick day. But if she succeeded in resting that day, she would try to make up any missed work, or she would plan a special activity with her children. Whenever **Gina** found herself experiencing freedom from pain and increased levels of energy, she almost immediately took on more obligations at school or at home.

I finally had **Gina** map a whole week, then a whole month, before **Gina** could acknowledge the pattern of recovery and overexertion and relapse. Even when **Gina** saw and understood the larger pattern, it was still apparent, when she spoke about upcoming obligations (Thanksgiving, the Christmas holidays), that she had great difficulty applying her insight to the future.

Almost as a game, I also asked **Gina** to write down next to the daily activities on her list what she would rather be doing at that moment. **Gina** would write next to, for example, "unloading the groceries" something like "sunbathing in the Bahamas" or "drinking brandy in a Parisian café." Partly this gave **Gina** and me a chance to cut the tension and seriousness by joking about escapist fun. But **Gina** herself began to see elements in her fantasies that she could actually realize. She clearly saw that they nearly always involved fulfilling herself or having fun with other people—the two areas of activity so underrepresented in her actual life.

She began to comprehend the desirability of including activities from each category, and she was also starting to clarify what was important to her in her life. Although it meant that she had to endure some grumbling from her husband and the kids, she used one long weekend to go to New York to visit her sisters. Sometimes she had the children stay in the after-school program so that she could go out for coffee with a couple of her close colleagues. She also began writing a journal. Although it began as a narrative based on her activity charts, she found that she started including more reaction material and more expression of her sadness, frustration, and grief at the changes in her life.

I welcomed **Gina**'s expressions of anger and grief at her present situation and helped her to identify new difficulties that emerged. I also encouraged **Gina** to indulge in activities that were particularly soothing or gratifying. **Gina** had loved children's adventure stories from the time she was a girl and had enjoyed reading aloud to her children when they were younger. When a teacher friend told her about a new adventure series, **Gina** started reading them while taking a warm bath before going to bed.

Sophia, given her past commitment to scientific methods, seemed on the surface to be an ideal collector of objective data about her life, but in fact the reverse was true. She had so intensely defined herself as an intellectual, and she had been such a high achiever that she found it nearly impossible to look at her current self in the harsh light of science. She experienced overwhelming shame when she considered what she had become and enormously painful loss when she realized that she would never accomplish the world-class research that everyone, including herself, had expected from her. To bear her pain and her loss, she jettisoned the life of the scientist altogether. This meant she did not want to collect data or write lists.

At the same time, **Sophia** desperately needed to examine the pattern of her daily activities because she was very limited physically, she regularly overextended herself, and she had suffered several relapses. To a certain extent, I was able to elicit practical information about **Sophia**'s activities during office visits. But to bring **Sophia** herself to understand how her current activity level was harming her, it was necessary to use metaphoric and symbolic discussions.

Philosophical discussions revolved around the hubris of, for example, grocery shopping, making a separate trip to the video store, and cooking dinner on the same day. Because **Sophia** could throw herself into an exhaustion that lasted well past what was in her cupboard—necessitating fast food meals that were nutritionally bad for her—I had to engage her in a metaphoric fiction. **Sophia** was to think of herself as a warrior heroine on a long, hard journey beset with difficulties. This heroine had to keep her body prepared constantly through disciplined attention to the practical. She had to train herself like a Zen novice so she would be constantly prepared to face whatever challenges arose before her. Symbolic language and metaphoric story reintroduced the discipline and structure that had gone out of **Sophia**'s life when she ceased to practice science.

Metaphoric language helped, but what really produced significant change, as is discussed later, was the reinvigoration and reintegration of **Sophia**'s spiritual life. Through her reanimated spiritual activities, **Sophia** was eventually able to accomplish many of the practical changes that helped to moderate her symptoms and make her life more manageable.

I worked assiduously with **Sophia** to teach her to express her grief, loss, and anger. **Sophia** was by nature an exceptionally sunny, good-natured person, and she had been brought up to be unfailingly polite. Her illness experience was, however, subjecting her to terrible losses and a great deal of trauma, which she had no way of expressing. I commented repeatedly that an experience such as **Sophia**'s with the disability company would anger me and that pain and confusion such as **Sophia**'s would make me very unhappy. I noted how upset I would be if my career and everything I had worked for had been snatched away by illness or any other cause. **Sophia** gradually began to understand it was acceptable for her to complain, rage, or grieve and that it might help her. At first, she would come into the office with a huge smile on her face as she announced how mad she had been all week, but in time true feeling backed up her statements. It was a tough fight to overcome the behavior of a lifetime, but **Sophia** found that she truly could say whatever she felt in my office. She also made these feelings part of her spiritual life by daily taking her case to God.

Kim took a positive delight in collecting data. It brought praise and compliments from me, and the discussion of **Kim**'s pains and discomforts, in association with her activities, seemed to encourage her to ever more detailed reporting. After a rather short time, however, it seemed that **Kim** had become focused on elaborating her difficulties and sufferings rather than on learning about the intersection between her activity and symptom patterns. It became obvious that insight-building was not taking place using these tools, nor was real comprehension of her suffering and losses. Moreover, the relationship with me was becoming skewed into one in which **Kim** attempted to please me by presenting me with the kinds of trauma she thought I wanted to hear.

I was in a difficult situation. I was developing negative countertransferential issues with **Kim**, which are discussed later. I did not want to engage in the kind of disbelief that patients often experience, but I also felt strongly that authentic reportage was not occurring, and hence no learning would occur either.

To deflect the focus of pleasing, I began praising **Kim** for things that were not related to suffering and not even directly related to activities—the choice of colors **Kim** was wearing, her humor about the weather, and so forth. By trying to refocus the relationship as one of caring about **Kim** as a person—not as a collection of symptoms—I hoped I could later open space to talk objectively about **Kim**'s activities.

TREATMENT: SOCIAL/INTERACTIVE DOMAIN

Teaching Family about Normalization Failure

The issues raised in the assessment section about the social/interactive domain include or suggest many of the interventions. Most importantly, however, if the Phase 2 patient is new to the clinician, the clinician needs to establish a relationship with the patient's family, as described in the Phase 1 treatment section. The clinician's relationship with the family is key to being able to intervene effectively. Clinicians working on the patient's social/interactive issues within the phase theory paradigm need extensive familiarity with family therapy techniques. They need to educate new families concerning the illness phases and the permanent reality of the patient's condition. Patients' families must become aware that patients will not return to their preillness state and that it can be harmful to encourage patients to perform more activities than their activity thresholds permit.

During Phase 1, clinicians have worked with family to teach them (1) that the patient is actually sick and not "crazy" or malingering and (2) how to become effective workers in the patient's crisis. In Phase 2, families need to learn how to rearrange their values and norms to accommodate the long-term nature of chronic illness. Unfortunately, many significant others become so overwhelmed by the prospect of permanent change that they leave. But many others want to stay. They just don't know how to go about the process of re-structuring their lives to make this work.

Family Roles and Responsibilities

When family members have become sufficiently comfortable with the clinician, they and the patient need to discuss the roles and responsibilities of the various family members (S. S. Travis & Piercy, 2002). Clinicians need to attend very carefully to cultural forms that are very different from the clinician's own. Not only do ethnic, religious, and racial differences matter here, but poverty itself creates a culture for patients and families, which the clinician needs to understand. These can be teased out of the family narrative or discussed as a separate subject and charted. In time, the clinician will demonstrate, by comparing the pre-illness roles and responsibilities with the patient's activity charts, that it is necessary for the family to rearrange these matters to use the patient's limited energy most effectively and meaningfully and without harm to the patient (Fennell, 2001).

Family Narrative and Traumas

The assessment of roles can often best be examined as part of the family narrative of the illness, for this story simultaneously acknowledges the vicarious traumas that family members suffer and the difficulties of their position. Ultimately, as with the patient and the patient's narrative, the clinician uses the family narrative to help family members learn to grieve for the losses and undesired changes in their lives.

As importantly, clinicians also employ the family narrative to help revise family roles, clarify needed changes in values, develop new family norms, and educate the family and patient to what may be called "illness etiquette." In time, the clinician hopes to help the family revise their illness narrative in a way that relieves them of stigmatization, false perceptions, and unrealistic expectations and that permits them to cope with the new situation.

Once the family members have actually articulated their preillness roles and responsibilities, it becomes easier for everyone to see why they feel life is so difficult now. It becomes obvious that the patient is not doing all he or she did in the past, which means the jobs either go undone or other family members have to take up the slack. The clinician discusses, with patient and family together, the patient's activity threshold and educates the family to the costs of the patient's attempting to exceed that threshold. The clinician might note, for example, that given the patient's other activities, he or she can prepare only three or four dinners a week. If other family members cannot make the remaining dinners, the clinician may suggest the family buy takeout meals. If financial considerations make this impossible on a regular basis, the clinician works with the family to establish a simple, unvarying set of healthy weekly dinner menus that use already-prepared ingredients. In this way, either the patient or another family member will be able to put the meals on the table easily and automatically.

Values Clarification and Norm Development

Family members need to understand that the old arrangements for living together will never return. The roles each member had in the past may be totally altered by the patient's illness. If the family's own particular traditional roles coincide with culturally traditional roles, this disruption is extremely distressing and confusing to everyone. For some families with highly structured family roles, it may be hard to even comprehend the scope of changes required. When families love and support their ill members, they usually realize that the patient's essential well-being is more important than who repairs the car or washes the clothes. Nonetheless, the family members need to clarify their bedrock values and put the illness experience into the context of those values. Once they have done this, family members can develop new norms for family roles and responsibilities (Fennell, 2001). They can learn, for example, that a father should not work full time at the cost of prolonged bouts of illness, nor should a mother keep the house and children neat and presentable at the cost of all personally rewarding activities.

Financial Issues

Families with significant financial resources may be able to buy household or child-care assistance. But when families cannot afford them, the clinician may be able to teach them how to do things completely differently. Perhaps they will have to limit doing the laundry to once a month. If so, they will first need to watch for sales to purchase enough underwear and other items of clothing to see members through from one laundry to the next. Some of these techniques can be helpful even for patients with very limited resources. Clinicians particularly need the assistance of social workers who keep abreast of community resourses in this area.

Reducing Keystrokes

Many of the clinician's interventions at this juncture concern learning to carry out life's basic maintenance activities with a minimum of effort. This often requires patients and their families to modify former standards, but doing so may then permit patients and families to hold firm on issues they do not want to compromise.

Suggested Reading

For some patients and families, clinicians can also recommend books for them to read, such as Sherry Register's *The Chronic Illness Experience* or Susan Milstrey Wells' *A Delicate Balance: Living Successfully with Chronic Illness*. These books contain not only a wealth of practical information, but also a perceptive, sensitive discussion of how patients and families can deal with ignorance or stigma they face in the outside world. They introduce their readers to what may be called *illness etiquette*.

Education to Illness Etiquette

Acquiring a new illness etiquette is essential to establishing a healthy, normal life. Patients and their families need to learn how to behave around others concerning the illness. They need to learn what to say, how to say it, to whom, and when. This can be particularly important with patients who do not belong to the mainstream culture or who are new to this country. They need to learn what it is possible to say to others, as well as to overcome shyness, embarrassment, or anger. Because these conversations or even confrontations are so individual, clinicians may wish to encourage their patients to bring in actual examples from their lives rather than dealing with the topic generally. Patients may need to say something to their boss, for example, or to their in-laws, or to a well-meaning but hurtful friend. Together the clinician and patient repeatedly role-play conversations that allow the patient to take a strong, unapologetic stance while at the same time imparting essential information that their audience probably lacks. Learning to speak for themselves is also important for patients concerning health care providers. The historical and cultural power distribution between patient and doctor can make it difficult for patients to question a doctor's decision, analysis, or behavior. But patients can learn that illness does not reduce their value as humans, nor does it remove their right to courteous professional treatment.

Couples Intervention

The assessment section of this chapter addresses the kinds of interventions that may help couples begin to navigate what is usually entirely new territory, including issues of sexuality, companionability, role changes, socialization practices, and so forth. Phase 2 patients and their partners are almost always under enormous strain because their lives have been so completely altered by the illness. Unfortunately, many marriages do not survive Phase 2 because the realities of chronicity are too much for one or both partners. But for couples committed to trying, clinicians can suggest that they enter couples therapy to learn new ways to relate to each other. Clinicians can also encourage the couple to be open to new modes of sexual, social, and companionable interaction.

Work Intervention

If Phase 2 patients are still capable of holding down a job, intervention takes the form of developing strategies for making the workplace and work environment as functional for the patient as possible. As mentioned in the assessment section, clinicians can often usefully intervene to educate the employer about the nature of the patient's illness and give a reliable account of the patient's actual capacities, describing what the patient will be able to do if certain arrangements are put into effect. The clinician can often suggest ways that the employer may best use the patient's skills and experience. An occupational or physical therapist may be able to suggest ergonomic modifications that will permit the patient to work with less strain and a more efficient expenditure of energy.

Disability

If Phase 2 patients cannot continue to work at all, even part time, clinicians need to help them obtain disability benefits. This is a highly complex, often frustrating process. Clinicians themselves, or their designees, need to guide patients and work with the patient's medical team so that patients present cases that enable them to receive the benefits to which they are entitled.

Examples

Christine and Michael had married with the desire and expectation that they would have children. Both had many brothers and sisters, and the family narratives clearly announced that the more members of a family, the better. At first, it seemed that **Christine**'s illness made a pregnancy unlikely, but she did, in fact, become pregnant. When she miscarried the child several months later, she wept in the doctor's office. This was taken as a sign of depression, and the doctor suggested that **Christine** take anti-depressants. **Christine** was furious at this inability to accept perfectly reasonable grief, and I had to do a good deal of trauma intervention work to keep **Christine** on track about seeing any doctors at all.

When **Christine** and Michael learned about an opportunity to adopt a Chinese baby girl, they were overjoyed. **Christine** had not been able to get pregnant again, and she recognized that even if she did, she might be subjecting her body to severe strains. She and Michael were becoming more comfortable with the changes in their roles and responsibilities, and they believed that even in their present situation, they would be good parents, if not precisely traditional ones. They had developed realistic norms for a life lived with **Christine**'s variable disability, so they began to prepare a concrete plan for including a child in their life.

I discussed with them what parenthood would entail and was finally convinced that they were developing a workable child-rearing plan. Michael moved to a 3:00 P.M. to 11:00 P.M. shift so that he could help in the mornings, and two of Michael's aunts made themselves available to care for the baby every afternoon so that **Christine** could rest. Michael's family proved to be increasingly helpful as time went on and strong supporters of the couple's adopting a child.

Christine and I had some difficulty transforming her unrealistic notions of what she could do as a mother. For example, **Christine** had always seen herself teaching sons or daughters her carpentry skills, but that was clearly no longer a possibility. She had to learn how to make herself into a meaningful and loving mother from her sofa. Their baby girl, Mei, was not quite six months old when she arrived. A beautiful child of happy disposition, she delighted everybody. The schedule created on paper worked out well in fact.

A serious and unexpected problem did, however, arise. When **Christine**'s disability company learned about Mei, their investigators declared that if **Christine** was well enough to adopt a child, she was de facto healthy enough to return to work. I helped **Christine** successfully fight this attempt to cut off benefits by demonstrating that **Christine** and Michael had made child-rearing possible by bringing in outside help, not because of a change in **Christine**'s health status.

Christine and Michael also found that their very limited intimate life was further restricted by the baby's arrival. But this happens in all families. With a certain amount of ingenuity, which they had already exhibited, they would find some, even if fewer, opportunities to be together sexually.

Everett and his family were experiencing an intergenerational rewriting of the family narrative. His sons and their families were deeply involved in their parents' situation and were struggling with the huge changes that had occurred in their father and in the parental household. I carried out one family intervention session focused on the family's loss, their pain, and their anger early in the course of seeing **Everett**. As time went on, however, it became important to bring the family into greater understanding and more supportive attitudes about the new dynamic in **Everett** and Joan's house. All the sons, wives, and grandchildren were invited to attend, but not all did. As is often the case, those more supportive came, while the more critical and angry stayed away.

I wanted to guide the younger generation into recognizing that the physical abilities of everyone's parents change as they get older and that it is simply a question of when. **Everett**'s "when" had come earlier and more extremely than they had expected. Working with the sons, I drew out expressions from them about what they had learned from their father. Their own healthy, happy children were obvious proof that, among other things, the sons had learned how to be responsible men. After one son was able to speak to me about his feelings for his father, I had him speak these same words directly to his clearly embarrassed but moved father.

I also asked questions such as whether their father was still important to them, even if he was in a wheelchair. Both the sons and the parents heard it said aloud that disability did not end their love. The sons' expressions of esteem for their father and their statements of his worth helped make real to **Everett** that physical vigor was not the sole constituent of manhood.

I noted how proud **Everett** must be of Joan, even though I knew perfectly well that **Everett** was often annoyed because Joan had to do things he'd rather be doing himself. I observed how running the parental household was now a team effort, with cocaptains. **Everett** and Joan had learned to adapt to new circumstances quickly, and they were doing a good job, even if they were doing it differently from the way it had been done in the past.

In all my efforts, I was modeling new attitudes for not only **Everett** and Joan but also their sons. One daughter-in-law was particularly helpful. She commented how much she admired what Joan was doing and how she felt closer to her now that she and Joan were living more similar lives. The daughter-in-law felt more in tune with a family modeled on team effort (or even matriarchy), rather than what had once been a fairly undiluted patriarchy.

In a separate session, I also began teaching **Everett** about illness etiquette with his friends and neighbors. Unlike many chronically ill individuals, whose conditions are often invisible, most of **Everett**'s acquaintances knew that he had suffered a stroke and had been disabled by it. Unfortunately, this did not stop them from sometimes saying thoughtless, hurtful things. One older neighbor, seeing **Everett** outside making his slow, careful trip to the mailbox, called out to ask if **Everett** would be out there raking leaves the following weekend. **Everett** was surprised at how upset this comment made him. **Everett** and I talked about what kind of events he should just walk away from and what behavior needs to be answered on the spot. The neighbor was clumsy and unthinking, but the comment was not worth taking personally. The man was making the sort of hearty, inane comment that had characterized most of their exchanges in the past.

A situation requiring a response was one with **Everett**'s youngest son, who lived at a distance. Perhaps because he felt helpless and guilty, this son was angry with the doctors, with his brothers and their wives, but most particularly with **Everett** for the amount of work being thrust on Joan. He had always been close to his mother when growing up and had long been angry with his father because he felt his father never appreciated how overworked his mother was. This son did not believe that his father was really so disabled and said that he just needed to work harder at rehabilitation. The young man needed accurate information about his father's condition, and he needed to understand that he was saying inappropriate things.

Sophia needed guidance when it finally became necessary for her to ask for help from her neighbors. Although **Sophia** felt she could call on her distant family, and although she was willing to enlist public services such as Meals on Wheels, she suffered great embarrassment at the mere thought of "burdening" her neighbors. Several people had actually offered her help early in her illness, but she had declined. Eventually, it became clear that **Sophia** had to ask her neighbors for occasional help. I helped **Sophia** create an actual script to tell her neighbors what her situation was and what to request from them, which I practiced with **Sophia** until she became comfortable with the words. Finally, **Sophia** overcame her chagrin and made the calls. Both neighbors were happy to help, especially because **Sophia** was both specific and limited in what she requested. In time, this slight connection strengthened. **Sophia** did not become bosom friends with these neighbors, but they became people she enjoyed seeing for a cup of tea when she was feeling lonely and isolated.

Gina needed to cut back to part-time teaching if she was going to establish an activity level she could sustain over time. She knew that the school would be willing to reduce her schedule if necessary to keep her services. The problem was her husband, Vince, who felt that her full-time salary was financially necessary, especially with his work potentially in jeopardy.

In a session alone with Vince, I empathized with his very real difficulties and losses. It is not easy to live with someone who is disabled and who can't carry a full adult load. Furthermore, people's sympathy tended to stream toward **Gina**, not Vince. On the contrary, he was supposed to make life comfortable for **Gina**, whatever the cost to him. I pointed out that both Vince and **Gina** were suffering. As a family, however, they needed to strategize. **Gina** would soon make herself totally incapable of working at all if she continued at her present pace. I showed Vince the charts of **Gina**'s condition and its relationship to her output of energy. It looked as though **Gina** could sustain household activities as well as part-time work, but that was probably the most they could hope for. Because Vince was troubled about the family's economic situation, perhaps this would be a good time to talk with a financial advisor. This would allow them to examine what resources they had, what they needed, and how they might budget more effectively. Rather than moralizing about Vince's behavior,

PHASE 2
Checklist for Treatment

Physical/Behavioral Domain

_____ 1. What medical protocols are now in effect? Is the patient's life structured so that these can be carried out?

_____ 2. What medication changes have been ordered? Have you asked the medical team about potential interactions between these medications or between ordered medications and others the patient is already taking?

_____ 3. Have you and the patient reevaluated his or her activity threshold?

_____ 4. Have you educated the patient about the personal energy process and about the four levels of activity?

_____ 5. Has the patient collected activity data and divided it among the four groups? Have you taught the patient about activity adjustment, making sure to include some activities in each of the four groups?

Psychological Domain

_____ 1. Have you done further work to help refine the patient's self-observation?

_____ 2. What activities have you recommended to help the patient maintain insight?

_____ 3. What activities/therapy have you engaged in to help the patient overcome his or her psychological defenses? Are characterological distinctions important here? What specific interventions have you made to fit these findings?

_____ 4. Have you encouraged the patient to express his or her feelings and to allow specific structured time for grieving?

_____. 5. Have you begun to help the patient clarify his or her values and begin the process of setting new norms?

Social/Interactive Domain

_____ 1. Have you begun educating the family/partner to normalization failure?

_____ 2. Have you discussed revision of family roles and responsibilities with the family/partner?

_____ 3. Have you reexamined family traumas and revisited the family narrative?

_____ 4. Have you begun discussion of revising family values and adjusting norms because of the changed situation?

_____ 5. Have you begun education in *illness etiquette?*

_____ 6. What specific couples interventions have you carried out?

_____ 7. If the patient is still working or is on sick leave, do you need to intervene with the employer, coworkers, or the physical work situation? What actions have been carried out?

_____ 8. If the patient cannot work, have you provided assistance or helped find expert assistance as to disability?

I empathized with him, pointed out the hard reality of **Gina**'s activity and collapse cycle, and offered practical strategizing for the family as a whole.

COUNTERTRANSFERENCE IN PHASE 2

The emotional reactions that assail clinicians with Phase 2 patients may very well include those they encounter with Phase 1 patients, including revulsion, fear, anger, and disbelief. As with Phase 1 patients, the clinician's Phase 2 patients may trigger traumas of their own. Clinicians may reject their Phase 2 patients or overidentify with them. But certain other issues come to have particular salience in Phase 2.

Conflict

Clinicians often experience conflict with their Phase 2 patients. As they work assiduously to teach patients the observation and differentiation skills the patients need to progress, it often seems that patients just do not seem to learn. They usually fail to understand the big picture and hence do not move forward the way the clinician is invested in their doing. Like the patient's family members, who do not want to accept their new fate, the clinician becomes

PHASE 2 **Countertransference**
Conflict Normalization failure Phase 2 seeking behavior Vicarious traumatization
Clinical Stance Compassion for suffering Engagement of grief reaction Coaching and restructuring Modeling toleration of chronicity Providing containment

exasperated by the patient's failure to improve. The family may see improvement in terms of return to preillness normal, and the clinician may see it when the patient acquires new insights and skills, but in both cases clinicians and families get annoyed at the patient for failing to meet their expectations (Alexandris & Vaslamatzis, 1993; Olkin, 1999; Pearlman & Saakvitne, 1995; J. P. Wilson & Lindy, 1994).

Clinicians frequently experience conflict with patients' families, whose behavior may reward patients for unhealthy behaviors and punish them for healthy ones. Laziness and selfishness may appear to motivate families when they insist that the patient must return to incapacitating former roles and responsibilities. To make matters worse, clinicians with Phase 2 patients often find themselves in conflict with their organizations—their HMOs, their hospitals, or their agencies. The organizations tend to want patients moved out of the system, when the clinician knows that the patients still need continuing support and education.

Normalization Failure

Like patients and their families, clinicians can also feel annoyance that patients fail to return to normal, even though clinicians know better in one part of their minds. Clinicians also participate in the culture's preference for acute illnesses that achieve eventual cure, and they sometimes cannot help wanting their patients to get better and move on (Figley, 1995; Marbach, 1999; Schlesinger et al., 1999; Schwartz-Salant & Stein, 1995).

Clinicians need to acknowledge these feelings of conflict and annoyance and use the experience to understand deeply how insidious and pervasive societal attitudes about chronic illness are. They need to examine their own issues with chronicity and ambiguity to better model them for their patients.

Phase 2 Seeking Behavior

When clinicians become angry or suffer burnout over cases that do not seem to budge, no matter how hard the clinician tries, the all-important bond with the patient can easily rupture. Moreover, in Phase 2, patients are in a seeking mode. They no longer accept whatever clinicians tell them but believe that perhaps their failure to improve is the clinician's fault. Sometimes they speak of this openly and announce that they are seeking a new clinician.

The clinician can remind patients that they have been working to turn them into wise health care consumers and that they should seek the best help available. It is often wise for clinicians to alert patients to the fact that not everyone offering help is equally qualified and some are not qualified at all, but they should always encourage patients to seek their own best interests. Clinicians should always leave the door open for patients to return and can follow up after some time has gone by to see whether patients who have left are receiving the services they need.

Vicarious Traumatization

With Phase 2 patients, clinicians often suffer the vicarious traumatization of practicing with marginalized or disregarded patient populations. The urgency of Phase 1 patients and the crisis situations they are in sufficiently mimics the acute model of illness that professional peers find treatment of them acceptable. But with the long-term commitment to Phase 2 patients, who clearly are not "getting better," professional peers sometimes regard clinicians working with these populations as choosing to work with undesirables. Because this professional traumatization occurs to the clinician at the same time the patient may be looking elsewhere for a "better" therapist, clinicians with Phase 2 patients can experience a real degree of frustration and pain.

Examples _____

As mentioned earlier, **Kim** activated a number of negative countertransference issues with me. Her dependent, approval-seeking behavior not only interfered with treatment interventions, but that kind of behavior had tended to annoy me from the time I was a child.

As to treatment, I began attempting to build a warm relationship with **Kim** that did not depend on ever-greater suffering and painful symptoms. Because tracking practical everyday activities seemed to bog us down, I tried to engage **Kim** more deeply in her life narrative. From this, I tried to draw attention to **Kim**'s strengths and abilities so that **Kim** might begin to see herself on an equal footing with me, not as a pleading petitioner.

I reflected on how much physical difficulty and pain **Kim** had experienced and on how much disbelief she had encountered over her lifetime of illness. It was hardly surprising that **Kim** might attempt strategies of pleasing to ingratiate herself and win help rather than anger people and cause them to dismiss her or hurt her further. The transformative step of Phase 2—meeting suffering with compassion—seemed called for here.

Sophia was an easy match for me because I felt her to have a loveable personality. But I found myself enormously frustrated at **Sophia**'s unwillingness to examine, let alone grasp, the practical changes that would help to stabilize her physically. Her overdoing of activities led to serious collapses. She would then be unable to maintain her ADLs, which meant that she ate poorly. This further exacerbated her physical deterioration. I found myself blaming **Sophia** for failing not so much to return to normal but to achieve the stable condition that she might seriously aspire to. I became even more annoyed when I realized that I was feeling professionally inadequate because my frequently successful methods were not working at all. First, I had to recognize that I needed to change my approach with **Sophia**. And to get in this frame of mind, I needed to practice compassion and to reflect deeply on the true tragedy that this brilliant, lovely woman had suffered. By seeking new ways to engage **Sophia** in understanding her condition and by constantly modeling the anger, grief, and sense of loss that I was convinced **Sophia** felt, I began to find other paths to treatment goals.

Everett's concept of masculinity and the patriarchal family he had established produced many negative knee-jerk reactions in me. Nonetheless, there was no question that **Everett** was suffering, that Joan and his children were suffering, and that he needed a new way to regard himself as a man and a human. Indeed, because I believe strongly in a different model, it was with real conviction that I could try to educate him to it. Learning how to empathize truly with **Everett** was more difficult, but it eventually became rather fun as I turned into a kind of honorary son.

Christine's family simply appalled me. What made this difficult for my relationship with **Christine** was that I needed to honor **Christine**'s affection for these people and her desire to maintain connections with them. I found that by setting up parameters of acceptable behavior with **Christine**, she was able to become her own judge of whether family members were behaving appropriately. Also, as her husband's family began to play a larger role in their life, **Christine** saw in daily ways how a more functional family supported rather than undermined one another.

Joshua aroused an immediate, uncritical admiration in me because he had made so much of his life despite living with daily exposure to racism. I also tended to idealize the warm, supportive community that he and Maybelle lived in. These feelings were amplified when I learned of the treatment **Joshua** had received from the neurologist. At some point, however, to carry out meaningful work, I needed to look at **Joshua** as an individual, not as an entire suffering minority.

TRANSFORMATION STEPS IN PHASE 2

Meeting Suffering with Compassion

The transformational step for clinicians dealing with countertransference in Phase 2 is to meet the suffering that they encounter with *compassion*. If the essential step in Phase 1 is to *allow* the suffering—to recognize or acknowledge its existence—the clinician now takes an active step forward to engage that suffering, but to do so with compassion.

Engaging the Grief Reaction

First and foremost, this means that clinicians engage the grief reaction. During all the work in Phase 2 that clinicians carry out with patients of observation and differentiation and the realigning of norms and activities, the patients are every day encountering the actuality of their own losses. While clinicians are telling patients that life can be better in the future, all the patients understand is that they must do less, cut back, have less. It is, therefore, essential for clinicians to regularly call attention to and encourage patients to express their grief and loss and discouragement as emotively as possible in a structured, almost formal way. Crying or raging are both healthy expressions of loss and may help prevent serious psychological problems such as severe depression. Obviously, if patients come to their illness with a prior personality or addiction problem, all the issues are intensified, and the expression of grief requires special consideration and containment. It becomes extremely important to differentiate illness issues from premorbid problems and traumas and to encourage relieving grief for the illness issues.

When patients can consciously process their suffering and loss, their suffering becomes conscious and known. If patients' suffering is not openly expressed, it does not disappear, but instead wells up in disparate, seemingly unrelated neurotic symptoms. To prevent neurotic suffering that can emerge as many other symptoms but will not be solved by attacking those symptoms directly by themselves, clinicians need to work assiduously to make patients conscious of their suffering and expressive of it. Doing this is one aspect of the development of new norms in Phase 2.

Examples

I sought to engage the grief reaction of all my clients and to meet their suffering with compassion. But individual cases draw attention to specific challenges. With **Sophia**, for example, it is possible to see how the patient may have difficulty contemplating her situation because her losses are so great and her nature and training have either suppressed or discouraged expression of the necessary emotions. For **Everett**, too, education into the permissibility of emotions and then into the necessity for expressing them formed a central part of my intervention effort. **Lewis** saw his difficulties as self-generated; hence, it did not occur to him to feel grief, but only horror. As he gradually came to understand how his physical and psychological difficulties fit together, he could also begin the process of grieving for the life he couldn't lead and honoring the suffering that he was actually enduring. **Kim**'s difficulty with focus and reflection characterized her expressions of grief as well. They were so generalized and nonspecific that she had trouble identifying where her suffering came from, let alone what she might possibly draw from it. **Joshua** needed to learn to express his profound grief, of which he was unconscious, as well as his very intense anger, which was often his defense against examining and experiencing his grief. Although the anger was real and essential to express, it was only through expressing his grief that he could begin to move toward meeting his suffering with compassion.

CLINICAL STANCE IN PHASE 2

Clinicians attend to their patients in two different but overlapping settings. They try to help patients deal with the practical issues of their new situation, whether this is learning how to allocate activities so as to stay emotionally healthy or speaking with an employer about a patient's work conditions. But increasingly as patients progress through the phases, clinicians address the large, overarching issues of meaning, or what might be called "the big picture."

Coaching and Structuring

In Phase 2, clinicians handle the practical world issues by coaching their patients in how to manage different scenarios and in helping them to structure a new life with new norms and values using a phase template. Coaching not only entails practical advice and suggestion, but also encourages and models the grief reaction for patients.

Modeling Toleration of Chronicity

Informing all the clinician's practical interventions are the big-picture issues, and central to Phase 2 is the clinician's modeling of toleration of chronicity. What is in the process of happening between the clinician and the patient is development of a lifelong solution because the chronic condition will likely last indefinitely. Given the longevity of people, patients are likely to experience additional chronic conditions as they age even if the first condition diminishes or plateaus permanently. Gradual acceptance of this basic truth occurs while patients and families change their norms and values, but it also helps to make such changes happen. The two are mutually reinforcing. Moreover, throughout the process, the clinician asserts that although suffering will be ongoing, it is not mutually exclusive with having a whole and meaningful life.

Providing Containment

Clinicians also provide containment for their Phase 2 patients. Although containment may seem a problematic term with its connotations of control and imprisonment, it is actually highly necessary for Phase 2 patients who would otherwise find themselves feeling adrift in the universe. All the rules have changed for them, and nothing is as it was. Their world has turned upside down, and they have no familiar or reliable reference points. Like a parent keeping outside bounds around a newly mobile child, the clinician provides trustworthy boundaries that assure patients that they can learn about their new world in safety. The clinician will further assert for them what they may not believe now but must take on faith—that what they learn now and how they come to live can be meaningful and fulfilling.

Examples

Christine required ongoing, simultaneous exposure to reflection about the big picture of her life and the practical activities of which it was composed. Particularly after she and Michael adopted Mei, she needed to be reminded of how all the meaningful large issues of her life—most especially Mei—were affected directly by how she conducted herself within the realm of practicalities. Coaching and structuring were essential with **Christine**, and I had to articulate boundaries for **Christine** because she, who had once been so capable and energetic, had great difficulty containing herself.

Coaching and structuring were also essential with **Everett** and Joan. They had no models for the new behaviors they needed to adopt, so they had to be taught them, but in a way that would preserve their dignity and self-respect. I also constantly modeled toleration of chronicity for **Everett**, who at first could not bear to contemplate living in his disabled state. It was important to bring **Everett** toward the notion that he was, in his current situation, exhibiting the finest qualities of his own definition of manhood—being strong, brave, persistent, responsible, and so forth.

Joshua, too, needed to begin learning how to tolerate chronicity, which was difficult for him because his symptoms were largely unfelt. Much of his considerable achievement in life had occurred because he had expended effort to make things happen. When he was faced with something that he could not alter and was potentially life-threatening, none of his previously successful methods of dealing with life helped.

Lewis responded quickly and well to coaching and structuring, both of which helped to contain him. He had much greater difficulty, as do most patients, learning to tolerate chronicity.

Sophia needed to have me model behavior so that she could learn some of the emotions she was feeling and how she might possibly express them. She was thoroughly conscious that her life was part of a bigger picture, although she had to realign her place in that big picture. She did, however, need to learn that how she lived in the practical world made a difference, even in her relationship to God and the meaning of life.

PHASE 2
Checklist for Countertransference

_____ 1. Have you examined your personal feelings about the patient?

_____ 2. Do you find yourself in conflict with your patient, particularly as to learning about self-observation, process and content, identification and differentiation, and so forth?

_____ 3. Are you beginning to tire of the fact that the patient is not getting better? Do you wish contact with this patient would reach a conclusion soon?

_____ 4. Is the patient disappointed with your failure to cure him or her? Is he or she seeking other help? How do you feel about this?

_____ 5. Are your colleagues sometimes dismissive of your work because of the patients you serve?

_____ 6. Are you able to regard suffering with *compassion?*

_____ 7. Are you able to engage your own grief reaction?

_____ 8. Are you able to coach and model behaviors that will help the patient and his or her family move through the phase process?

_____ 9. Are you able to help restructure the patient's life so that it will be manageable but also meaningful?

_____ 10. Are you able to help the patient erect new life boundaries that provide containment?

_____ 11. Are you able to model toleration for ambiguity and chronicity?

SPIRITUAL/PHILOSOPHICAL PERSPECTIVE IN PHASE 2

Absent or Indifferent Deity

Patients in Phase 2, like those in Phase 1, still believe that the locus of power concerning their lives and particularly their illness resides outside themselves. For those who believe in God, their relationship to God mirrors their relationship to their illness. In Phase 1, these patients regard God either as absent altogether or as actively punishing them with their illness and pain because they are or have been bad in some way. When patients arrive at the greater containment of Phase 2, they no longer feel God is punishing them precisely, but rather as though God has turned his attention elsewhere.

PHASE 2
Spiritual/Philosophical Perspective

Experience
      Absent or indifferent deity
      Hierarchical, patriarchal beliefs
      Seeking behavior
      Influence of others of like kind

Clinical Action
      Passive support of patient's choices/actions if not harmful

---

Hierarchical Religious Belief

In Phase 2, the illness experience draws many patients back into the practice of religion, especially if the institutional form that the religion takes is highly structured and hierarchical. Many clear, invariant rules and rituals help contain the world for these patients, whose lives have been completely overturned. It also relieves them from the burdensome issues of ambiguity. Because Phase 2 patients usually feel better than they did in Phase 1, they often believe that they will return to their former state of health if they perform prayers and practice rituals sincerely, properly, and over a long enough period of time. On the basis of their plateau experience, they feel that eventually God will reward their compliant behavior. In this hope, they are usually strongly encouraged by family and members of their congregation (Allport & Ross, 1967; Payne et al., 1991; Peck, 1987).

Seeking Behavior

But Phase 2 is also a time of seeking, and it can include seeking new, more satisfactory spiritual connections. The newly aroused critical faculty in Phase 2 patients can often make them reject the God of their past because that deity was apparently willing to subject them to gratuitous pain and suffering. At the same time, the need for unambiguous rules and emotional containment is so strong that Phase 2 patients frequently choose new organizations or spiritual settings that offer firm, unambiguous, hierarchical structure.

Influence of Others of Like Kind

In many cases, Phase 2 patients are influenced spiritually by the new friends they are making who suffer from conditions like their own. These others of like kind treat them empathetically and understand their suffering. If, in addition, a new friend seems to be emotionally supported by active religious practice, the patient may be attracted to that friend's church, synagogue, or congregation.

Clinician's Role

Where the patient's spiritual life does not hurt the patient or others, it is usually best for clinicians to passively support whatever course the patients choose. The highly structured religious settings that Phase 2 patients usually prefer actually aid clinicians in the work of containing patients' nearly boundaryless world. Later, in Phase 3, the clinician will encourage patients to begin exploring their own individual thoughts about spirituality, but that does not usually occur in Phase 2. Phase 3 patients undertake to explore the basic human questions: Why am I here? Why am I conscious and thinking? Why do I suffer? What is the meaning of existence? But during Phase 2, these issues emerge only tangentially, in the course of other interventions such as reallocating activities to include, among other things, ones related to personal fulfillment and growth.

Examples ———————————————————————————

Sophia had lived in a deeply spiritual world all her life. Even when she enthusiastically took up the tools of modern scientific investigation, she still devoted time to daily prayer and meditation. As mentioned in the previous chapter, she had needed to strengthen the inner connection to this spiritual practice after she became ill because, over her years of study and professional practice, it had become somewhat rote. She had, however, the tools to reignite her spirituality. She also learned that offering her complaints, her angers, her losses, and her griefs to God was one way she could improve the quality of her life. Doing this fit into **Sophia**'s conception of what an individual might say to God; therefore, although she had trouble speaking about such things to other people, she did succeed in articulating them to God.

Joshua and his wife had been life-long churchgoers and were very active in church activities. It came as a profound surprise to Maybelle when **Joshua**, who was to her thinking so clearly in need of the Lord and the prayers of the congregation, began to resist attending services. He was angry with God, whom he'd served honestly and enthusiastically, and who he believed was treating him shabbily in return. **Joshua** had met a couple of other men in his community who also suffered from persistent high blood pressure, and he was more interested in talking to them and finding out where they worshiped or what they thought of God. I talked with Maybelle, who was deeply pained by **Joshua**'s behavior. I reassured her that **Joshua** was engaging in a healthy and positive action—that he was seeking to truly understand what role spirituality played in his life. Rather than engage in practice that was at least temporarily empty for him, he was seeking spiritual attitudes that meant something to him now.

Christine had grown up a practicing Catholic, as had Michael, and they continued to attend church sporadically, as **Christine**'s health and their schedules permitted. **Christine** was getting no meaningful comfort or understanding from these forms, however. She even joked about it, treating church as simply a cultural expression of her family and community, not as a serious spiritual activity. With the arrival of Mei, she thought about her religious life more closely. She could see no other church to attend, and she wanted Mei brought up in her cultural traditions, but she also wanted religion to have more meaning for herself and for Mei than it had so far. I suggested that **Christine** read the writings of various church mystics whose relationship with God was profound and not merely formal. But **Christine** had a good deal of difficulty reading. Eventually, in a group meeting at my practice, **Christine** became friends with two women who belonged to an ecumenical prayer group. They invited her to join and even held meetings at **Christine**'s home when she was unable to get out. The variety of prayers

PHASE 2
Checklist for Spiritual/Philosophical Perspective

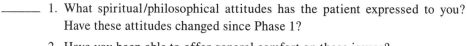

_____ 1. What spiritual/philosophical attitudes has the patient expressed to you? Have these attitudes changed since Phase 1?

_____ 2. Have you been able to offer general comfort on these issues?

Again, it is important to note that spiritual/philosophical issues come most actively into play in Phase 3. During Phases 1 and 2, the clinician attempts largely to provide comfort and containment, passively assenting to the patient's actions as long as they are not harmful to the patient.

and prayer traditions that the group brought to **Christine**'s attention began to give her some of the emotional substance that she needed to flesh out her nascent spiritual life.

See Table 5.1 for a summary of Phase 2.

Table 5.1   Phase 2: Stabilization

1. *Course of Illness*

  Physical/behavioral domain
    Plateau
    Stabilization
  Psychological domain
    Increased caution/secondary wounding
    Social withdrawal/social searching
    Service confusion/service searching
    Boundary confusion
  Social/interactive domain
    Interactive conflict/cooperation
    Vicarious secondary wounding
    Vicarious traumatization manifestation
    Normalization failure

2. *Identifying Characteristics*

    Some control and ego strength regained
    Seeking behavior: others of like kind, other treatments or clinicians
    Low tolerance of chronicity
    Reduced self-pathologizing
    Fewer ideations
    Normalization failure

  Clinical Goal
    Stabilization and basic activities restructuring

  Clinical Summary
    Collect data
    Differentiate
    Develop insight
    Develop norms and goals

3. *Assessment*

  Physical/behavioral domain
    Medical/medications review
    Activity threshold review
    Medical and rehabilitation coordination
  Psychological domain
    Phase placement
    Personal narrative
    Trauma assessment: premorbid, comorbid, iatrogenic, disease/syndrome, cultural

(continued)

Table 5.1 *Continued*

Social/interactive domain
  Effect failure on family of normalization
  Review of family roles and responsibilities
  Family narrative
  Vicarious trauma evaluation
  Couples evaluation
  Work evaluation

4. *Treatment*

Physical/behavioral domain
  Medical protocols
  Activity threshold modification
  Education on personal energy process, four activity groups
  Data collection
  Education on activity adjustment
Psychological domain
  Self-observation refinement
  Insight maintenance
  Overcoming psychological defenses
  Characterological interventions
  Expression of feelings, grieving
  Clarification of values/norm development
Social/interactive domain
  Education of family about normalization failure
  Revision of family roles and responsibilities
  Family narrative/traumas
  Clarification of values/norm development
  Education to illness etiquette
  Couples interventions
  Workplace interventions/strategy development/disability

5. *Countertransference*

  Conflict
  Normalization failure
  Phase 2 seeking behavior
  Vicarious traumatization

Clinical Stance
  Compassion for suffering
  Engagement of grief reaction
  Coaching and restructuring
  Modeling toleration of chronicity
  Providing containment

6. *Spiritual/Philosophical Perspective*

Experience
  Absent or indifferent deity
  Hierarchical, patriarchal beliefs
  Seeking behavior
  Influence of others of like kind
Clinical action
  Passive support of patient's choices/actions, if not harmful

Chapter 6 ———————————————————————

PHASE 3: RESOLUTION

DEVELOPMENT OF MEANING

The single most important intervention activity with Phase 3 patients concerns the development of meaning. In Phase 2, patients expanded and refined the insight into their illness and activities that they began in Phase 1. This is an essential kind of insight, which is both difficult to achieve and hard to maintain. But even this kind of insight is not enough to sustain them for the long haul (Prochaska, DiClemente, & Norcross, 1992; Prochaska et al., 1994). Patients also need to place their lives in a wider context of meaning, first about the illness experience that has been imposed on them, but more importantly about what makes a life, even one as constrained as theirs, worth living (Biordi, 2002; Johnson-Taylor et al., 1995; Kahn, 1995; Schirm, 2002). The success patients have in achieving the resolution that allows them to integrate their illness into their lives depends largely on the exploration of meaning (Frankl, 1983; Hellstrom, Bullington, Karlsson, Lindqvist, & Mattson, 1999; Jobst, Shostak, & Whitehouse, 1999; Kissane, 2000; Magid, 2000).

Most thoughtful people, at some point in their lives, reflect on the large philosophical or spiritual questions that concern being and existence, purpose and meaning. They ask what they are, why they exist, and whether they exist for any purpose. They seek broad explanatory answers that will help them understand and contain what they know and the varied experiences of their lives. They may do this within the context of a formal religion, or they may draw eclectically on a variety of secular and spiritual traditions. Ultimately,

---

PHASE 3
Course of Illness

Physical/Behavioral Domain
    Improvement
    Plateau/stabilization
    Relapse

Psychological Domain
    Grief reaction/compassion reaction
    Identification of pre-crisis self
    Role/identify experimentation
    Locus of control returning to self
    Awareness of societal effects
    Spiritual/philosophical development

Social/Interactive Domain
    Breaking silence/engulfment in stigma
    Confrontation
    Role experimentation—social, vocational
    Integration with new supporters/separation from nonsupporters

---

their search allows them to establish a framework of meaning that makes their life supportable and worthwhile.

There are many people, of course, who never contemplate these issues. For some, their lives are sufficiently stress-free that they are able to pass easily from one experience in life to another without attending to more than the practical activities required to maintain their happy existence. Others are far less fortunate. Their lives are so stressful and subject to such dislocation and threat that they never have any opportunity to reflect on issues of meaning. Their every waking hour is spent dealing with the difficulties and crises at hand.

But most people require and make the effort to find some sense of meaning in life. They do this to avoid existential despair and survive emotionally the difficulties that disrupt the lives of most individuals. Illness, whether acute or chronic, often stimulates the desire to find meaning because it threatens the individual with pain, suffering, and sometimes even death. It is possible for individuals to pass through episodes of acute illness and forget, once the crisis has passed, the questions that arose while they were sick. But for those with chronic illness, the previous state of well-being never returns, even when chronic illness patients achieve a plateau state.

Meaning Development for Chronic Illness Patients

It is a basic tenet of the Four-Phase Model that chronic illness patients must contemplate issues of meaning and attempt to formulate their own individual philosophies or spiritual answers if they wish to integrate their illness into their lives. It is also a tenet of this model that integration is the only effective solution for living with a chronic illness.

Meaning in Phases 1 and 2

Patients in Phases 1 and 2 are deeply preoccupied with the practical realities of their troubled world. The chaotic search for diagnosis and relief that characterizes Phase 1 patients permits almost no thought about meaning. Many patients tend to fear that their condition is some sort of specific or nebulous damnation, and any philosophical or spiritual response they have is, at worst, primitive or magical and, at best, placatory. Phase 2 patients are capable of greater attention and reflection, but initially they, too, are preoccupied with the practical, and they still hope for a cure. They need to learn to understand their illness, their boundaries, and how to rearrange their lives. As a sense of control begins to return to Phase 2 patients, however, and as they find others who support and empathize with them, the search for emotional and spiritual containment draws many into fairly hierarchical, authoritative religious structures. They do not usually attempt to develop individual or specific meaning for themselves but use traditional formulations that already exist. Often they find help in the religion of their childhood or sometimes in the religion of a sympathetic person of like kind.

Meaning Development in Phase 3

In Phase 3, by far the most significant work patients accomplish is the exploration of their own personal, individual conceptions of meaning. Whether patients continue to practice within an established religion or not, it is essential for clinicians to lead patients into a deep investigation of their actual, personal thoughts about the nature of life and where they and their experience fit in the great scheme of things. Patients may ultimately choose to affirm the meanings defined by an established religion or philosophy, or they may come to assert belief in an assorted collection of personally meaningful ideas. Whatever form meaning takes for patients, it must arise authentically out of their feelings and their understanding. It is not something they subscribe to because they are told to but because it answers truly to what they feel on the deepest level. The role of clinicians is not to select or evaluate the beliefs of patients, but to guide them into a significant, truly authentic examination of the larger order and their place in it. Clinicians do this at the same time they are continuing to help patients observe and analyze the practical issues in their daily lives.

IDENTIFYING PHASE 3 PATIENTS

Increased Internal Locus of Control

When patients arrive at Phase 3, their presentation has visibly shifted. They may or may not be physically compromised, but their social and emotional presentation is qualitatively different from individuals enduring the crisis of Phase 1 or struggling to stabilize their lives in Phase 2. Patients exhibit a

---

PHASE 3
Identifying Characteristics

Increasingly internalized locus of control
Increased awareness of societal effects
Differentiated responses and increased self-esteem
Increased tolerance of ambiguity/chronicity
Respect for suffering and development of meaning
Creative process engaged

Clinical Goal
Development of meaning and construction of new self

Clinical Summary
Grieve
Maintain
Reframe

---

much greater internalization of locus of control. More and more, their sense of control firmly resides inside themselves.

Increased Awareness of Societal Effects

At this point in their experience, as demonstrated in their individual phase narratives, they have learned about the causes and effects of societal response to chronic illness and about stigmatization. This understanding helps keep them from entirely internalizing negative social experiences. They can now differentiate between things over which they can exert real control—such as their attitude toward themselves and their self-respect—and things they cannot control—such as other people's opinions.

Differentiated Responses and Increased Self-Esteem

At the same time, they can differentiate things to which they must respond in others—such as job discrimination—from things that they should disregard—such as a relative's foolish comments. As a result, they are far less self-pathologizing, and they have much greater self-esteem.

Increased Tolerance of Chronicity and Ambiguity

Phase 3 patients have also learned how to do some of the emotional heavy lifting required to tolerate both chronicity and ambiguity. Some of these new emotional muscles and strengths come from surviving the grief reaction that they processed during Phase 2 when they attempted to return to their previous precrisis selves and found they could not. During Phase 3, they engage the very deep grief they feel for losing that preillness self. They pass through what may be called a "dark night of the soul" in the effort to arrive at the philosophical or spiritual grounding of a sturdy new self.

It is important to remember that medical understanding is changing all the time. Very possibly, some conditions that have no cure now will one day have a cure. Patients with chronic illness should always keep informed about advances in understanding of their disease. It is, however, the point of this book that many conditions persist for the rest of any individual patient's life and that a good quality of life comes only to those who find a way to accept and live meaningfully with the chronicity and ambiguity of their condition.

Moreover, many conditions impose either static or dynamic disabilities on people and require the same sort of integration into the patient's life.

Respect for Suffering and Development of Meaning

In Phase 1 and Phase 2, patients learned to allow their suffering and then to address it with compassion. In Phase 3, they learn to respect themselves for enduring their suffering. There may or may not be positive lessons they can learn from their suffering, but simply by virtue of enduring it, they deserve respect. This respect finds expression in articulated self-compassion, which is one of the identifying characteristics for clinicians of Phase 3 patients. By expressing the compassion they feel for themselves, patients show that they are now standing with themselves rather than fighting against an alien self that the sickness has made them. One other necessary aspect of this compassionate, respectful response to patients' experience of suffering is the development of meaning.

Creative Process Engaged

The process of patients' respecting their suffering, perhaps learning something useful from it, and developing meaning often occurs as part of or concurrently with some form of creative action (Schirm, 2002; Johnson-Taylor et al., 1995). The creative process helps further facilitate the internalization of locus of control, which in turn permits patients to achieve a personally meaningful, socially enabling illness narrative. With this kind of resolution of their experience, patients are fully prepared to carry out the integration activities of Phase 4.

Mixture of Phases

It is important for clinicians to remember that patients can simultaneously exhibit traits of different phases as to different aspects of their experience. This can be confusing to clinicians who see for the first time, for example, patients who have developed a profound personal sense of meaning before their illness. Such patients are strongly grounded for the eventual illness integration of Phase 4, but they may still have much work to accomplish in Phase 2 aspects of activity analysis and behavior modification. Or, for reasons totally other than illness, a new patient may have developed a Phase 3 understanding of social stigmatization but still be coping with Phase 2 issues of passing for normal.

Patients even in Phase 3 and Phase 4 can easily be thrown back into Phase 1 crisis and chaos by a serious new illness or trauma. Although they have achieved deep insight and understanding about their original chronic illness, and although they have found a way to incorporate their illness into a new, authentic self, this does not inoculate them against all of life's other hazards. Death or tragedy will afflict them with crisis, just as it does other mortals. And crisis may seriously exacerbate their original illness symptoms. New illnesses or even severe relapses in the original illness, especially if these involve prolonged pain, frequently push well-integrated patients back into a crisis state. These patients are, however, better positioned to process the new trauma. They understand how to do it, and they know where to look for help. The phase process may perhaps be conceived as analogous to a rising spiral, in which patients who have worked through the phases once may find themselves cycled back into crisis, but at a higher level of understanding and very likely with higher levels of later integration as well (Fennell, 1995a, 1998; Jason, Fennell, et al., 2000).

In their stage model of behavioral change, Prochaska and colleagues have argued that people do not move directly forward through the stages, but rather they recycle, usually many times. But they also assert that individuals learn from their experiences in the earlier stage so that when they move forward the subsequent time, they do so more rapidly and effectively. This gives their progress forward a kind of upward spiral pattern (Prochaska, DiClemente, & Norcross, 1992; Prochaska et al., 1994). In their model, individuals can reach an end point. They can complete the stages and exit the process altogether. With chronic illness, however, patients do not exit the phase process. Successful navigation brings patients into Phase 4, and there they attempt to remain. It is an ongoing process.

Examples

All the cases discussed earlier in the book entered into Phase 3, although they were not all able to progress through the work of the phase. **Sophia**, **Everett**, **Christine**, **Lewis**, and **Kim** had been with me from Phase 1. All in their own way had contained the crisis of Phase 1 and engaged in the hard analytical stabilization work of Phase 2. They had attacked the practical problems that their conditions had caused and knew many of the tools and techniques that could help improve the quality of their day-to-day lives. They learned how to observe their own behavior and how to modify their expectations, attitudes, and norms. In other words, they ultimately learned how to modify their relationship to themselves. All had done some conscious grieving for their losses and had worked with their families and friends to readjust their roles and responsibilities. I recognized that all five were entering Phase 3 when they began displaying a greater internalized locus of control as they began to see their practical interventions having a greater effect on how they felt. As the patients worked through exercises aimed at readjusting their home, friendship, and work relationships, they developed greater conscious awareness of how societal attitudes affected their lives. They all learned to differentiate their responses depending on whether stigmatizing attitudes occurred in a setting where they had to fight back or represented merely irritating behavior that they could ignore. All began to demonstrate a growing ability to live with the ambiguity of their ever-shifting situation and to accept its chronicity as well. They were starting to feel genuine compassion for themselves, which found expression in their reconceptions of their illness narratives.

After being helped to manage her medical and employment crises, **Sophia** used my metaphoric stories to start exerting some control over her activity levels. She learned—very slowly at first—that she could provide the most supportive environment for her body if she restricted her activity level before she collapsed rather than being forced to rest because of collapse. At the same time, she recognized that her symptoms took many and varying forms that she could not predict but could only handle as they appeared. Encouraged by my active modeling, **Sophia** was also beginning to express first her rage and then her deep grief at the horrific losses that her illness had gouged from her life. The passage of time and the response of the medical professionals she saw convinced her that her condition was permanent, at least in the present state of medicine. But, fortunately, **Sophia** had a strong spiritual base from which to start the difficult business of building a new self and a new life.

Everett had a difficult time coming to the recognition that his stroke had left him with permanent disability. However, simultaneous with the process of learning practical ways to restructure his life, he also gradually began to comprehend how he could be a man who incorporated at least parts of his former self. In the stressful process of rearranging family roles and responsibilities, **Everett** was both benefited and hindered by an attentive, largely loving family. During the hard work of Phase 2, many of the most vexed family issues received airing and began gradually to resolve. Even through **Everett** had originally regarded autobiographical activities as complete nonsense, he had even embarked on that new adventure by taping stories of his childhood, his growing up, his war experiences, his marriage, and his family life. In the course of reflecting on his own life, he surprised himself by what he recalled and what he realized it meant to him.

Christine had clear clinical knowledge about the chronicity of her MS and the ambiguity of its symptoms. The most painful thing for her and Michael to recognize was that she was not one of those MS patients who spontaneously remit for years at a time. Everything indicated that she was deteriorating, slowly but apparently relentlessly. Being action-oriented, however, **Christine** tended to live in the now. She consciously reorganized her activities to give her the most efficient use of what energy she had, and she adapted to the ups and downs in her symptoms. Her unhappy relations with her birth family continued to bother her, but when she adopted her baby, thereby creating a family of her own, **Christine** found a whole new way to express herself. Having a child gave her a way to tackle the serious existential questions that were about to come crashing in on her.

Lewis had come to recognize that his horrors were the product of a disease that could be difficult to live with but not impossible. Achieving his diagnosis of Tourette's and obsessive-compulsive disorder was probably the single most important factor in **Lewis**'s being able to move forward through the phases. Diagnosis relieved him of his greatest fears and anxieties. In addition, however, the regular self-reflection of Phase 2, with its processing of activity and symptom data, gave **Lewis** the sense that he now had a way to exert maximum control over his life.

Kim gradually came to process her daily symptoms and activities without exaggeration or attempts to curry interest by embellishment. Because she had a great variety of conditions—some from childhood—it was nevertheless difficult for her to grieve in a focused way. She lashed out in rage and suffering when she was in pain, but she had trouble reflecting specifically on the nature of her losses. It appeared, however, that she had gained some understanding of the chronicity she would experience and, particularly, of the ambiguity of her conditions. By adopting good sleep hygiene techniques, effective methods for dealing with her restless legs at night, and better activity management, **Kim** felt that she was beginning to gain control over her life. During Phase 2, she had also enjoyed a fairly long plateau period. Her symptoms had by no means disappeared, but they had not increased, and she suffered neither relapse nor the onset of a new condition.

Gina and **Joshua**, the patients who came to me in Phase 2, also moved into Phase 3. **Gina** overcame her own negative evaluation of her FM and CFS largely through her very real experience of symptoms. She had come to me to try to find better methods of living with her illness, and in this she was at least partially successful. After several sessions, she could chart her well-trodden road to collapse in her activity and symptom charts. She had even mapped longer term cycles of overexertion and exhaustion. To engage in serious norm readjustment and life alteration, however, **Gina** needed to acknowledge deeply that her condition was permanent, with symptoms that might appear and disappear, diminish, or flare up suddenly. During Phase 2, **Gina** arrived at this state of understanding. She realized that she was not going to get better and be able to resume her preillness life. Her husband, however, had not accepted this, and **Gina** was still trying to behave in ways that would meet his expectations. She felt she knew how to manage her life, but she could not face arguing with Vince about her needs. She suspected and feared that he would want a divorce rather than rearrange his life so completely.

Joshua recognized that his hypertension was chronic. Because high blood pressure is painless and usually controlled by medication, this might have made no difference in his life. But medication was not controlling the problem sufficiently, and **Joshua**'s additional symptoms frightened and angered him. Activity data collection and symptom analysis helped **Joshua** identify more successful behavior patterns. Sleep hygiene and some simple meditation techniques also improved **Joshua**'s condition. His blood pressure came down somewhat, although not as much as his doctor wanted. It was enough, however, for **Joshua** to begin to hope that some combination of self-monitored activity and medication might work. He suffered fewer headaches and had better techniques for stopping those that started before they became debilitating. **Joshua** was finely tuned to societal stigmatization, particularly as expressed in any racial fashion. Because his condition is common among African American men, **Joshua** was alert to all issues of discrimination or inadequacy in medical understanding because of the afflicted population. He was also frankly open about his anger with God. It took more time to get to grief and loss, but rage was a good place to start.

New Example

I had the fairly unusual experience of treating a new patient who was clearly in Phase 3. **Erin** was a White woman in her late 30s, who had suffered a succession of mystery illnesses during her late childhood and young adulthood. In addition, as a young woman, her appendix had ruptured, but this was not diagnosed and treated until several days after it had poisoned her entire body cavity. **Erin** had also experienced the death of her parents, a beloved grandmother, and a young man with whom she'd been deeply involved. She thought that she had been tempered in the furnace of these devastating events and had formulated what she believed was a strong, supportive philosophical stance. But when she had a complete physical collapse, which was ultimately diagnosed as lupus, she felt herself falling completely apart emotionally.

Erin comprehended the chronic nature of lupus and could accept the ambiguity that it would impose on her life. She even recognized that she could rearrange her activities to support a vastly different life from the one she had intended. But she couldn't make sense of things any more. Why was this happening to her and what was the point of living? What conceivable deity would permit such miseries as she had seen and experienced? How could she possibly go on? In other words, **Erin** was wide awake, struggling desperately with her dark night of the soul.

ASSESSMENT: PHYSICAL/BEHAVIORAL DOMAIN

Most Phase 3 patients came to their clinicians originally in either Phases 1 or 2. It is uncommon for clinicians to see patients for the first time when they are in Phase 3. Physical signs that patients are entering Phase 3 can include a leveling off of symptoms and/or a distinctly improved quality of life. The

PHASE 3
Assessment

Physical/Behavioral Domain
    Medical/medications review
    Activity threshold review

Psychological Domain
    Phase placement
    Personal narrative
    Existential questions

Social/Interactive Domain
    Family/couples case management review
    Review of wider social world issues
    Work evaluation

interventions of Phase 2, especially concerning patients' analyses of their own activity process and their balance of activity types, combined with their observations about how their symptoms present when they engage in different activities, have led them to make sufficient adjustments to improve their overall sense of well-being.

This is not to say that Phase 3 patients may not suffer relapses. On some occasions, relapses may be triggered by severe but unrelated illness or trauma. Clinicians and patients should always remain mindful that relapses may occur at any time in chronic illnesses. At the same time, however, patients in Phase 3 have usually come to process pain and suffering in a different way. In addition, they often find that the changes they have made in their values, expectations, and activities reduce the opportunities for relapses to occur.

Regular Medical Review

If a Phase 3 patient is, as a matter of fact, a first-time patient, the clinician should make sure that a complete physical and medications assessment is carried out. With ongoing patients, regular medical reviews, including medication reviews, continue, but these are not as global as the examinations in Phases 1 and 2 unless there is a distinct change in patients' symptomatology.

Patients as Medical Coordinators

As patients progress through Phase 3, clinicians train them to become their own medical coordinators, that is, to assume the management function that the clinician has carried out thus far. In time, patients cease to have regular visits with the clinicians who are helping them learn to manage their chronic illness experience, and they need to maintain the medical oversight function themselves in the future.

Activity Threshold Review

Clinicians conduct an activity threshold review in Phase 3, but this is now carried out in partnership with the patient. By Phase 3, patients have located their benchmark physical capabilities and determined their general emotional hardiness. They have learned to observe themselves objectively and analyze and differentiate their observations, and they are reasonably successful at maintaining their insights over time. They understand the four general areas of activity—personal maintenance, personal fulfillment, social and familial, and work or occupation-related—and they know that their emotional well-being depends on maintaining a balance of activities among the four groups. They have learned to monitor their symptoms so that they recognize when they must reduce or modify their activities. They have also learned to examine the things they want to do, those they feel they should do, and their responsibilities. They know that if their expectations exceed what they are actually able to accomplish, they must reevaluate their values and priorities or court the possibility of relapse or debilitating grief. In Phase 3, patients consolidate their capacity to monitor their activity threshold themselves, with the clinician now acting as coach or guide when they have questions.

Static versus Dynamic Disability

Increasingly during Phase 3, clinicians mentor patients so that they can deal on their own with the manifestations of their illness and its disabilities, whether these are static or dynamic. The physical disabilities resulting from, for example, multiple sclerosis may include periodic need to use a wheelchair. During times of wheelchair use, it might be said that the patient's disability is clear-cut and static. But over a longer period, the disabilities produced by MS are not static, and they require flexibility of response on the patient's part. Patients need to be prepared to adjust and shift with the changes that life and their illness bring. As they absorb and process the interventions of Phases 2 and 3, they gain reasonably effective methods for doing this (Bezard, Imbert, & Gross, 1998).

Examples

For a while, **Sophia** maintained a plateau of symptoms, but her condition was very gradually deteriorating. **Sophia** comprehended that she had a dynamic disability, the character of which would change over time. She knew that she had to remain flexible about solutions because what worked now might be insufficient later. She managed to achieve a modest level of functioning, however, by carefully monitoring her activity. Moreover, having been guided through a maze of medical and disability issues when she first came to me, **Sophia** had gradually learned how to coordinate her own medical needs. She grew to recognize what kinds of symptoms required immediate follow-up, and she was particularly alert to reactions to new medications. She understood what elements were essential to her physical safety plan and what kinds of help she needed to have on call. She and I talked in detail about how she would carry on in the future, particularly if she moved out of state, which was likely.

Everett and Joan also now understood how to keep track of **Everett**'s condition, his physical therapy, and his medications. Both had learned to be more assertive about **Everett**'s needs and how to be more specific about them. **Everett** knew that he had a permanent disability, but one that was, by and large, static. If he could adapt his life to present conditions, he had every reason to believe that things would not get worse. He also hoped to improve in small ways, but at least he and Joan knew fairly clearly the boundaries of his physical potential.

Both **Christine** and **Gina** comprehended the medical aspects of their conditions. **Christine**'s greatest difficulty came from her hostility toward doctors, which iatrogenic traumatization had generated in her. She had, however, with my help, located physicians with whom she had good rapport. She also became more outspoken when she felt that personnel in medical offices were behaving inappropriately toward her. **Gina** had a good relationship with her doctor. Her experience with her children's condition had taught her a great deal, and she also learned how to oversee her overall medical situation.

Having access to a Tourette's specialist gave **Lewis** the medical reassurance both he and his primary physician needed. Both felt that they had an excellent resource, should anything unexpected occur.

Joshua got along satisfactorily with his primary physician, who had recommended that he see me. His strong objections to the cardiologist he had seen were overcome when we were able to locate a cardiac specialist out of the area who was African American herself and who was carrying out research on hypertension among Black men. **Joshua** mostly needed to learn how to discuss his condition with medical personnel without having to accept inappropriate behavior from clinicians.

Kim had experimented with a variety of alternative therapies. She did maintain contact with a credentialed allopathic doctor, but the variety of **Kim**'s complaints and the pain that plagued her sent her searching for any new treatment that promised to relieve her altogether. From her stories, I gathered that **Kim** followed each new experiment faithfully—maintaining the special diet, consuming the vitamins and special supplements, practicing the special meditation techniques, smelling the selected aromas, or engaging in imaging. For a while, she nearly always experienced some overall improvement. Her pain diminished, and her agitation settled somewhat. Inevitably, however, some new physical problem would erupt, and the alternative therapy would cease to provide any benefit.

I hoped that **Kim** was genuinely developing insight and good self-management techniques, but I suspected that **Kim** might be relating to phase treatment as just another in a succession of alternative treatments. Although her sleep had improved, her pain had lessened, and her activities were not excessive and were fairly well distributed, I felt the real test would come with a relapse or a new crisis.

Erin, as a new patient, required a full physical review. Her diagnosis of lupus was firm, borne out by numerous tests, and her clinicians all agreed on the diagnosis. She was having a problem with medications, however. She reacted badly to the various anti-inflammatories her clinicians felt were essential to containing her condition. Up to this point, **Erin** had had good relations with her medical team, probably in part because she was unwilling to accept harmful treatment or attitudes from anyone, but the medications issue was straining her relationships with the doctors. They were beginning to act as though they regarded her adverse reactions as psychological in origin rather than physiological.

ASSESSMENT: PSYCHOLOGICAL DOMAIN

Revisiting the Personal Narrative

At the start of Phase 3, the illness narratives of most patients reflect a good deal of sophistication about the practicalities of living with their chronic illness. By now, patients have usually been working with a clinician at least a year, and they are now able to incorporate into their daily lives the interventions they learned in Phase 2. They have committed themselves to new values and norms, which permit them to live with a slowly growing sense of self-esteem and without a constant threat of relapse.

Existential Questions

Because patients now have the tools to cope with daily life, however, the questions of why this entire experience has happened to them is thrown into stark relief. For some patients, even their best quality of practical life is not very high. They regularly suffer considerable pain, disability, and social isolation. Having done everything practical they can to ameliorate their condition, and for many having gained nothing resembling their former healthy lives, they often ask why they should bother to live at all? Why continue? What is the point? This is patients' dark night of the soul, and it is one they must traverse to attain integration of chronic illness into their lives.

Examples ———————————————————————

All of the patients faced serious existential work in Phase 3. Details of this work are discussed in the treatment section. The new patient, **Erin**, bonded quickly with me. Her experiences had given her a great deal of insight, and she was able to examine the content and process of her life nimbly. Her exposure to death had developed in her an openness to the concept and expression of grief.

ASSESSMENT: SOCIAL/INTERACTIVE DOMAIN

Family Case Management Review

The most significant interventions in family case management usually occur during Phase 2 as patients and their families undertake the difficult process of identifying and revising their values, norms, and responsibilities. It is, therefore, also common, when the participants cannot understand or accommodate the new situation, for families to dissolve during Phase 2. When the members have a strong desire to preserve the family, however, they usually continue to attempt to adjust family expectations and distribution of roles and responsibilities. For some, however, this is an impossible task, even with the best will in the world. It may be beyond the emotional or cognitive abilities of significant family members. They may not have the skill base or sometimes the financial resources. Even with understanding, patience, desire, and the necessary finances, bringing about significant change may be a prolonged activity.

Empowering the Family to Manage Themselves

During Phase 3, clinicians should review the family adjustment process with both the patient and family members to see whether they are continuing to incorporate the new values and norms required by the chronic illness and whether they are continuing to establish new family roles and responsibilities. In Phase 3, clinicians act primarily as facilitators, helping to guide family members toward becoming their own case managers. Clinicians focus on teaching the family how to manage the new situation by themselves.

Patient as Burden

During Phase 2, patients who developed the skills of observation and analysis, and who have become able to maintain their insights, learned through numerous failed attempts that they will never return to their preillness state. As a consequence, throughout Phase 2 and at the start of Phase 3, they often regard themselves as nothing but a burden to their partners or their families (Canam & Acorn, 1999; Faison, Faria, & Frank, 1999; Hall, Stein, Roter, & Rieser, 1999; Helseth, 1999).

Changing this perception comes about in a number of ways; an important one is the family's discovering gains that may have occurred. These are rarely anticipated but come about as both patient and family develop insight into the new situation. It is often hard to avoid silver-lining platitudes in such discussions, but couples and families frequently develop a heightened awareness of one another and their various qualities through the illness experience. Sometimes, the changes necessitated by illness slow a family down in a way that all the members appreciate, even though they are not happy about, the reason for the change. The sense of being only a burden to others is also powerfully alleviated by the development of meaning.

Wider Social World

During Phases 1 and 2, clinicians primarily addressed the social/interactive issues of patients within their families. Whereas clinicians encouraged patients to understand society's attitudes and social stigmatization arising from their illness, interventions focused on applications of this understanding within the patient's intimate group. In Phase 3, however, patients increasingly take what they have learned and, with the support they now derive from others of like kind, they often confront societal attitudes actively, breaking silence about their illness.

Work Evaluation

It is not uncommon for patients in Phases 1 and 2 to have taken extensive sick leave from their jobs. At first, the crises associated with the onset of their disease usually force them to take time off; then they frequently take further time from work in their attempt to determine what is wrong. When they arrive at a plateau of symptoms, their efforts to return to their preillness work schedule may cause relapses, forcing them to take yet more time off. In some cases, clinicians are able to help Phase 2 patients make workplace adjustments or educate employers to the patient's illness so that the patient is able to continue working. But if it has not happened already, by the time many chronically ill patients reach Phase 3, their employers may want to terminate them. This may occur even though the employer has full knowledge of the patient's illness, is aware of the issue of discrimination, and knows that the patient-employee has rights as a disabled person.

Examples

Sophia lived at too great a distance for her family to provide meaningful assistance in a regular fashion. She recognized that she frequently needed help and had finally learned how to ask others for it. **Sophia** was in great need of a richer community of friends, however. During Phase 3, she achieved this through her spiritual activity, which came to be a defining aspect of her new self. This is discussed later.

Everett and Joan resolved many of their family issues during Phase 2. Although awkward moments continued to occur, the couple managed to deal with their changed roles and responsibilities. Their sons and daughters-in-law could see that the new arrangements were working reasonably well. They learned that they had to help only when help was requested. Because they were not required to care for their parents full time, they gradually reverted to a pattern of social visits as well as assistance visits, which brought a great deal of joy back into their parents' lives. Joan especially was happy to see her grandchildren regularly. **Everett** needed additional contacts, however, and a broader social world. What he found is discussed later.

Everett could not return to work. He received a small pension from his former employer, and both he and Joan began collecting Social Security. Although their income was small, their financial needs were not great, and they owned their house outright.

Christine found a new passion in raising her daughter, but she also made new social contacts. She became part of a prayer group and formally joined an MS support group. Not only did her new friends give her life added emotional richness, but also the members of both groups understood her condition and would meet at her house when she was unable to get out. They also made themselves available to help when **Christine**'s regular helpers were sick or otherwise unable to come. Although **Christine** felt that she had forced Michael to take on more burdens in the marriage than were "fair," she knew that he loved her, still desired her company and companionship, and rejoiced with her in their newfound parenthood. They faced ongoing struggles with the disability company, but **Christine** and her doctors, with the assistance of her social worker, had learned how to present a strong case in her favor.

Lewis realized that he could lead a "normal" life despite his condition. He could seek the love and companionship with a woman, he could have friends, and he could join clubs or groups. Although he knew that stress (good or bad) would almost certainly generate an increase in his disturbing ideations, they no longer frightened him as completely as they had in the past. Moreover, when he felt doubt, he knew that he could discuss his fears openly with me. **Lewis** was thoroughly involved in his teaching, which he loved, and was able to maintain a full-time schedule.

Kim found companionship among the other students in her degree program. She lived in an apartment by herself, but her parents lived nearby and provided both financial and physical assistance.

Gina had to face the daunting task of discussing with Vince the person she had now become. She knew that they had to establish different roles and responsibilities in their marriage and life together. Although **Gina** could not help believing that she was now a burden to Vince, she had to accept the reality of her situation. She also knew that she had to ask for part-time teaching.

Joshua's anger at what had happened to him and at a lifetime of working to overcome the obstacles of racism were the catalysts in a new activity that came to fill his life. He began to make friends with other Black men with hypertension. They found him to be such an articulate spokesman for the problems they faced with doctors and in the workplace that he came to be in demand to give formal presentations. He continued to work at his old job, but as his public speaking engagements began to demand more of his time, he asked to work part time. He was near retirement age, his wife earned an adequate salary, and their major expenses were past, so **Joshua** did not feel driven financially. He had not, however, discussed his condition and his fears with his wife, and he needed to do this.

Erin, a public interest lawyer, had battled ill health and the deaths of loved ones while getting through college and law school. Although she had almost no immediate family living now, she had a strong cadre of friends. After passing the bar exam, **Erin** worked for Legal Aid, taking the cases of people too poor to afford legal counsel. She then joined a legal policy organization, which helped defend the interests of the poor by examining programs intended to serve them but often poorly administered. The group provided legal analysis to lawyers working in the public interest sector. **Erin**'s work absorbed all the time she could devote to it, but it also provided her with an enormous sense of satisfaction and

PHASE 3
Checklist for Assessment

Physical/Behavioral Domain

_____ 1. Has the patient received a medical review? Have the patient's medications been reviewed?

_____ 2. Have you reviewed the patient's activities with him or her?

Psychological Domain

_____ 1. What indicators place this patient in Phase 3?

_____ 2. Have you asked the patient to provide/update his or her personal narrative?

_____ 3. Has the patient begun to express existential concerns? Is the patient despairing? Is the patient potentially suicidal?

Social/Interactive Domain

_____ 1. Have you conducted a family/partner case management review? What were the results?

_____ 2. Have you begun to discuss the patient's wider social world?

_____ 3. Have you conducted a work evaluation? Are there issues with the patient's employer or fellow workers?

---

introduced her to many people who became stout friends. She felt she was helping to make policy that established some social justice in an often unfair and cruel society. Her physical collapse required a complete reevaluation of her future. It also required her to call extensively on her busy friends for help and support. **Erin** had always been a fighter, but she was now tired to death of fighting. The trouble was that she didn't know how to do otherwise.

CLINICAL GOAL AND TREATMENT ISSUES IN PHASE 3

The overarching clinical goal of Phase 3 is to help the patient develop meaning and construct a new self.

The major treatment issues of Phase 3 are to facilitate patients' processing of the deep grief resulting from the loss of their precrisis self and to help them develop personally significant spiritual or philosophical meaning in their lives. This usually takes the form of what may be called a "vertical" search for meaning because it focuses closely on the patient's individual place in the universe. In Phase 4, this search for meaning expands "horizontally" to include discovering meaning that defines a broadly engaged life. On the practical level, the major treatment activities involve teaching patients how to coordinate their medical requirements and to maintain successful monitoring and analysis of their activity thresholds. Clinicians also seek to teach patients and their partners or families how to maintain their own case management, and they work with patients to modify their work situation appropriately or to help effect the most supportive job separation. They may also provide guidance in the process of applying for disability benefits.

TREATMENT: PHYSICAL/BEHAVIORAL DOMAIN

Learning Medical Coordination and Advocacy

For the most part, intervention concerning the physical issues of Phase 3 patients takes the form of education. Patients are now ready to begin learning how to be their own medical coordinators and advocates. Not all patients can. The level of disability in some requires that another person act as coordinator. But for those who can, Phase 3 is where their education in these areas begins. They now accept that they are not going to return to their precrisis normal, and they recognize that, practically speaking, they need to assume responsibility for their health maintenance process. Clinicians begin to teach patients about the various elements of their medical profile and the issues likely to be most pertinent. They discuss the desired effects of the protocols the patient now undertakes. This includes the side effects of medications, the results of physical or occupational therapy, the improvements or lack thereof from nutritional therapy, and the reasons for continuing the protocols or perhaps eventually eliminating them. In other words, clinicians start teaching patients to take over management activities that clinicians have up to this point coordinated.

If patients have internalized the lessons and activities of Phase 2, they have begun to acquire competence in speaking for themselves with medical and other health care professionals. They are becoming active consumers of medical care and hence will avoid or leave harmful or ineffective practitioners.

PHASE 3
Treatment

Physical/Behavioral Domain
    Education as own medical coordinator
    Education as own health care advocate
    Education as own activity monitor

Psychological Domain
    Maintenance of insight and issue reframing
    Expression of grief for lost self
    Existential dilemma
    Definition of pre-crisis self
    Analysis of actual losses
    Commitment to "time in the tunnel"
    Baseline authenticity
    Antithetical intervention
    Creative process and activities
    New societal attitudes
    Exploration of different traditions
    Meaning development
    Faith and humor

Social/Interactive Domain
    Education of couples and families in self-management
    Patient political action
    Change of supporters
    Work interventions

Attention to Activity Threshold

Phase 3 patients have the skills now to monitor their own activity thresholds and to assess how well they are maintaining their physical equilibrium. They understand how they personally experience the arc of any activity they perform, and they are familiar with their basic physical and emotional constitution. They know that they need to monitor their symptoms, engage in activities from all four different areas when possible, and assert values and norms that best support their greatest level of health and functioning. They have learned how to trade off activities. They know, for example, that they may engage in occasional strenuous exertion if they make up for it later by rest and subsequent restorative activities in other areas. By Phase 3, clinicians perform only an oversight function concerning activity thresholds. They answer questions and make suggestions when patients ask for them.

Examples

As noted in the assessment section, all of the patients developed the ability to manage their health needs and to review their activity thresholds. Most were living in a plateau of symptoms, but even those who were gradually deteriorating, like **Sophia** and **Christine**, had a fairly sophisticated knowledge of how to follow through during the investigation of new problems. Most of the patients had suffered at least one relapse, so they were aware that it could happen again. Most also had come to recognize at least intellectually that they would eventually suffer other crises, whether related to their current condition or totally separate.

TREATMENT: PSYCHOLOGICAL DOMAIN

Maintaining Insight and Issue Reframing

Given the intensity of the new psychological work in Phase 3, it is important for clinicians to check with patients regularly to see whether they are maintaining insight and continuing to reframe daily events in terms of all they have learned about their bodies, their minds, and society's attitudes. Clinicians must provide constant reinforcement on the practical issues of chronic illness as they and their patients move forward into a more profound grieving for the patients' lost self, the development of a new identity, and an exploration of spiritual or philosophical meaning development.

Deep Grief for Lost Self

The grief over the lost precrisis self that patients experience in Phase 2 tends to happen because it has been encouraged by the clinician. The patients infrequently will this grief to occur or consciously and actively mourn their loss. Instead, patients usually suppress such feelings because that is what society prefers. Moreover, patients in Phases 1 and 2 often refuse to accept the idea that the precrisis life is gone forever and hence refuse to acknowledge any permanent losses. By Phase 3, however, they know the old life and the precrisis self will never return. Their grief is profound, and in Phase 3 many will, with support, choose to engage it intentionally because it is difficult, if not dangerous, for them to suppress it.

Existential Dilemma

With the death of the self that they perceived themselves to be and the end of the life they had intended to live, chronically ill patients and those around them usually experience great dread and confusion. Phase 3 patients are thrown into a severe existential dilemma as they try to determine why they should live and how. From their point of view, they have fallen into a dark pit. They are in the depths of despair.

Dark Night of the Soul

Many clinicians find this period difficult to treat, both because of the countertransferential issues it generates and because it strongly resembles clinical depression. Indeed, it can be considered a form of depression. Medication may be necessary because it can help to moderate patients' emotions and help them to think more clearly. But medication is not sufficient, and it will not resolve the underlying cause. The only effective method of dealing with the problem itself is for clinicians and patients to work through this dark night of the soul together. What patients need now from their clinicians is a deeply compassionate response and an open, articulated willingness to accompany the patient on the journey through this painful, dark, frightening tunnel toward finding a new self and a new life. Many clinicians find this experience too intense because it can easily release all their own personal fears and terrors about the meaning of existence. Some try to move their patients to other practitioners or primarily treat the patients with medication for depression. But if patients fail to negotiate this difficult path, develop a new identity, and locate some personally meaningful concept of life, however much the concept may shift and change over time, they nearly always slip back into a perpetual vicious cycle alternating between Phase 1 and Phase 2. Out of despair and hopelessness, they can fall victim to fraudulent practitioners or even commit suicide.

Defining the Precrisis Self

While engaging the patient's grief reaction with a compassionate response and allowing and welcoming the most profound kind of mourning, clinicians also begin to elicit very specific characteristics of the patient's precrisis self. This self involves two aspects, an external one involved in the roles the patient performs in life and an internal one often characterized by descriptions such as extroverted or introverted, boisterous or quiet, assertive or passive.

When first asked to describe their precrisis self, patients sometimes state only that they were happy before they were ill, they liked who they were, and they believed that they had a future. Now they dislike what they have become and have little hope of fulfillment in life. Clinicians must tease out details. Did the patients like being the center of attention or did they prefer to observe quietly what was going on around them? Did they speak up and take charge of situations, or did they tend to defer to the wishes and opinions of others? Were they fearless or anxious? Were they emotional or stoic? Did they take pride in being physically or emotionally strong? Did they value being able to support their families? Were they figures of importance in their business? Did they take pride in being quick-witted and clever? Did they love sailing? Did they plan to have children? Had they always been athletic, especially enjoying tennis and dancing? Were they deeply involved in community activities?

Other questions place this illness struggle in context. Have the patients struggled to overcome other adversities? Had they perhaps just gotten their lives in order, only to have this illness make pointless all their hard work? If patients are young people, have they even begun to have an adult life? What did they hope to be and do, or were they completely confused about the future even before their illness?

Analysis of Actual Losses—External

Clinicians help patients identify and then analyze the specific qualities and roles that the patients felt defined them. With changes to the external self, it sometimes becomes clear that qualities necessary for the roles have not, as a matter of fact, been lost absolutely, but only in the particular guise that patients experienced them before illness. Patients may still be perfectly capable of raising healthy, happy children even though they must use a wheelchair and rely on the spouse's income to supplement their own disability payments.

Socially active patients may still participate meaningfully in the life of their church or community organization, for instance. But they may have to limit their activities to one or two committees and participate in meetings only every two months or so.

Internal Changes

Internal changes are often even more distressing to patients and seem far more indicative of fundamentally undesirable change than external role changes. When patients have always been assertive and outgoing, they can feel enormously diminished in their current fearfulness and introversion. When they have prided themselves on their self-control, they can feel hopelessly betrayed by how easily their emotions now break through. But patients can form no new attitudes or evaluations until they have actually contemplated specifically what they felt they were before and what they think they are now.

Using the Clinician's Faith

Whereas some aspects of self have not actually been lost altogether, others are truly gone forever, including a relative freedom from pain and the density of experiences that can give a healthy life much of its richness. Nearly all patients find themselves trying to deal with new personality characteristics or with aspects of themselves that had never been significant in their lives before. In their external world, some patients will have lost friends, jobs, or even partners. Some will have lost their entire old world. All patients need a great deal of support and guidance as they come to terms with their new personality characteristics, make new friendships, and create new structures for living. At the very start, they especially rely on the clinician's abiding faith that they will be able to build a meaningful life.

Committing to Time in the Tunnel

Clinicians have to be painfully honest with patients at this point. The work ahead is not easy, and there are no guarantees about particular outcomes. At the same time, clinicians must profess profound faith that patients will ultimately benefit from the process and will come through to a better life.

Metaphor is almost the only way to convey what patients now face. They must commit to endure a difficult term of imprisonment; they are going to do hard time. They will experience discomfort as they search for a new self, and, at the same time, they will have no clear sense of direction or even illumination of the scene itself. Despite the fact that few things or people outside themselves, other than the clinician, encourage them, they must bravely persist in the process. Clinicians must assure their patients that unlikely as it seems, they will, nevertheless, be able to do this.

Phoenix from the Ashes

Most Phase 3 patients know all too well that their old lives have burned to the ground. What clinicians are asking them now is whether they will commit to a process of trying to find something better than their current situation, even though they must endure daily pain and difficulty. Clinicians must assert with conviction that a phoenix can arise from the ashes. Although a few patients may just wish to die at the beginning of Phase 3, clinicians must emphatically assure them that it is worthwhile to them as clinicians, and will be to the patients as well, to invest the time and energy necessary for the patients to create themselves anew.

Importance of Countertransference

Satisfactory resolution of countertransferential issues is of the utmost importance in Phase 3. Patients can borrow faith only from clinicians who continuously acknowledge and process their own terrors and inadequacies. During Phase 3, clinicians must not only convince patients of their faith that the patients can win through to a better life, but also teach patients how to respect their suffering, creatively learn from it, and bring value from it. This faith is something the clinician must feel. It cannot be faked.

Baseline Authenticity

To create the new self, patients must build on a solid base. Patients often say that they don't know how to feel authentic or how to do this thing of finding authenticity. Actually, there is no "doing." They observe and note how they feel and what they think right now. They accept as true of themselves only those feelings and thoughts that are genuine, real, and authentic. It is essential for patients to carry out this process safely in a safe place with a safe person or people. They must reject all the pretenses that they have maintained up to now to meet societal or family or even their own inner expectations. All feelings are acceptable expressions as long as they do not actually hurt the patient or other people.

At first, the authentic Phase 3 self may be simply a miasma of rage, pain, grief, and misery. But clinicians should assure patients that even these emotions have real value simply because they are genuine. With nearly everything from the old life stripped away, it may seem to leave patients only bare stony ground, but clinicians point out that the ground is real and provides a solid base. Throughout patients' journeys toward discovery of a new self and some form of life meaning, clinicians constantly ask them to test any new assertions about themselves for personal truth and genuineness.

These Phase 3 activities would be impossible for patients in Phases 1 or 2 because in those phases patients openly or privately believe that eventually they will find a cure and be returned to their former life. Phase 3 patients no longer think they will be cured or cured in any foreseeable future. And they are usually relieved to stop pretending. They are tired of struggling vainly to pass and attempting to meet impossible desires or expectations. Such behavior has not returned them to their prior state, but instead has consistently depleted their limited energy. As Phase 3 patients begin the very gradual process of creating a new, authentic identity, they also usually begin making wholly new choices about their mix of activities from the four groups. Establishing what is truly meaningful to them often radically revises their priorities about how they will expend their practical energy.

Antithetical Experimentation

One opening strategy some clinicians use involves encouraging patients to experiment with totally antithetical roles or identities or emotions. Sometimes this can happen very easily because the patients have actually been thrown into those identities, albeit against their will. Clinicians can guide them to see or imagine benefits from these new personality characteristics or to see the purposes and satisfactions that can arise from different roles. Without getting into simplistic notions of using the lemons of life to make lemonade, patients can be guided toward understanding potentialities that they have never before considered. The individual who was once highly active may learn satisfactions that can be gained from quiet, but intense, contemplation or observation. The person who used to take charge may find rewards in learning how to be more receptive. Eventually, and most importantly, clinicians help patients to see and to realize that even their suffering, once the thing they most rejected, can be productive and worthy of their respect.

Creative Process

Creation of a new identity occurs most smoothly when patients deeply engage their creative processes in some manner that is personally rewarding. Some use writing, but others paint, carve, compose, dance, sing, or build. The activity need not be anything traditionally considered creative. It may consist of tying fishing flies, training dogs, designing a new fall wardrobe, or becoming involved in political activities. It may simply involve making a collage out of magazine photos or knitting a scarf. Even those patients with very limited resources need to be helped to find a way to express themselves creatively. What is important is that the activity be personally meaningful and that it engage the patient's imaginative and creative energies. Ultimately, patients use their awakened creativity to construct their illness narrative as a proud story of heroism, but getting to this may be a long, circuitous process (Aberbach, 1989; Edwards, 1993; Holm-Hadulla, 1996).

Reading Materials

For patients who read, clinicians often find it helpful to recommend accounts by prisoners such as Nelson Mandela or Martin Luther King, who used their time in jail to grow politically, socially, and spiritually. They can also call attention to culturally familiar stories such as Christ's 40 days in the wilderness or the story of Job. All stories of people coming through difficulty and adversity to meaningful lives serve to strengthen patients' resolve to continue through to a new life. If the patient comes from a very unfamiliar tradition, the clinician can try to elicit from the patient equivalent stories from his or her culture, or the clinician can, with a librarian's help, try to locate material that might be meaningful.

Clinician as Storyteller

If patients are not readers, clinicians must become storytellers. Some stories recall to patients the folk stories they have probably known since childhood, in which heroes suffer difficulty, pain, neglect, or hostility but persist in their quest until they succeed, sometimes with the help of apparently insignificant others whom they themselves were once able to help. Some stories should honor unrecognized heroism. Clinicians can point out, for example, that by the Catholic Church's own assertion, most saints in history have never been recognized but have led their lives of heroic virtue totally unknown. Clinicians must continuously acknowledge that patients cannot possibly see to the end of the journey, but that the journey itself has significance and value. It is a mystery worth living in.

The Noble-Disabled Danger

Clinicians tread a fine line here. They do not want to project their patients as examples of heroic stoicism set on earth solely to enlighten those members of the public who are not suffering as the patients are. Rather, clinicians want their patients to recognize that they are, as a matter of fact, exhibiting enormous bravery daily, that they are heroes, even though their outward activities appear ordinary and often very limited. They encourage patients to honor their suffering because they have endured it and sometimes, perhaps, they have learned from it. In any case, honoring of suffering is made concrete by patients' expressions of compassion for the suffering self.

Nonverbal Creative Activities

It is important to note here that nonverbal creative activities often build significant meaning, even though it cannot be conveyed in words. Music, particularly, but also the experience of nature, can directly affect a patient's spirit and generate a profound sense of meaningful place in the cosmos. Because the relationship between clinician and patient is mediated through words and written material is a most useful way to convey many different ways of thinking about issues, it is easy to fix on verbal expression to the exclusion of equally important methods of reaching for meaning. But for many patients, clinicians need to help them find nonverbal forms both to communicate and to express themselves.

Clinician Share Activities

Where possible, clinicians should share activities with patients to get the creative process started. They and patients may find themselves eating together or squashing play dough into shapes together. One clinician recommended that a patient buy cheap crockery from garage sales and joined her in dramatic binges of smashing as a way to express rage and grief.

New Vision of Societal Attitudes

As patients assemble a true, authentic self, they become aware in an altogether new way of societal attitudes and how damaging they can be. Although they have learned about social stigmatization and traumatization in Phases 1 and 2, in Phase 3 the falsity of societal attitudes becomes transparent. Patients now refuse to collude with the culture, either consciously or unconsciously. Most of the time, they manage to stop explaining, excusing, or defending themselves to others, but stand proudly with themselves as being valuable human beings just as they are. It is this solid awareness of how wrong and hurtful the culture can be that impels many chronically ill Phase 3 patients to take up political or social action.

Exploring Different Traditions

In Phase 2, many clinicians draw successfully from the methods of the cognitive behaviorists, grief strategists, solution-focused therapists, to name a few. But Phase 3 interventions require other resources. Clinicians must use an array of creative expressions and help their patients explore meaning as it is expressed in many different cultural and philosophical traditions.

Meaning Development

At the same time that patients are using antithetical experimentation and creative expression to help find authentic elements that will help to form their new self, they are also pursuing an investigation of existential meaning and purpose. Clinicians should develop a rich library of materials and maintain a strong network of spiritual/philosophical contacts so that they can make available to their patients the widest possible array of thinking and contemplation on the subject. The development of meaning is further elaborated at the end of this chapter.

All these activities tend to return a sense of control to patients, and they also permit and encourage expressions of compassion for the self. Moreover, they reveal and at the same time support a growing tolerance for ambiguity and chronicity. The new self lives in a universe where physical, mental, and emotional characteristics change and shift all the time. Phase 3 patients become matter of fact about the ambiguities and chronicity of their situation, which are simply givens in the world that the new self is learning to manage.

Faith and Humor

One vitally important aspect of the relationship between clinician and patient—humor—is absolutely essential by the time that patient and clinician travel together through the dark tunnel toward meaning. Faith and humor, even black humor about how horrible the situation is, can sometimes help move the work forward significantly. The darkest time is not necessarily when clinicians should introduce humor into their relationship with patients, but they certainly want to have some lightness and the ability to joke by the time they get to Phase 3. And long before Phase 3, clinicians must have impressed on their patients their total faith that the patients will come through to a better life (P. L. Berger, 1999; L. Brown, 1991; Hassed, 2001; Rodning, 1988; Samra, 1985; Yates, 2001).

Examples

Sophia recognized that her condition was permanent early in her sessions with me. It contributed to her despair and her turning away completely from thinking along scientific lines. During Phase 2, she could also see that she was not even always maintaining a plateau of symptoms. When she was finally able to take in information about her activities management and carry out some changes, she hoped that her altered behavior would improve her condition. She did learn to use such energy as she had more efficiently, but even when she began asking others for help, she did not improve markedly. She felt better, however, and was not deteriorating at the rate she had been.

She also began approaching her enormous grief in Phase 2, so by Phase 3 she was truly able to mourn the world and hopes she had lost. She had been completely wrapped up in her research, and her accomplishments had been groundbreaking. All her mentors and colleagues expected her to continue excelling as she had throughout school, college, graduate education, and early professional career. Although **Sophia** was a lovely, friendly individual, her close connections were almost entirely collegial. Losing her work—and her cognitive impairments made work impossible—was apparently to lose everything.

But **Sophia**'s strong religious upbringing and daily practice of prayer and meditation gave her a place to begin looking for help and comfort and, ultimately, for meaning. Initially, I encouraged her to complain to God, to rage and suffer in her prayers. This did help **Sophia** begin expressing her feelings authentically. A great transformational moment came for her, however, when she decided to attend a professional clinical conference on death and spirituality. Getting to the conference and staying at a hotel were a major production for **Sophia**. But she wanted to listen to scientists talk about an issue that was vitally important to her now.

What she found was a completely involving emotional and intellectual event. At several panels, she was asked to contribute as an audience member with highly relevant experience. She was so exhausted by talking that in one instance she had to lie down on the floor of the conference room to recover. The speakers and audience did not regard this as embarrassing or unseemly but came to her assistance with sympathy and understanding. They made her feel that she had done exactly the right thing at that particular moment. More broadly, they made it clear that she was offering them information of great importance to the work they were pursuing. When she returned home, she was alight with ideas about helping people in pain and disability, like herself, find a supportive, spiritually oriented community of friends and supporters. She began creating prayer and meditation groups via the Internet with people like herself—scientists, academics, thinkers. Because people like **Sophia** are dispersed all over the country and the world, it is sometimes hard for them to find others like themselves who talk and think like themselves.

Sophia is without question fortunate in having been raised by a loving family that supported her as best they could when she became ill. She did not suffer erosion of her self because of her family. But she had certainly been damaged by the way everyone at work seemed to turn on her when she became ill. Somewhat naively, she had believed she had made a new kind of family. When her illness interfered with ongoing profitable research, however, she discovered that those who watched the bottom line just wanted to get rid of her, and the rest were not going to risk promotion or even their jobs by coming to her defense. With the prayer circles, however, she found like-minded people again, but this time she was forging links to people who genuinely had minds and souls that she could admire.

Sophia did not believe that her prayer circle activities would change her condition, but she felt that living authentically with genuine people who also felt love and connectedness with her and each other was doing something meaningful in the universe, or, as **Sophia** put it, they were performing what was in "God's mind."

Kim suffered terribly as she attempted to grapple with the work of Phase 3. Probably because she had experienced substantial benefits in the prior work she had done—she had overcome crisis and internalized a significant degree of control—she sincerely wanted to move forward. She conscientiously tried a variety of creative activities, including writing her autobiography and illness narrative. She did find some calm and a temporary sense of emotional expansion when listening to music. I tried to involve **Kim** in antithetical exercises, but attempts to locate a basic, authentic **Kim** proved unsuccessful. **Kim** could not tolerate authentic feelings of emotional pain for any period of time.

It also proved impossible for me to help **Kim** break a pattern that had characterized her response to a variety of therapies. **Kim** would commit herself to a new technique or new therapy with a high degree of optimism. She would assiduously follow instructions, especially if she experienced some relief by doing so. But when the necessary work began to create emotional difficulty, pain, or suffering, she would lose all the insight she had developed as to why the difficult work was necessary to help her improve and how the pain she felt now was temporary. It was as though **Kim** were in physical therapy, and when attempting to extend her range of motion caused her pain, she quit exercising altogether. Moreover, each time that **Kim** quit a therapy, she was completely convinced that the fault lay in the technique, not in her unwillingness to pursue it.

Kim tended to seek out friends who also believed in a wide variety of alternative approaches and promised cures. They kept track of all the new allopathic or alternative methods that were enjoying current popularity and encouraged those in the group who needed help to seek rescue in the new therapy. As with many Americans, **Kim** and her friends wanted quick, total results. They would follow a new program attentively for a short period of time, but when a brief expenditure of effort did not produce complete cure, they would become discouraged. Soon another method or cure would appear, and they would flock to it in hopes that here was the fast miracle method they needed.

Thus, although **Kim** had seemed on the verge of understanding the chronicity of her condition—one characteristic of a person entering Phase 3—she slipped back into a Phase 1-Phase 2 cycle when she found that the work was too difficult for her to carry out. Once again, she grasped at the hope—strongly supported in this by her friends—that a therapy existed that would cure her altogether. She had only to find it.

Each time **Kim** pressed against the limits of her ability to benefit from a therapy, she would began to experience a sharp rise in anxiety and desperation. This growing panic would stimulate her search for the new therapy, but it also marked a slipping back into the crisis situation of Phase 1. Unfortunately, **Kim**'s desperation and disillusion appeared to grow with each succeeding phase cycle. Her anxiety increased, but her compliance with successful therapies or techniques declined, exacerbating her physical symptoms.

When **Kim** left my practice, she said that she had heard of a new clinician who was achieving cures for people like herself. It was probable that this new program will stabilize her into Phase 2. However, unless she actually does achieve a cure, **Kim** will probably endure repeated cycles of Phase 1 and Phase 2 as she lives in chronicity but attempts to find a magic bullet cure.

Without consciously planning it, **Christine** began a completely authentic, antithetical experiment when she took on the role of mother. Instead of behaving as her own family had behaved toward her and demanding the sorts of responses her own family did, **Christine** was able to create for Mei a very different reality—a childhood and family that was loving and supportive of the individual that Mei was. In the multitude of creative acts that made up **Christine**'s parenting, she gained insight and was able to reframe her own experience. She had to struggle to maintain these insights about her birth family and also those that she had learned in conversation with me. But in her efforts to reframe events in terms of what she had learned since becoming ill, **Christine** received help from Michael, from her MS friends, from me, and even from Mei.

Every day, **Christine** learned that regardless of what she had lost—and she was constantly aware of how limited her physical parenting was compared to what she had once imagined—she had gained riches from Mei that she never imagined. At first, merely holding the baby and enjoying Mei's smiling response were miracle enough. But as Mei got older, **Christine** found that she loved answering the little girl's perpetual questions because she could do that from the couch. Indeed, the couch became part of the game. Sometimes it was an island, sometimes a ship or a car or a house, on which Mei and her mother had imaginary adventures. Mei loved showing **Christine** her toys, playing in front of her, having an audience. **Christine** was the perfect listener because she moved around very little. Mei's enjoyment of Michael's physicality pleased **Christine** as well. If she couldn't be as boisterous as she wanted with her baby, Michael could. **Christine** felt that the three of them were a real team. Despite the fact that she tried to grieve her losses, **Christine** mostly found herself delighting in her extraordinary gains.

Christine did, however, have pressing fears in relation to Mei. She was greatly concerned about Mei having a disturbed childhood or becoming neurotic because she was growing up so deeply embedded in an illness experience. I reminded **Christine** that Mei had come from a situation where she probably would not have had as good a life as that she was now living. In addition, **Christine** and I discussed how many people grow up in complex situations with challenges. Mei would doubtless experience good and bad effects from her particular childhood, regardless of what **Christine** and Michael did to mitigate the situation.

Christine also knew that she might not live to see Mei reach adulthood or have children. The sorrow and dread that this produced found some expression in her prayers, where she placed herself in the hands of God. God's reality for her, however, was largely manifested in the kindly, loving involvement of the prayer group members, so **Christine** for the most part believed that God would permit her to live as Mei's mother for as long as Mei needed. She still attended the Catholic Church when she was well and enjoyed the music and ritual of the services, but she paid little heed to spiritual or metaphysical directives from the Church. Her meaningful spiritual center was located in her prayer group and her new family.

Lewis worked assiduously to maintain insight into how his condition affected his life and how it could generate disturbing ideations. Although few others realized **Lewis**'s problems, he had tended to judge himself by attitudes he'd learned from the general culture. Now he consciously attempted to reframe issues that seemed to threaten or stigmatize him. He was worried about whether he had the stamina, however, to continue this for the rest of his life. Sometimes, it just seemed too much.

He began to examine what he had learned in his illness and the misery it had caused him. Was there a real and valuable **Lewis** who could emerge from this? I called attention to **Lewis**'s own heroic past and how he had struggled out of poverty to achieve an education and then a profession in which he shared the benefits he had gained with others. Because he had never read many stories as a child, I gave him a collection of folktales from around the world, which dramatize stories such as his. I then encouraged him to read biographies, particularly of Black men, who had struggled against near insuperable odds to achieve benefits for themselves and their people. **Lewis** had never conceived that the descriptive terms of heroism and courage might apply to him, and he very slowly began to develop a respect for all that he had done in his life.

Everett was loath to engage in any self-examination, which he had always regarded as a boring thing that women did among themselves. Nonetheless, he was slowly brought to examine his losses and eventually to express some grief. It was very hard, however, for **Everett** to move beyond a lifetime of considering strong, silent behavior as defining the most worthy sort of man. Listening to his family express their gratitude and admiration helped him see that it was not his stoicism that they admired, but his active love and engagement with them. He discovered that his strong, silent behavior had tended to keep his family at a greater distance than either he or they desired. **Everett** was also touched and strengthened by the utter indifference of his young grandchildren to his condition. They asked him questions, hung on his answers, laughed with him, and told him about their activities, all with total disregard for his limited mobility. **Everett** even came to see that his condition kept him fixed in one place for them, unlike their fathers, who could brush the children off to go mow the lawn or wash the car.

Although **Everett** wasn't much of a reader, he became interested in watching history programs on TV. When he saw a documentary on captured American flyers in Vietnam, he suddenly had a way of understanding what I had been talking about when I had spoken of his time in captivity. He found himself looking for other programs about imprisoned soldiers and even began reading some books that I located on the subject. Although he felt he was in a much better situation than the captive soldiers, he also recognized that, in some ways, it was worse because he now acknowledged his situation wasn't going to change. All the same, the courage, persistence, and concern for others that these soldiers expressed gave him models that he took to heart.

Everett also learned that part of his pleasure when he used to go camping and fishing with his sons occurred because of the beauty of the places they went. Even with his disability, this natural scene was not lost to him. Joan or one of his sons would sometimes take him by car to one of the more accessible mountain lakes where he used to fish. There they would just sit with him quietly, absorbing the surroundings. In a confidence that I treasured, **Everett** revealed his belief that in the works of nature, he could see the hand of God. On some level, as **Everett** accepted the permanence of his disability, he also felt raised out of despair because he believed that a God who troubled to make such grandeur as the natural world offered had a purpose for him as well.

Gina's careful examination of her activities brought home to her consciously that she was chronically ill and that her symptoms would probably shift and change over time, not necessarily for the better. Having lived with her children's difficulties, she was intellectually open to the chronicity and ambiguity of her condition. What she had to face now, however, was that she couldn't continue trying to be her old self. The practicalities of this were daunting enough, but emotionally **Gina** was devastated. She felt like half a person at best, like someone hardly worth bothering with. She was also confronting a real problem in her marriage just at the point where she desperately needed support. Only her responsibilities toward her children, she said, kept her from seriously contemplating suicide.

I offered **Gina** my own faith that she was going to find a way to live that was not only possible but also fulfilling. I noted that **Gina** would probably find relief when she finally acknowledged to herself, but also to those around her, that she was not who she had been. But more than relief, I asserted, **Gina** would gradually discover a self who was truly

Gina, not a construct of her parents' expectations, her husband's expectations, her school administrators' expectations, and so forth. Moreover, **Gina** would not need to abandon everything about the past. Probably what she valued most in her old self would appear, perhaps transformed, in the new self as well.

Gina felt that being a successful mother was of primary importance to her, followed by being a good teacher. Not long ago, she noted sadly, she wanted to be a good wife as well, but increasingly now that seemed to her to be a meaningless one-way street. As she and I discussed what constituted being a good mother and a good teacher, **Gina** realized that it need not depend on exhausting physical output. What her children most needed from her was not guided activity but love and attention. She could sit at the kitchen table and listen to them. Teaching necessarily demanded more physically, but she could still be a good teacher teaching fewer classes.

Gina was embarrassed to admit it, but the children's adventure stories she had taken to reading actually spoke to her about courage and persistence and bravery in the way that adult books and conversations didn't. The central figures in the stories had not had their honest reactions trained out of them yet, nor had they lost their desire to do good, to care for people, to love. **Gina** realized that deep inside she sometimes still felt like one of those children. It was these emotions that animated her deep desire to protect and help her own children. **Gina** began to believe that she had to become completely honest about herself to herself. For strategic reasons, she might pretend with other people sometimes, but with herself she had to become completely authentic. This meant that she examined just about everything that happened to her during the day as well as everything she did and thought to see what it meant to her.

As discussed earlier, **Joshua** took creative action by engaging in what was essentially political action. He might be stuck living with this problem—and he was still scared—but he was going to fight all the problems surrounding it as long as he could. It became clear to **Joshua** that although he'd lost, for example, the freedom to travel because of his worries about his health, he had gained new friends and a new sense of purpose.

Erin, the new patient, needed to express and explore her deep grief, not only for her life now, but also for all the losses she had mourned in the past. She could do this, but the tunnel in which she now found herself was so black, so devoid of the possibility of light anywhere, that she still felt utter despair. **Erin** loved music, so I suggested that she listen for at least an hour a day to her favorite composers. **Erin** must have spent a month with Bach's Brandenburg Concertos. Their beauty and balance went directly to her emotional center, causing her to weep and then to calm afterwards and rejoice, for no reason that **Erin** could articulate. She felt they put her in touch with something larger and more impersonal than herself, but something that was also beautiful in a way that flooded her with a sense of gratitude.

As **Erin** began to be able to talk, she discovered an unexpected bond with me. We both had a very unorthodox, black sense of humor. **Erin** had seen so much death and trouble and cruelty that sometimes all she could do was laugh about it. When I wasn't shocked, as **Erin**'s colleagues often were, but instead genuinely joined her, **Erin** realized that she'd found a way to throw up her hands without giving up. She was tired of always fighting, even fighting the good fight, and humor relieved her. It also gave her a different way of observing how she felt.

Erin became thoroughly involved in two projects simultaneously—her personal narrative and the definition of her preillness self. She teased out early attitudes and defining experiences with all the relentlessness of a well-paid tax lawyer and reevaluated and reframed them with all the skill of an ill-paid public interest lawyer.

The questions still remained of why **Erin**? Or indeed why anyone? **Erin** came to the conclusion that the answers for her had hovered just beneath her consciousness all her life. Her sheer output of work, she felt, was her attempt to do what God or whoever should have made unnecessary in the first place. She was out to save her bit of the world despite God. Contemplation led her to certain insights, although she could keep them in mind only momentarily. Most important was the notion that in caring about others in the world, particularly others who are unable to care properly for themselves, people enter a place where a good God either exists or could exist, and it doesn't really matter which. What is important are the good human actions. Some evils that happen to people, she decided, were the products of human action—and people must fight to change that. Other things happened arbitrarily, such as hurricanes or the flu. To some extent, people may prevent the harmful effects of such things, but for the most part, they are able only to succor those who suffer because of the arbitrary events.

TREATMENT: SOCIAL/INTERACTIVE DOMAIN

Empower Couples and Families

Phase 3 interventions as to family and couples concern transfer of case management from the clinician to the participants. Considerable practical work with a patient's family and partner occurred during Phase 2, and by Phase 3 they have often revised roles and responsibilities into a workable system. But when families or partners achieve a Phase 3 recognition of what chronicity means—that is it not simply a long time, but forever—it can sometimes force them to experience their own dark night of the soul, just as the patient does. Families create the world of the patient, and they may find it very difficult to live philosophically or spiritually with what is happening to the patient and to themselves. Clinicians may need to address these issues or guide the families toward professionals who can help them.

Maintenance of the family responsibility systems now begins to devolve to the participants. Where before they have come to the clinician for help, they now learn how to handle new or changed situations themselves. Clinicians help them begin to create ways to review their situation and intervene only when the patient, a family member, or the patient's partner requests advice.

Patient Political Action

The most striking aspect in the social/interactive domain of some Phase 3 patients is their engagement in social action and political activity. In keeping with their unwillingness to accept whatever ill treatment society metes out to them, patients can often become confrontational. If patients are going to become politicized by society's reaction to their illness, this transformation occurs in Phase 3. As they locate an authentic new self whom they value intrinsically, patients now consciously refuse to accept stigmatization and often feel strongly motivated to work for the betterment of others like themselves. In Phase 2, patients often made contact with organizations composed of people with the same illness because they found there emotional support and understanding and sometimes the answer to questions about their condition. Empowered by their new sense of self, some Phase 3 patients volunteer to promote better knowledge of their illness and improved social attitudes and treatment.

Change of Supporters

Phase 3 patients no longer dissemble with those around them. If family or partners do not accept patients as they are now and the new situation as it is, patients are more willing to try to build lives with others who will support them. But their growing confidence and commitment to their new selves also allow them to attempt to reconnect with previously distanced friends and family. Their clear vision of who they are enables them to act more confidently and without pretense, and this sometimes makes it possible to renew relationships that broke under the strains of Phases 1 or 2.

Work Interventions

Phase 3 patients react to their workplace situations in much the same way as they relate to the outside world in general. Whereas in the prior phases they often sought to continue in their jobs, even though its conditions made it extremely difficult for them to perform, they now take a more assertive stance. Some demand the necessary adaptations to their particular job environment, citing the Americans with Disabilities legislation. Others acknowledge that employment is more than they can handle in their condition and seek disability. Still others seek entirely different work or different work arrangements. Clinicians can provide invaluable information and advice to patients in all these endeavors. They can help with job negotiation, job separation, or job modification. They can guide patients through the complex disability application process. They can help patients sort out the pros and cons of other employment possibilities or work arrangements. Once again, however, clinicians step back into a more advisory role as the patients themselves take charge of reorganizing their employment life or negotiating its closure.

Examples

Most of the patients described in this book worked out solutions to living with their families or friends in Phase 2. Moreover, the activities they carried out at that time gave them a template for dealing with new or changed situations. As with their own interior lives, patients and their families needed to maintain insight and remember to reframe new issues as they came up. As a consequence, my principal interventions in Phase 3 were to remind patients and their families that they had acquired the tools they needed to manage their own affairs.

Gina was one exception to this. It was during Phase 3 that she and her husband separated and ultimately divorced. As **Gina** tried to become more frank and open with Vince about what she needed and how she had to live, he grew more and more distant. He did not like their changed life and barely recognized the woman he had married. He found her now strident, aggressive, and demanding, and at the same time less and less available to spend time with him or show an interest in his activities. **Gina** became increasingly angry at what "for better or for worse, in sickness and in health" apparently meant to Vince, but she also found she didn't care personally if he left. She was terrified, however, about what this would mean for her and the children financially. She couldn't work full time any more, and she knew she needed more than a part-time salary to continue living the way they had. This upheaval sent **Gina** on a downward spiral of debilitating symptoms. I worked to bring **Gina** through this new Phase 1 crisis and to reestablish Phase 2 stabilization. Because of our prior work together, processing the cycle took far less time than it had taken to go through Phase 2 the first time. I also helped **Gina** locate a good lawyer. In addition, I again offered to speak with **Gina**'s school administrators about her condition, but **Gina** had already found that the administration was willing to be flexible about her work schedule. **Gina** knew that attitudes can change with changing administrators, but at that point she was able to pursue satisfactory work arrangements on her own.

Joshua was the clearest example of a typical Phase 3 action in the social/interactive domain. Energized by his own experience—his suffering and his stigmatization—**Joshua** began working with a new group of people to change the way the world around him treated African Americans with his condition. Eventually, as he informed himself further, this political effort encompassed other illnesses besides heart and hypertension conditions.

Joshua still needed to talk candidly with Maybelle about his fears. She needed to understand what he was feeling and why sexual activity

PHASE 3
Checklist for Treatment

Physical/Behavioral Domain

_____ 1. Have you begun educating the patient to become his or her own medical coordinator?

_____ 2. Have you begun educating the patient to become his or her own health care advocate?

_____ 3. Have you begun educating the patient to become his or her own activity monitor?

Psychological Domain

_____ 1. What activities have you recommended to help the patient maintain insight and carry out issue reframing?

_____ 2. Have you encouraged the patient to express grief for the lost self?

_____ 3. Have you helped the patient to define the pre-crisis self and to analyze what actual losses the patient has suffered?

_____ 4. Have you educated the patient to authenticity as the bedrock of the new self?

_____ 5. Have you explored antithetical experimentation with the patient?

_____ 6. Have you encouraged the patient to engage his or her creative processes in whatever area he or she chooses? It is important to have the broadest possible conception of how creativity may be expressed.

_____ 7. Have you explored with the patient new ways of looking at society and at reacting to social attitudes?

_____ 8. Have you encouraged the patient to explore many different traditions to help develop meaning?

_____ 9. Have you exhibited faith and employed humor?

Social/Interactive Domain

_____ 1. Have you begun educating the family/partner in self-management?

_____ 2. Have you encouraged the patient in taking an active role concerning his or her illness?

_____ 3. Have you encouraged the patient to enlist supporters and not to struggle to retain nonsupporters?

_____ 4. If the patient is still working or is on sick leave, do you need to intervene with the employer, coworkers, or the physical work situation? What actions have been carried out?

_____ 5. If the patient cannot work, have you provided assistance or helped find expert assistance as to disability?

scared him. Because the prospect of such a talk humiliated him, **Joshua** took some time to recognize that such a conversation was necessary and important for the survival of his marriage. They also had issues relating to their church life, which are discussed later.

Everett also broadened his social contacts because of his illness, much to his surprise. He and Joan had occasionally used the transportation services provided by the local senior citizens' organization. During trips, he had become acquainted with some older men who also suffered a variety of disabilities. They had found a way to remain active and social by volunteering time at the senior center. A couple of them answered phones or helped with the transportation schedule, but several others ran a small repair shop where they fixed lamps and toasters and whatnot. **Everett** loved this kind of activity. The fine motor skills required for most of the jobs totally eluded him, but everyone enjoyed having him around to kibbutz, and he was able to help with repairs that required less dexterity. He also felt more comfortable with these men who liked and accepted him the way he was now than he did with some of his old acquaintances who he believed were frightened or put off by his condition.

COUNTERTRANSFERENCE IN PHASE 3

Probably no countertransferential feelings are stronger or more upsetting to clinicians than those that occur during Phase 3. Before this, clinicians have consistently had a sense of being in charge of the situation even as they strive for an egalitarian relationship with their patients. The work of Phase 3, however, magnifies distressing emotions, which clinicians feel independently of any particular patient. These emotions put them very personally and particularly in the same situation as their patients.

Inadequacy

Few human beings, let alone clinicians, have thoroughly stable philosophies that account satisfactorily in their minds for life's horrors and suffering. Few are totally convinced about the meaning of life and the purpose of their own particular existence. Often, they feel conspicuously inadequate not only to resolve their own existential quandaries, but also to take on the task of helping

---

PHASE 3
Countertransference

Inadequacy
Terror and depression
Withdrawal and rejection
Resolution
Clinical Stance
    Respect for suffering
    Heroic captivity
    Antithetical interpretation
    Engagement of creative process
    Standing with self
    Parallel process
    Witnessing

---

patients explore theirs (Figley, 1995; Kissane, 2000; Pearlman & Saakvitne, 1995; Schwartz-Salant & Stein, 1995).

Terror and Depression

Some clinicians are frightened by existential questions, which arouse in them a kind of terror. Some move almost instinctively into unconscious denial when such issues present themselves. Others feel consciously depressed when they themselves contemplate how suffering characterizes the experience of people all over the globe and how much of this suffering is not even attributable to human behavior, which might be amenable to correction. If clinicians are feeling inadequate, terrified, and depressed, what, they imagine, can they possibly offer patients? At least, such clinicians know how these considerations reverberate in a person's mind. Those who deny these feelings in themselves are likely to harm others who are grappling with them (Figley, 1995; Kissane, 2000; Pearlman & Saakvitne, 1995; Schwartz-Salant & Stein, 1995).

Withdrawal and Rejection

Some clinicians resolve the problem by unconsciously withdrawing from their patients. More thoughtful ones may recommend that their patients seek help from clergymen or other cultural specialists in such matters. But some clinicians simply reject the patient or the necessity to search for meaning, or both. If they keep the patient, they medicate for depression, leaving the underlying problem unresolved. They stand behind the cloak of science and assert that addressing spiritual or philosophical problems is outside their professional mandate (Figley, 1995; Kissane, 2000; Pearlman & Saakvitne, 1995; Schwartz-Salant & Stein, 1995).

Resolution

For clinicians who find this phase method effective, however, and for those who have learned to recognize, process, and use their countertransferential reactions, they see opportunity here as well. They attempt to resolve their countertransferential issues and grow philosophically themselves, as they journey with their patients. When clinicians openly acknowledge having questions and doubts of their own, they actually give significant aid and comfort to their struggling Phase 3 patients. Many clinicians move toward different resolutions than those of their patients, so they must remember that their obligation is to help their patients on the search, not select particular outcomes. Both clinicians and patients usually learn in the process that few people ever arrive at a totally articulated stance on existential issues. New experiences and new ideas often generate subtle or major alterations in individuals' spiritual or philosophical positions. But getting into the frame of mind where they think about these issues and finding some ideas that are personally sustaining transforms life, whether of patient or clinician.

Examples _____

I have experienced all of these emotions and will again in the future. Few people resolve the big existential questions in a way that persists through every turn of fate. Everybody gets knocked off base by his or her own experience or witnessing the experience of others. Because the very business of clinical work puts clinicians in the way of all kinds of loss and suffering and despair, it's not a surprise that they can feel battered. No clinician should do this work alone, without the support of trusted colleagues and advisors.

Kim aroused strong feelings of inadequacy in me because I could find no way to harness this bright, intelligent young woman's qualities to help her help herself. That was my job and I was transparently failing at it.

That **Gina**'s growth and understanding should result in the end of her marriage, with all the attendant financial insecurity, was not a surprise to me, but I again felt overwhelmed by a sense of inadequacy to help **Gina** weather this passage.

As I came to appreciate **Everett**'s past and everything that he had built in his life, I felt truly inadequate to help him find spiritual or philosophical solutions.

Erin's black hole of despair inspired me with terror, especially because I responded so strongly to her personality and admired how much she had done to incorporate and accept all her prior experience. If **Erin** could suffer such emptiness and lost reason to live, what chance did I have if anything serious befell her?

The prospects that **Christine** and **Sophia** faced, each slowly deteriorating before my eyes while trying to guide them toward positive acceptance of their suffering, depressed me unutterably at times. In self-defense, I frequently wanted to withdraw. I felt enormous guilty relief at times when **Gina** or **Sophia** would cancel an appointment. I felt even worse because I knew that I was not properly performing my work as witness if I was preoccupied with avoiding or escaping from the testimony. In all these cases, perhaps particularly with **Erin**, I learned to expand my own worldview from witnessing the struggles of my patients and the diverse ways they found to come to terms with their lives. Even **Kim** taught me important things about the tremendous difficulty of the work and the strong pull that the desire for miracles or a quick fix exercise over everyone. Statistics are always hard to grasp emotionally. Someone wins the lottery, people say, why not me?

TRANSFORMATION STEPS IN PHASE 3

Meeting Suffering with Respect

The transformative step in Phase 3 is to meet the suffering experienced by patients with *respect*. In Phase 1, clinicians and patients have learned to allow the existence of suffering; in Phase 2, they have come to regard it with deep compassion. They now completely reverse the patient's initial feelings. Where the suffering was originally hated and rejected, it is now regarded with appreciation as a painful place but one from which patients, by virtue of their endurance, may gain unexpected benefits, insights, and depth.

Heroic Captivity

One of the most important insights is the heroic character of the person who lives with suffering and still finds the courage and persistence to search for purpose and meaning in life. The painful prison to which illness committed the patient becomes a sort of holy ground because it is here that the patient searches and finds a new self and a new understanding of life.

Antithetical Interpretation

Guided by the clinician, the patient experiments with ideas, roles, and identities that once seemed completely antithetical. Although those roles and identities may not be where the patient ultimately comes to rest, the investigation opens new worlds of understanding and allows patients to reframe experiences that seemed capable of only one interpretation originally. The suffering that has been loathed may no longer seem solely hateful, but rather a vehicle for transformation.

Engaging the Creative Process

Clinicians also start patients engaging their creative capabilities. Using whatever medium appeals to them, even many different ones, patients begin making things that satisfy their esthetic and emotional senses. This activity in turn provides both useful content and a kind of training for employing the same creative powers in the construction of the new self and the development of meaning.

Standing with Self

Over the course of Phase 3, as patients survive their dark night of the soul and in so doing find meaning and purpose for the new self who they know profoundly that they are, they learn to stand with themselves. They do not hide who they are or apologize for their existence. They value themselves as worthwhile human beings, even heroic souls, who have many things to contribute to their world.

Examples

These issues have been discussed at some length for the individual cases in the psychological treatment section. What is important here is that clinicians engage in the same activities for both their patients and themselves and actively model them for their patients.

CLINICAL STANCE IN PHASE 3

Parallel Process

Clinicians carry out an important parallel process as their patients construct a new self and search for meaning. Some clinicians think they need not join in this effort, much less investigate their own existential issues. But it is very hard for anyone to evade these issues forever. Moreover, when clinicians go through the patient's meaning development process, they usually feel honored to have participated in such an arduous effort. For many patients, it is not a pretty journey or even necessarily successful. Satisfactory meaning may elude the patient altogether. Patients may never get to the end of the tunnel or even see a light at the end of it. Nevertheless, by experiencing the process, both clinician and patient learn to honor as worthy the time they have spent searching and the nobility of character that it took to pursue the effort. Working together honorably provides its own kind of light in the tunnel.

Witnessing

Clinicians also act as witnesses. The patient's journey may not be the clinician's personal struggle or agony, but clinicians are the ones who see it and who reflect it back to the patient. They validate the patient's experiences, they acknowledge the patient's mourning, they witness the patient's painstaking construction of a new self, and they honor the patient's bravery and persistence. The act of witnessing is powerful and can be transforming in and of itself.

Examples

Clinicians cannot help but feel honored when people as brave and persistent as **Sophia**, **Christine**, **Lewis**, **Joshua**, **Everett**, **Gina**, or **Erin** commit their confidence to them. This is a rare gift, and clinicians need to reflect that fact back to their patients. Even **Kim** struggled honestly and openly to deal with her difficulties. Sometimes failure deserves even more honor than success.

PHASE 3
Checklist for Countertransference

_____ 1. Do you feel inadequate in the face of the patient's existential anxieties?

_____ 2. Do you feel anxious about your own existential questions?

_____ 3. Are you sometimes depressed when considering existential issues?

_____ 4. Do you want to discharge this patient?

_____ 5. Do you feel that some other specialist trained in the field should take over on issues of meaning?

_____ 6. Do you believe that you have yourself grown philosophically and refined your own existential perceptions as you have worked with your patient?

_____ 7. Do you _respect_ what suffering can do in life?

_____ 8. Have you been able to use techniques such as heroic captivity, antithetical experimentation, and engagement of the creative process for the good of both the patient and yourself?

_____ 9. Do you regard yourself as having made a parallel journey with your patient?

_____ 10. Do you regard yourself as a witness?

For all of these patients, my witnessing meant that their thoughts, sorrows, despair, and hope were not occurring in a forest where no one heard. I heard. I knew what my patients had done, how difficult it was, and how brave they were. They had not gone unheard and unseen.

SPIRITUAL/PHILOSOPHICAL PERSPECTIVE IN PHASE 3

Search for Meaning

Patients need to engage in a search for meaning to validate their existence in the universe and to find reasons for their suffering and struggle. They need to find or approach some explanation for what has happened, even though that explanation may be that such things are totally random and without any intention, divine or otherwise (Johnson-Taylor et al., 1995; Schirm, 2002). They also need to generate for themselves a genuine sense of purpose—not simply some traditional bromide foisted off on those the society regards as damaged, but something the patient can sincerely and personally commit to (Allport &

PHASE 3 Spiritual/Philosophical Perspective

Experience
    Search for meaning
    Authenticity
    Increasingly internalized cosmology
 	
Clinical Action
    Introduction to various traditions
    Introduction to nonverbal, nontraditional sources
    Helping locate additional resources
    Nondirective assistance

Ross, 1967; Keefe, 2001; O'Neill & Kenny, 1998; Payne et al., 1991; Peck, 1987; Relt, 1997).

Authenticity Drives Change of Spiritual Attitude

Until Phase 3, patients are usually so preoccupied with their immediate physical and social condition that they can rarely engage very effectively in meaning exploration. They sometimes fear their illness is some form of divine punishment, and if they seek help spiritually, they usually embed themselves in a structured religious setting to contain their fears. To attempt any serious investigation of these matters in Phases 1 or 2 would be to mismatch phase and intervention. Besides being ineffective, it might well discourage necessary exploration of the issues when the time was ripe. Phase 3 patients, however, have changed. They now cease to pretend and no longer try to make themselves fit what they perceive as society's demands. They become committed to truth and authenticity about themselves as they try to construct their new self. Inevitably, this drive for truth extends to their spirituality or philosophy. Where the tenets of their religion or their prior beliefs seem inauthentic or inadequate for their new self, they look to new resources.

Introduction to Various Traditions

Patients are not helpless creatures incapable of action without the clinician's direction, but clinicians can be helpful in the patient's search for authentic meaning. They can expose patients to a variety of unfamiliar traditions, which may give their patients a new angle of vision on the essential questions of human existence. Most patients in this country are at least thinly acquainted with some Western traditions, usually either Christianity or Judaism. But they may be completely unaware of how Buddhists conceive the purpose of suffering or how secular philosophers from the ancient Greeks and Chinese to present-day ethicists and psychologists regard the meaning of human existence. A Christian may well benefit from reading the ways certain Jewish philosophers frame the purpose of existence, and a Jew may benefit from considering the insights of certain Hindu mystics. For those who eschew the traditional religious framing of purpose, psychologists such as Carl Jung or philosophers such as Martin Buber may offer suggestive conceptions. Atheistic humanists propose that people themselves develop definable humanity as they assert meaningfulness to their short stay in existence by behaving in certain ways that make life better for themselves and those around them in the world. Folktales from all over the globe present wonderfully various insights into how it is to be human, what is valuable about being human, and why a person should live at all.

Nonverbal, Nontraditional Sources

Nonverbal experiences build significant meaning for some individuals. And this is not limited to people for whom reading is difficult. Music can reach directly into a person's visceral perception of the universe and transform it in much the same way that mystics are said to be transformed by momentary perceptions of Oneness or God. For some people, contemplation of the natural world offers a transcendent majesty and beauty that suffuses them with respect for their existence. For some chronically ill patients, words and rational discourse have tended to cause pain and misunderstanding, whereas nonverbal experiences come pure, without diminishing or disappointing associations.

Clinician's Role

Clinicians and patients should have formed such a strong bond by Phase 3 and clinicians should be so well acquainted with their patients that they should have fairly clear notions about what writers or traditions would likely appeal to their patients and build on their strengths. Clinicians should also have a range of personal contacts who can help them find reading for patients who indicate interest in ideas totally unfamiliar to the clinician.

Calling on Additional Help

Without abdicating responsibility or closing off their own personal interest in patients, clinicians can also suggest that patients discuss these matters with their priest, rabbi, pastor, or other spiritual advisor. They can suggest that patients with the time and energy consider courses in philosophy or religion that deal with issues of meaning and purpose. Courses not only introduce students to new ideas, but also gather together a group of people who are interested in the same concerns. Having new friends to discuss existential ideas with can be powerfully stimulating to Phase 3 patients.

Nondirective Help

It is important to stress that clinicians should not guide patients toward philosophies or spiritual traditions the clinician personally favors, but rather should attempt to help patients locate traditions or ideas that are personally meaningful and relevant to them. Clinicians should also encourage patients to constantly test the existential ideas they explore to see whether they fit with what the patients regard as authentically true for the new self they are constructing.

Internalized Cosmology

If Phase 3 patients found solace in strongly hierarchical religious institutions during prior phases, it is necessary and desirable for them to examine how elements of that tradition match with their newly developing ideas. They may continue to feel strong personal and emotional allegiance to their religion and its tenets, or they may supplement those with private beliefs as well. Some may find they need to seek a different, more satisfactory spiritual institution or outlet. Again, the clinician does not choose or direct in this activity but simply tries to alert patients to potential conflicts between patients' personal beliefs and those of any institution they are involved with.

Patient's Self the Measure

While respecting the thought and wisdom that have gone into the creation of every spiritual and philosophical tradition, Phase 3 patients locate the ultimate responsibility for determining the truth and meaningfulness of spiritual and philosophical ideas within themselves. During the first two phases, they experienced life as they tried to fit it into conceptions created by other people, which may not have coincided with their own personal reality. Phase 3 patients know they must live according to what they know to be true and possible for themselves and according to beliefs that they deeply, genuinely, and personally commit to.

Examples ──

Sophia's spiritual renewal was detailed earlier. She was able to draw on the powerful, rich base of her childhood religion, which she had continued to practice, if somewhat mechanically, during her adult years before her illness. **Sophia** did not find herself struggling against particular doctrines but drew from the well of her church those waters that sustained her. Whether it was her church's doctrine or not, **Sophia** included as part of "her" church all people who believed in a good God who cared for all his universe, however mysterious the workings of this were. For **Sophia**, people had been enabled by God to help one another survive all anguish and despair by loving kindness and shared prayer. With what energy she had, she set herself to making such a loving community among the people to whom she related best—the bright, intellectual, questioning individuals who found themselves for whatever reason in need of spiritual reassurance and help.

　　Everett had practiced a form of social religion all his life. He came to question this deeply after his stroke. In part, he was embarrassed to struggle into church, but that superficial shame was insignificant compared to his anger at the frivolous nature of social church-going when he was in such misery. For the first time ever, **Everett** needed to think about whether the beliefs articulated at Sunday service spoke to him. Did these beliefs fit with the self that he was gradually discovering he was? His work was complicated, as is frequently the case, by Joan's strong commitment to the church and her belief in its benefits for **Everett** spiritually. She was very upset when **Everett** did not want to attend services and particularly when he refused to have his name inserted into the general prayers for recovery.

I talked with Joan about letting **Everett** work this out on his own. I emphasized how important it was for **Everett** to come to conclusions that truly spoke to him personally. In time, **Everett** did resume church attendance. He even felt a stronger, more thoughtful connection to the beliefs and prayers. But what really transformed his spirit was the affection and involvement of people who related to the person he was now. It seemed to **Everett** that such generosity and love could come only from God, and he was willing, in return, to engage in rituals that God might like.

Christine's spirituality was taking the form of motherhood. She felt herself translated by the experience into something far greater than people had always seemed to her. Although there is no question that motherhood gave **Christine** an opportunity to explore qualities in herself and others that she never had before, I had to remind **Christine** that Mei was an individual who would have a life of her own. She did not exist to serve **Christine**'s spiritual growth, however happy a concurrent effect that might be. **Christine** acknowledged this and tried to bear in mind that Mei was her own little human self. But her delight, easily abetted by Mei's funny affectionate character, taught her so much about the nature of joy that it was hard for me to continue being a spoilsport.

Lewis had left religion behind when he escaped the community where he was born and went to college. Intellectually, he found no substance in the doctrines of his youth, preferring instead the elegant order and structure of mathematics. But math provides little emotional support when a person is suffering, so **Lewis** began to rethink matters spiritual and philosophical. He remembered with enormous affection the pastor of his church. This man had not only helped protect him against abuse at home but also defended his desire to complete high school. He had even helped raise money to send **Lewis** to college. So whereas **Lewis** had little respect for the beliefs of the church, he had admiration and gratitude for the minister's greatness of spirit. Moreover, he realized that he had entered high school teaching—rather than college teaching or research work, either of which would have paid him more—because he wanted to give something back to others like himself. This he felt he had decided because of the example of his pastor. The more he considered it, the more he believed that good generates more good. **Lewis** might not have developed an elaborate cosmology, but he had articulated for himself a reason to live and a source of meaning in life.

Joshua put God on trial and God lost. **Joshua** was furious that a man could work the way he had to better himself, to raise a good family, to serve his community—all in the face of discrimination and racism and the genuine danger it posed for himself and other Blacks—only to be struck down by an arbitrary, capricious God. **Joshua** never thought much of Job, whom he felt God just bashed into submission. Getting other wives and children and herds wouldn't sit well with Maybelle, he used to joke. The interrogation of God actually clarified for **Joshua** what he thought and felt about many issues that he had never consciously thought out before.

Maybelle was appalled by what was happening. The two had been pillars of their church for decades. It was the centerpiece of their social life, and at the same time, they both had often expressed sincere commitment to church doctrines. They had brought up their children in the church because they believed it preached the actual truth of God. Now **Joshua** was just throwing it away in the face of what Maybelle perceived as a minor physical ailment. Even when she came to appreciate the seriousness of his condition, Maybelle could not understand **Joshua**'s anger. It took time for her to realize that it came with enormous grief, not just for himself but for all the struggling Black men that he knew.

When **Joshua** began speaking out, first about African Americans and heart disease, but then in terms of broader medical issues, he began to find where meaning really dwelt for him. He decided he didn't know about God. Perhaps there was a purpose and plan here. But what mattered for **Joshua** was bringing justice to the world here and now. This was what gave his life meaning.

Gina was largely preoccupied with the immediate practical problems in her life. Insofar as she was able to consider issues of meaning, she did so through the children's fiction she read. She was embarrassed by this, but in her heart of hearts—which is what matters—she felt that these stories told her what was important in life. The stories also carried assurances that eventually the good and heroic triumphed. Often, she felt a bit cynical about this—evil and cruelty seemed to do very well—but she liked good better, and good was all that she believed made life worth living.

Erin also came to rest on a bedrock belief that something inherently meaningful exists in the good that people create for one another, for no reason and no personal gain. Despite losses, despite suffering, this space

PHASE 3
Checklist for Spiritual/Philosophical Perspective

_____ 1. Have you helped the patient engage in an authentic search for meaning?

_____ 2. Have you suggested exploration of various different traditions?

_____ 3. Have you suggested nonverbal, nontraditional sources of meaning?

_____ 4. Have you been willing to help the patient find others who can help in his or her search for meaning?

_____ 5. Have you provided nondirective assistance, letting the patient find his or her own meaning?

where doing good took place was where meaning existed. God ceased being particularly relevant to **Erin**. She was not an atheist, because God might well exist. But what was important for her was the good people did in the here and now. Beyond that, she was willing to live in the mystery.

See Table 6.1 for a summary of Phase 3.

Table 6.1 Phase 3: Resolution

1. Course of Illness

Physical/behavioral domain
  Improvement
  Plateau/stabilization
  Relapse
Psychological domain
  Grief reaction/compassion reaction
  Identification of pre-crisis self
  Role/identify experimentation
  Locus of control returning to self
  Awareness of societal effects
  Spiritual/philosophical development
Social/interactive domain
  Breaking silence/engulfment in stigma
  Confrontation
  Role experimentation—social, vocational
  Integration with new supporters/separation from nonsupporters

2. Identifying Characteristics

Increasingly internalized locus of control
Increased awareness of societal effects
Differentiated responses and increased self-esteem
Increased tolerance of ambiguity/chronicity

(continued)

Table 6.1 *Continued*

Respect for suffering and development of meaning
Creative process engaged

Clinical Goal

Development of meaning
Construction of new self

Clinical Summary

Grieve
Maintain
Reframe

3. *Assessment*

Physical/behavioral domain
Medical/medications review
Activity threshold review
Psychological domain
Phase placement
Personal narrative
Existential questions
Social/Interactive domain
Family/couples case management review
Review of wider social world issues
Work evaluation

4. *Treatment*

Physical/behavioral domain
Education as own medical coordinator
Education as own health-care advocate
Education as own activity monitor
Psychological domain
Maintenance of insight and issue reframing
Expression of grief for lost self
Existential dilemma
Definition of pre-crisis self
Analysis of actual losses
Commitment to "time in the tunnel"
Baseline authenticity
Antithetical intervention
Creative process and activities
New societal attitudes
Exploration of different traditions

Table 6.1 *Continued*

Meaning development
Faith and humor
Social/interactive domain
Education couples/families in self-management
Patient political action
Change of supporters
Work interventions

5. *Countertransference*

Inadequacy
Terror and depression
Withdrawal and rejection
Resolution

Clinical Stance

Respect for suffering
Heroic captivity
Antithetical interpretation
Engagement of creative process
Standing with self
Parallel process
Witnessing

6. *Spiritual/Philosophical Perspective*

Experience
Search for meaning
Authenticity
Increasingly internalized cosmology
Clinical action
Introduction to various traditions
Introduction to nonverbal, nontraditional sources
Helping locate additional resources
Nondirective assistance

Chapter 7 ─────────────────────────

PHASE 4: INTEGRATION

Phase 4 patients integrate their illness into a whole and meaningful life. They no longer live merely as an illness writ large, but as individuals with a variety of interests and engagements, despite how limited they may be physiologically. Their illness is just one aspect of their being. And by reengaging in a variety of areas in their lives, Phase 4 patients persuade family, friends, and coworkers as well to regard them as individuals for whom illness is no longer their only defining characteristic (Baker & Stern, 1993; Michael, 1996; Willems, 2000).

This is not to say that Phase 4 patients arrive at a perfect life, without pain, suffering, frustration, or stigmatization. What it means is that much of

| **PHASE 4** |
| **Course of Illness** |
| *Physical/Behavioral Domain*
    Recovery stage (integration as cure)
    Improvement/plateau/relapse

Psychological Domain
    Role/identify integration
    New personal best
    Continued emotional/spiritual/philosophical development

Social/Interactive Domain
    New/reintegrated supporters
    Alternative work/vocation activities |

the time they manage to live graciously despite the rigors of both life and their chronic illness. They have developed an understanding that doing this—living graciously in the effort—is worthwhile. Even when the effort is very difficult, they attribute high value to the sheer process, which in turn nurtures a renewed sense of self-esteem.

Very few individuals are so fortunate as to live in Phase 4 constantly. Most experience it transiently, at best for extended periods. Pain, exhaustion, or multiplying problems related to their original illness can wear them down, making them reexperience some of the confusions and distress of earlier phases. Despite their awareness of media stigmatization or instances of iatrogenic traumatization, these issues can nonetheless deeply distress patients and call into question the understandings and positions they thought they had reached at the end of Phase 3. In addition, life often brings events or other illnesses that knock patients back into prior phases, even though the new crisis does not pertain directly to the original illness. Living with chronic illness is a dynamic process, not a static one, even when patients have successfully moved through the phase process. Unlike what is posited for some stage models of behavioral change (Prochaska, DiClemente, & Norcross, 1992; Prochaska et al., 1994), even those who navigate the four phases successfully do not exit the process. Rather, they maintain themselves in Phase 4 as much of the time as they can.

For those periods of time, however, Phase 4 patients can experience true transcendence of an illness that they have processed. They are able to inhabit a three-dimensional life, which includes relationships and social engagements as well as personal fulfillment. They do this despite consciousness of their suffering, the never-ending nature of their condition, and the ambiguity this generates in everything from their understanding to their hopes and plans.

IDENTIFYING PHASE 4 PATIENTS

Individuals in Phase 4 rarely come as new patients to clinicians. Patients who have been in therapy with a clinician have usually gained what they need from formal intervention by the end of Phase 3 and the beginning of Phase 4. At this point, they are usually planning to live independently of regular therapeutic visits, although they often stay in touch with the clinician by e-mail or calling periodically.

PHASE 4
Identifying Characteristics

Understanding of the phases
Integration of pre- and postcrisis self
Reconstructed roles and relationships
Broadened sense of meaning
Quest for full life

Clinical Goal
Integration

Clinical Summary
Integration

Understanding the Phases

Phase 4 patients grasp that recovery, stabilization, and relapse are all parts of the normal cycle of chronic illness. They recognize that integrating their illness into a complete life is a dynamic process, not a static state at which they arrive and remain forever. They understand that they have learned techniques that they can use by themselves to contain future crises, achieve stabilization, and progress through resolution to integration again. They also know when they should seek professional help and how to do that.

Integrating Pre- and Postcrisis Self

Phase 4 patients consolidate a new self by integrating aspects of their precrisis self with a new, authentic self that they have gradually developed during the phases of their illness experience. They have, in fact, constructed a new definition of themselves. They have discarded the harmful scripts that the culture has thrust on them, rewritten their illness story, and embraced this new narrative as their own.

Reconstructed Cultural Roles and Relationships

As a result of their reconstructed definition of themselves, patients have a vastly different relationship to their community and culture, yet one that is usually congruent with the person that they were before their illness. When Phase 4 patients describe themselves, they include the reality of their chronic experience and their disabilities. When they speak of their new or reconstructed relationships with others, these relationships are intact and encompass an active awareness of their condition.

Broadening Meaning

Phase 4 patients continue to explore meaning development, but in Phase 4 they focus outward on the world at large as well as inward on their own personal relationship to the universe.

Seeking Fuller Life

Phase 4 patients seek to lead life as fully as possible. They do not wish to be limited simply to issues of their illness. They reexamine the four kinds of activities that they learned about during Phase 2 and attempt to derive meaning beyond practical accomplishment from the energy they expend in each area. They find ways to expand their practical lives without exhausting themselves and to infuse their entire life with meaning.

Understanding Likelihood of Future Crises

Phase 4 patients also know that their experiences of integration and even transcendence will likely come under assault from other life crises or different illnesses. They know they may have to process the phases all over again in some new context. But they also know they have learned a powerful and, for them, successful technique for moving to integrate future crises. Given the longer lives that most Americans may now expect to live, Phase 4 patients understand they will probably become sick with other illnesses. They know that, like everyone else, they are vulnerable to accidents and can lose crucial loved ones. None of these prospects fill them with joy. They are as scared and apprehensive about such matters as other mortals and perhaps with better reason given their prior experiences. But they know how to live daily in the present and to work with their fears and their griefs. On good days, they are able to do just that. On bad days, they hang onto their new faith that they can work toward better days (Fennell, 1995a, 1998; Jason, Fricano, et al., 2000).

Examples

Sophia entered Phase 4 as she poured what energy she had into constructing and expanding her prayer circles. She developed a great sense of calm about her condition, even during bad days, because she felt deeply that out of herself she had created something that would help herself and others to be strong, brave, supportive, and good. This, she felt, was the Lord's intention for her. The activity itself brought out all her old capacities to analyze, organize, and assess, so that from her point of view she was able to meld the former scientist with the new spiritual being she had become. Pain, suffering, and even exhaustion kept her in touch with the needs of all these new people she loved, and she knew that they supported her when she was down, just as she supported them. Although **Sophia**, like everyone, had her days of deep discouragement and trial, she tended to live more of her life in Phase 4 than not.

Everett also entered Phase 4 when he came to see that who he was now contained who he had been in the past. All the people he really cared about believed deeply that he was, in all important ways, the same person, and they showed this by how they behaved around him. Before his stroke, **Everett** had never paid much attention to his personal thoughts or feelings. He was surprised to realize that things he assumed must be important didn't actually matter to him that much. He recalled the intense physical life he had led with fondness, but he now found himself enjoying the companionship of the other volunteers at the senior center, even though it was different from physical activity. Moreover, he felt consciously that he was doing something good for other people. He had taken great pride in raising his family—a pride they reflected back to him with gratitude—and now his volunteering seemed to spread some of the same qualities over others in the community, including people he didn't even know. Believing this made him feel profoundly peaceful in the way that he felt sometimes when he witnessed the beauty of the natural world. **Everett** intellectually acknowledged that he could face crises again, but he was not strongly prepared to do so.

Christine had moments of Phase 4 integration because of her joy in her new family. She applied herself to injecting the best qualities remaining from her old energetic self to her severely circumscribed role as mother. With my guidance, she conscientiously kept up with her MS friends as well as her prayer group so that she would not place the whole burden of meaning in her life on Mei and Michael. **Christine** had difficulty articulating her feelings about meaning, and it seemed likely that she did not actually spend much time thinking about it. She felt good and hopeful and able to absorb the suffering caused by her MS because she had something else so good in her life. Her infrequent conscious self-examination did not bode well for future crises, but **Christine** did understand the practical processes of crisis containment and stabilization. It seemed probable to me that while **Christine**'s health remained stable or declined very slowly, she would waver between Phases 3 and 4. If, however, she faced a severe relapse, became sick with something else, or something bad happened to Mei or Michael, it seemed likely that **Christine** would be thrown into serious chaos.

Lewis benefited enormously by focusing on the exercises in authenticity that Phase 3 requires. He learned to pay attention to what he really felt and who he really was. He recognized that his condition would put many people off, particularly women, he felt, and he wanted to form a permanent relationship. But he knew that he must not fake, and he actually no longer even wanted to. By thinking deeply about his past and his work, he also understood where much of his happiness in life could come from. The greatest hurdle **Lewis** faced in the near future concerned his forming an intimate relationship. He had not yet come to a place where he could imagine life lived without a wife or partner, so it was possible that failure in this area might lead to crisis and despair. Like **Christine**, **Lewis** seemed likely to waver between Phase 3 and Phase 4 unless he was able to expand his sense of meaning.

Gina had not entered Phase 4 by the writing of this book. She was maintaining very good insight and was struggling to construct a new, authentic self. But the chaos caused by the collapse of her marriage and the increased responsibilities this created concerning the children kept her distracted from any significant progress on issues of meaning and from the creative activities that might help stimulate such thinking.

Joshua entered Phase 4 as he discovered how meaningful to him his speaking to African American groups had become. The other essential component was his overcoming his embarrassment and discussing his fears and reactions candidly with Maybelle. At first, this was awkward and **Joshua** revealed his feelings only partially, but both partners found they were beginning to relate to each other in a new way. By proceeding very carefully, their intimacy once again expanded. This became especially important when **Joshua** was diagnosed with prostate cancer. The new crisis rocked **Joshua**'s confidence, but he had made so many gains that he rebounded faster than either he or I believed likely. There is no question that his apparently successful treatment—he is still free of cancer two years later—played a great role in his emotional recovery.

Erin also moved into Phase 4 more quickly than I expected. Her total despair was hardly surprising given the events of her life. What **Erin** didn't recognize when she found herself in the black tunnel was that she had actually done far more of the processing work in her life than she thought. My most valuable contribution was to give **Erin** access to my faith temporarily and to witness and reflect back to **Erin** her bravery, her excruciating hard work, and her suffering. As meaning began to flow back into **Erin**'s life, she worked with me in constructing a new life and self who could continue her old commitments in a way that the chronically ill **Erin** could sustain. **Erin** also learned to broaden her activities so that her life was not entirely composed of social advocacy and personal physical maintenance. She came to see that she needed to have non-work-related social activities and time for fulfillment of other aspects of herself besides a social conscience.

Erin was swift to comprehend the cyclic nature of crisis, stabilization, resolution, and integration. She could see from her own life that unforeseen disasters could utterly flatten even those who had attained a reasonably high degree of emotional balance and meaning, but she also recognized from her work with me that she was learning ways to deal with these setbacks.

New Example

I had the unusual experience of receiving a new patient who was in Phase 4. **Father Stephen**, a Catholic priest and psychologist in his early 70s, came to me because of severe sleep problems, which did not respond to the conventional medical treatments he had attempted. **Father Stephen** had combined a lifetime of intense personal spiritual inquiry with an active therapeutic practice for individuals with serious illnesses. He had deep experience of practical observation and differentiation and a profound, constantly questing faith about the meaningfulness of life. He had witnessed great suffering in others and had seen it produce terror and misery, but also occasional strength and faith. His sleep problem exhausted, confused, and disoriented him in a way that he could not process. Although **Father Stephen** was deeply distressed, he nevertheless had a stubborn faith that there must be some way for him to resolve the sleep problem or else to integrate it into his life.

ASSESSMENT: PHYSICAL/BEHAVIORAL DOMAIN

Phase 4 patients often experience continued plateau or even improvement, but relapses are always possible. Some chronic conditions are progressive, and patients with these physical conditions eventually worsen. Clinicians' physical and behavioral assessments during Phase 4 are aimed primarily at determining patients' preparedness for managing on their own. Some individuals are never able to do this, and they require someone to carry out these activities. The clinician should help to identify and train that person.

Examples

As a new patient, **Father Stephen** required a full medical workup, with particular attention to his medications. His physicians were fairly sure

---

PHASE 4
Assessment

Physical/Behavioral Domain
    Recognition that plateau, improvement, relapse all possible

Psychological Domain
    Role and identity integration
    Maintenance review protocols
    Ongoing creative activity and meaning development
    Ongoing personal narrative and emotional development
    Integration assessment

Social/Interactive Domain
    Family, couples, friends maintenance protocols
    New and reintegrated friends
    Workplace review
    Alternative jobs/vocations

that his problem was a sleep disorder, but with a man of **Father Stephen**'s age and medical history, it was important to rule out a host of serious illnesses that could be fatiguing him. Also, given the fact that **Father Stephen** could fall asleep in the middle of a conversation, it was necessary to rule out narcolepsy.

When **Joshua** was diagnosed with prostate cancer, I helped Maybelle and him deal with the emotional turmoil this caused. I also talked with **Joshua**'s doctors about how to best integrate his blood pressure medications and sleep protocols with the interventions recommended by the oncologist.

With the other patients, I reviewed their physical status to make sure that they would be able to monitor their physical and psychological health issues.

ASSESSMENT: PSYCHOLOGICAL DOMAIN

Role and Identity Integration

Clinicians witness patients' clarification of their new identities and roles. To the bedrock core identity of self that patients retain from before their illness are added the understandings they have gained from their self-analysis and their new comprehension of the illness from which they suffer, both in itself and as a chronic condition.

Maintenance Review Protocols

Clinicians observe what constitutes patients' new "personal best" and then help patients to establish self-review systems so they can stay on track in their future lives.

Ongoing Creative Activity and Meaning Development

During Phase 3, patients have usually discovered the transformative power of creative activity. They continue to engage in creative work because of these benefits, even though the activities may change over time, which in turn helps to inspire their further development of meaning.

Ongoing Personal Narrative and Emotional Development

Clinicians review patients' ongoing personal narratives and urge the maintenance of this activity even after regular meetings with the clinician cease. The written narratives permit former patients to look somewhat more objectively at changes, insights, desires, accomplishments, and other aspects of their lives.

Integration Assessment

In preparation for ending regular sessions with patients, clinicians observe how well patients have integrated their illness into their lives and whether they are able to live meaningfully despite chronicity and ambiguity.

Examples _____

I could see that **Father Stephen** was prevented from analyzing his situation primarily out of exhaustion. He had obviously established a self that was authentic and supportive. His confusion and trouble seemed to stem almost entirely from the physical effects of insufficient and nonrestorative sleep.

Sophia and **Everett** were acting in accordance with their growing sense of their new selves. They held themselves to high new standards, but these standards fit with what was possible for them to accomplish. They took genuine pleasure in the new worlds they were creating. Although they knew well what they had lost and what they had suffered, they preferred to focus on how they could live now and in the future. **Sophia**, in particular, needed to be reminded to maintain her activity review protocols because she always tended to overdo. Now, however, overdoing usually related to her enthusiasm for her new activity rather than to her embarrassment at causing people trouble. **Everett** needed to be encouraged to find modes of creative expression and to continue his taped reflections on his life and how he felt. Both these activities helped keep him actively self-aware.

Lewis and **Christine** were both consciously committed to acting their new personal best. **Lewis** needed to remind himself regularly to process his experiences with all the techniques he had learned in Phase 2 and consolidated in Phase 3. He felt that some of his characteristics might make it difficult to find a partner, but he learned that he had other characteristics that were very appealing. His commitment to teaching and his desire to help others were more powerfully attractive than he had imagined. **Christine** needed to remember to work at broadening her sources of emotional support beyond her nuclear family, and she required strong encouragement to continue thinking about issues of meaning.

Joshua initially needed emotional support and understanding to deal with his new medical problem. Perhaps because it was an acute episode—or at least that is how it appears to be working out—**Joshua** was able to incorporate this new factor into his life fairly expeditiously.

Erin began locating the boundaries of her practical life as soon as she managed to ascribe some meaning to her existence again. She had already in her life developed a good deal of personal insight, and she was quickly able to differentiate the effects of current difficulties from premorbid traumas. She had a strong desire to continue her professional activities, but she did not feel an overwhelming urge to pass for normal for social reasons. Her friends and associates tended to accept as worthy and valid whatever self she presented; that is, they believed what she told them about her illness and behaved supportively. **Erin** also truly understood that she could worsen her condition by overdoing. Mostly, she wanted to learn what she could reasonably expect of herself and how she could tell what was reasonable and what wasn't. She did, however, need to attempt to broaden her life activities—which of necessity meant scaling back even more than she anticipated on work commitments—to create a more completely fulfilling existence.

ASSESSMENT: SOCIAL/INTERACTIVE DOMAIN

Family, Friends, and Couples Maintenance Protocols

By Phase 4, the families, friends, and partners of patients have usually learned how to live successfully with the patient's illness. Partners, friends, or family members who cannot deal with the patient's illness problems have usually left the patient during Phases 2 or 3, or else the patient has left them. In Phase 4, clinicians make sure that the friends, partners, or family have developed ways to review regularly how things are going and how to manage changes that they may need to make. Clinicians also remind these significant others that like the patient, they have learned what they must do when new problems or crises assault them. Again, the clinician's effort serves to prepare families and couples to live successfully on their own.

New and Reintegrated Friends

Beginning in Phase 2, as a result of seeking, and subsequently in Phase 3, patients have usually created new networks of friends. In Phase 4, these are consolidated, and patients may be able to reintegrate some old friends temporarily lost during earlier phases. In Phase 4, social life has become important to patients once again because they want to live in and of the world. Because they are open about their condition and do not dissemble or permit discrimination concerning their condition, they choose friends who are supportive. Some patients become involved in advocacy work for their illness or for the disabled in general. This advocacy world distinctly expands the lives of patients—it is both a cause and effect in this regard. For the most part, clinicians simply observe the expansion of patients' social lives. They may give advice on ways to deal with the awkwardnesses that arise occasionally, but mostly they celebrate from the sidelines.

Workplace Review

Before patients leave the regular therapeutic situation to manage on their own, clinicians usually make a last review of the patient's work situation, if the patient is still employed. Clinician and patient discuss whether the work is appropriate or overly taxing and whether it takes place in a physically and psychologically supportive environment. In concert, patient and clinician determine what changes may need to be made now and discuss what future changes in the work environment would require a new response. If it has not happened earlier and it is appropriate, clinicians give patients guidance on seeking disability.

Alternative Jobs or Vocations

Phase 4 patients who are able to continue working sometimes cease to settle for reduced hours at the old job or altered workplace conditions. They change the kind of work they do altogether. This comes as part of restructuring the self and refusing to countenance inauthentic, meaningless activity. Having transformed themselves internally and in relation to their social world, Phase

4 patients often see that it is possible for them to perform work that means something to them. Even those on disability may discover that they want to volunteer their services to support activities they think are valuable (Howard & Howard, 1997).

Examples

Father Stephen had to contend with administrators who wanted to make sure that his professional work was being continued while he was unable to work effectively. Because much of his effectiveness lay in the personal relationship he established with the people he cared for, this was hard to accomplish. As a consequence, **Father Stephen** pushed himself to work rather than cause any breaks in continuity with his patients. In doing this, **Father Stephen** was involved in a complex variety of passing that occasionally occurs in Phase 3 and Phase 4 patients. It comes from the patient not yet adequately balancing two well-thought-out but competing interior demands. In this case, **Father Stephen** fully recognized that he needed to help himself by doing what was necessary to resolve his sleep difficulties. But he also had a profound commitment to his patients, and serving them validated deep issues of meaning for him. Although he knew that his patients were not being well served by him in his present condition, he also knew that their bond with him as an individual was sometimes all that sustained them.

Lewis's work contributed to his sense of meaning. His principal problem was a tendency to overwork, but exhaustion increased his symptoms. He was learning, however, from these experiences that he had to pace himself so that he did not put the activities that were important to him in jeopardy. Also, although he did not share a complete medical history with every acquaintance, he became more candid with intimates. His own understanding of his condition helped him with this enormously.

Sophia found a new relationship context, and **Everett** completely revised his old ones so that these became supportive and helped expand their lives. Although **Sophia** and **Everett** could not work, they were able to pursue vocational activities.

Christine still struggled with her relationship to her birth family, but increasingly, she truly understood that these people might never be able to take the necessary steps to understand her or her condition. Fortunately for her, she not only had her own small nuclear family, but also, increasingly, she had become involved with Michael's family, who mostly accepted her for what she was. She also enjoyed her new friends and periodically sought to reincorporate old friends into her life. Some of these old friends found they liked the new **Christine** and were able to reestablish intimacy.

Joshua had to stop all activities during his cancer surgery and post-operative treatment. After he recovered, he decided to quit his job, although he agreed to do occasional consulting work for his old firm. He did gradually return to public speaking, however, because it gave him great satisfaction and put him in contact with new people who were concerned about the same issues he was.

Erin's friends were a thoughtful group who were highly attuned by their work to stigmatization and discrimination. When they acted inappropriately, it was usually out of ignorance, and they were happy to change when they understood what **Erin** needed. **Erin** wanted to continue

PHASE 4
Checklist for Assessment

Physical/Behavioral Domain

_____ 1. Is the patient cognizant that he or she may experience plateau, improvement, or relapse?

_____ 2. Does the patient know what to do medically in the various eventualities?

_____ 3. Can the patient competently be his or her own medical coordinator and health care advocate? If not, does the patient have someone the patient trusts who can act as such?

Psychological Domain

_____ 1. What indicators place this patient in Phase 4?

_____ 2. Have you reviewed the patient's role and identity integration?

_____ 3. Does the patient have adequate maintenance review protocols?

_____ 4. Is the patient continuing to update his or her personal narrative?

_____ 5. Is the patient continuing to engage in creative activity?

_____ 6. Is the patient continuing his or her exploration of meaning development?

Social/Interactive Domain

_____ 1. Do family, friends, and partner have adequate maintenance protocols?

_____ 2. Does the patient have supporters and reintegrated friends?

_____ 3. Is the patient considering a work or vocation change?

_____ 4. Is a work review necessary?

_____ 5. Is help with disability necessary?

to work part time, but this was somewhat more difficult than she thought it would be. Her organization, much as they wanted her to continue, had no structural way to incorporate consulting or part-time members. She also would not be able to help with any litigation because they needed individuals who would be available full time for the duration of any important case.

CLINICAL GOAL AND TREATMENT ISSUES IN PHASE 4

The overarching clinical goal of Phase 4 is integration of the patient's suffering as part of a meaningful, sustaining, and even rewarding life. The ideal moments, though they may be transient, occur when the patient transcends the illness experience altogether.

One major treatment issue of Phase 4 is to ensure the amalgamation of desired elements of the patient's precrisis self with the newly constructed self. Patients have gone through the entire paradigm shift from the cultural construction of illness as acute and unidirectional to one in which illness is cyclic, chronic, and inherently ambiguous. This is a tremendous change, and clinicians need to ensure that patients have a firm grasp of the insight and intervention techniques they learned throughout the phase process. Given the cyclic nature of their condition, patients need to return to these techniques when the crises of life require. Clinicians review to see that patients know how to monitor their health care needs and how well they, their partners, and their families understand the ways to maintain and review their roles and relationships. Clinicians also assist their patients, as much as they can, in the patients' further development of meaning, particularly as it refers to the broad range of their practical life activities.

TREATMENT: PHYSICAL/BEHAVIORAL DOMAIN

Checking Maintenance Protocols

During Phase 3, clinicians began training those patients who could in how to become their own care coordinators. In Phase 4, they actually pass on the mantle of responsibility. Initially, patients may find this very challenging, so

---

PHASE 4
Treatment

Physical/Behavioral Domain
    Review of maintenance protocols
    Review of relapse/stabilization/integration cycle
    Transience of Phase 4

Psychological Domain
    Maintenance of new self
    Free will
    Continued creative work and narrative
    Continued and broadened meaning development

Social/Interactive Domain
    Continued social action
    Recruitment and maintenance of integrated supports
    Workplace modification or work change

---

clinicians set up a structured review for a certain period of time and eventually transition to making occasional spot checks. Patients now schedule their own ongoing medical reviews, with the clinician offering advice or suggestions primarily when asked. The clinician may also help patients review their various maintenance protocols, and the clinician reminds patients of the medical data that must be kept up-to-date for disability. This may, for example, require patients to have periodic neuropsychological reviews.

Relapse/Stabilization/Integration Cycle

As patients prepare to leave therapy, clinicians need to make sure that they clearly grasp the cyclical nature of their illness and the likelihood that, like everyone else, they will be subject to non-illness-related crises and other illnesses. Clinicians emphasize the importance of checking medical changes with health care professionals immediately. They remind patients that when they find themselves in chaos again, they should immediately begin the work that they understand about containing the crisis, stabilizing their situation, and then working to resolve the new situation and integrate it in a meaningful way into their lives. They alert their patients to those things that should make them seek professional help again.

Transience of Phase 4

Clinicians remind patients that most people attain Phase 4 integration for periods of time at best. Often, patients find themselves struggling with old demons that plagued them in Phases 2 and 3, and life or illness crises can throw them back into Phase 1. The death of a partner or their own heart attack will require major recovery work on their part. Nonetheless, patients have learned how to do this and where useful and supportive resources may be found.

Examples

In conjunction with **Father Stephen**'s physician, I sent him to a sleep specialist. It was very important to establish a physical safety plan for **Father Stephen** because he was actually suffering even greater cognitive impairment than he had thought and was in some danger of injuring himself or others accidentally. I had him map his activities closely. We also discussed how his age, apart from his current sleep problem, would soon require that he begin to cut back. Although **Father Stephen** understood the desirability of establishing quiet periods in his day to help the sleep interventions do their work, he found it very difficult to decrease his activities. He did agree, however, to limit the number of new patients and to move some who were able to accept the change to other practitioners.

With **Erin**, I set up a medical monitoring checklist and a physical activities review system.

The other patients had been with me long enough so that they had already worked out such checklists and review systems.

TREATMENT: PSYCHOLOGICAL DOMAIN

Maintenance of New Self

Before patients go unaided in the world, they need to have a firm grasp on the new self they have constructed. They need to feel completely comfortable with that self and with the elements of the old, preillness self that they have retained. Clinicians can help them establish ways to maintain this new amalgam of self and to review its viability when it comes under stress.

Free Will

Clinicians emphasize to patients that they daily exercise their free will in committing to the phase processes they have learned. Their choice involves an enormous amount of hard work, which will almost certainly go unrecognized by the outside world. But the effort is worthwhile because of the better life it makes possible. By now, patients have absorbed into themselves and feel for themselves the faith they originally borrowed from their clinicians, especially in Phases 1 and 2.

Continued Creative Work and Narrative

Clinicians encourage patients to continue their creative activities or initiate new ones. Creativity in any area opens the mind and imagination to new understandings of the world and can stimulate a greater sense of meaning and purpose in life. Once patients have opened their eyes and begun to search for authenticity and meaning, they most often continue to seek and grow for the rest of their lives. Clinicians predict for patients that their creative impulse and drive will follow a cyclic period of its own, an ebb and flow. There will be times of great imaginative richness but other times when the impulse slacks off and there is no particular drive to create. Clinicians also recommend that patients continue to compose and revise their private illness narrative even after they leave formal therapy (Axtell, 1999; Longmore, 1995; Pastio, 1995; Wade, 1994a, 1994b).

Continued Meaning Development

Clinicians also support patients in their ongoing spiritual or emotional growth. They remind patients that, periodically, they should review and renew the conclusions they have reached so that meaning in their lives does not become flat or stale. It has to enrich them as they live in the ever-changing present. In Phase 3, and even at the end of Phase 2, one way patients move toward the development of meaning is by focusing on the most basic activities of daily life. In such apparently simple tasks as making their beds or preparing their meals, patients gradually learn to find value and even honor. If nothing else, in doing these tasks, patients recognize that they are doing no harm. The discipline resembles that of a monastery or a Buddhist temple, where neophytes focus on the value of each small activity in itself and of carrying it out with full attention and application.

Horizontal Meaning Development

In Phase 4, the search for meaning spreads over patients' entire lives and into all four areas of activity. They no longer concentrate solely on their personal place or meaning in the universe, but seek to locate the meaning of everyday activities. They explore what they contribute in family and social relationships. They consider why these relationships are important and what about them makes them special or desirable or meaningful. They examine their employment or their volunteer work to see whether it is meaningful and whether it contributes to life in some significant way. They examine their activities of personal fulfillment to see how these contribute to what they think is important or whether they want to do other things instead or as well. They also look at how their sense of meaning applies to others in the universe. They have become seekers in every sense of the word, especially seekers of meaning (Axtell, 1999; Longmore, 1995; Pastio, 1995; Wade, 1994a, 1994b).

Examples

With **Father Stephen**, I reinforced his belief that he would eventually be able to incorporate his immediate problems into an overall pattern of a meaningful life.

Sophia was expanding her meaning development to include others. She seemed to be strongly established in her new self, yet, at the same time, aware of the fact that fate might jolt her life again in some unexpected way.

I suggested that **Christine** might like to take up creative handwork of some sort, and **Christine** found that she enjoyed knitting. By using large needles and thick wool or cotton yarn, she was able to overcome some motor difficulties. She joked that this was her new "construction" activity, and she delighted in being able to make people gifts of her handiwork. **Christine** liked her new roles even though she chaffed at her limitations.

Everett seemed to be making his way on his own now that he had a new sense of himself. I worked to keep him thinking consciously about what was going on in his life, but even if he didn't, the quality of **Everett**'s life had improved a great deal.

Through an agreement with his high school, **Lewis** began contributing one morning a week at a Head Start program, where he started introducing simple mathematical concepts to the children. He found himself overflowing with inventive ways to do this, which I pointed out was his creativity going into high gear. **Lewis** discovered working with young children to be an amazingly healing activity for his own childhood traumas. He also found a potential companion in the woman who ran the program.

Erin and I discussed how she could continue to contribute her legal skills without exhausting herself or exacerbating her symptoms. **Erin**'s friends helped her apply for a grant that would support research into areas of public housing law. Going through this procedure acquainted **Erin** with the world of research grants, and she came to believe that she might be able to continue supporting herself in work that she thought was important. She also discovered that her name was getting around. Several organizations requested her help on special projects, and although she could not accept all the offers, she felt further confidence in her professional future. She also recognized that incorporating her illness experience into her already complex life and history would be an ongoing project. She recognized that the symptoms of lupus can vary radically and that she might become seriously ill sometime in the future. With this in mind, she began to work with friends about what she called her future safety plan—whom she would be able to call on for help and heavy-duty emotional support if she should suffer a serious relapse.

Erin had come to see that she needed not only meaning in terms of her personal relationship with the universe, but also a life in the daily here and now that included meeting her ADLs with grace and enjoyment, seeing friends for fun, and developing personal satisfactions not related to social welfare issues. She set aside time every day to either meditate, listen to music, or read materials related to philosophy and spirituality, but she also made more room in her life for chatting with friends, going on walks in the country, and watching videos or movies.

TREATMENT: SOCIAL/INTERACTIVE DOMAIN

Continued Social Action

Phase 4 patients usually continue to pursue social action around their illness or issues related to it. This meaningful engagement to improve the experience of others who suffer and to change negative cultural perceptions and activities tends to invigorate even those who are severely disabled. Clinicians applaud this involvement, which provides meaningful activity, friendships, and an opportunity to change society.

Recruitment and Maintenance of "Integrated Supports"

Even when Phase 4 patients are not involved in illness advocacy, they are active in maintaining and expanding their new or reintegrated network of friends. Again, clinicians support and applaud such activity. These new friends acknowledge and accept the real life that the patients live now. They understand whatever limits may circumscribe the patients' lives, but consider this no impediment to intimacy and engagement. Indeed, they may particularly value patients' hard-won wisdom and courage. With such friends, patients do not need to pretend or to try to pass. When these friends do not understand something that is happening with their chronically ill friend, they ask for explanations rather than making unwarranted assumptions.

Work Environment

Clinicians and patients have attended to work issues from the very beginning, but it is usually not until Phases 3 and 4 that patients approach total honesty with themselves about what they can sustain and what they want to do. In this society, it is very hard for people who are employed to give up wage-earning that supports them for less adequate part-time work or disability. By late in Phase 3 and Phase 4, however, patients have anchored themselves in truth as they best understand it, and they no longer try to fool themselves about whether they can work full time or continue to work even part time in occupations that worsen their overall health. Obviously, work is not even under consideration with some severely disabled patients. As in earlier phases, clinicians work with their patients to achieve the best employment ends for them, whether that means helping them to secure necessary modifications in the workplace or to apply for disability.

Examples

Sophia, **Everett**, and **Lewis** all consciously began engaging with new people in new activities that were meaningful to them. They remained in contact with supportive family and former friends, but they also expanded their worlds to involve active social connection.

Christine worked to maintain her insight about family and former friends whose behavior caused her pain and suffering. She tried to come to a place where she would open the possibility of reconnecting, but where she would be willing to forego the relationship if the individuals were not willing to change their behavior toward her. This was very hard for her because she wanted so desperately for certain people to change who probably never would. Insofar as she could, she tried to support MS advocacy work. Sometimes, this was no more than stuffing envelopes for the local group, but she also found that she was a helpful presence at meetings when new members joined. Her struggle with the disability company was ongoing, so **Christine** had to keep assiduous track so that her medical records supported her claims.

Joshua had entered Phase 4 with the expansion of his speaking work, and he returned to this activity as soon as his health permitted it. Both he and his wife could see how it brought together so many threads from both their lives. **Joshua**'s experience with prostate cancer simply increased the scope of his interest and, ultimately, of his talks.

Erin also suddenly found herself involved in patient advocacy. While working on her housing grant, she had growing awareness of the extraordinary difficulties faced by poor people, especially single mothers, when they suffered chronic illnesses. She found that she had an intense interest in this area, especially because she, as a middle-class White woman, had benefited so many times in her life from access to good health care. She saw how the inability to acquire adequate care produced a vicious downward spiral of problems, including unemployment, loss of housing, drug or alcohol addiction, and failure to care for children adequately. **Erin** actively began seeking ways to contribute her legal expertise in these areas.

PHASE 4
Checklist for Treatment

Physical/Behavioral Domain

_____ 1. Have you reviewed the patient's medical maintenance protocols?

_____ 2. Have you reviewed the relapse/stabilization/integration cycle?

_____ 3. Have you discussed the likely transience of Phase 4? Is the patient prepared for recycling through the phases?

Psychological Domain

_____ 1. Does the patient feel confident about maintaining the new self?

_____ 2. Does the patient feel he or she is exercising free will?

_____ 3. Is the patient still involved in creative expression and in meaning development?

Social/Interactive Domain

_____ 1. Is the patient continuing in social action?

_____ 2. Is the patient recruiting and maintaining supporters and reintegrating others from the past where possible?

_____ 3. Have you helped in whatever way necessary on work issues, with disability, or in locating new vocational activities?

COUNTERTRANSFERENCE IN PHASE 4

Happily, the countertransferential issues in Phase 4 emerge primarily from the success of the patient-clinician relationship. The emotions are those stimulated by the approaching end of formal therapy sessions. The clinician has been genuinely attached to the patient and deeply involved in their common activity. Frequently, clinicians have grown with their patients and feel a strong bond with them. Sometimes, they simply enjoy their company. Naturally, clinicians feel grief that this intense collaboration is coming to a conclusion. They can suffer a sense of loss as their patients embark on independent lives. But clinicians also feel great pride. They have been witnesses to so much that their patients have endured. In the darkest times, their patients have courageously continued. They have believed in the clinicians' faith that the process would work for them, even though they had little personal faith that it would (Nouwen, 1972).

PHASE 4
Countertransference

Attachment
Grief
Loss
Pride

Clinical Stance
Integration of suffering
Free will
Daily acts of bravery
Societal action
Creative action
Living with paradox
Parallel integration
Release

Examples

I felt enormous affection and pride in all these patients. I was tremendously pleased with their insights, their accomplishments, their bravery, and their commitment to live life as fully as they could. I liked working with them all and knew I would truly miss having regular conversations with this lively, diverse group. Although living without regular therapeutic intervention was the end everyone had sought and achieved, I knew I would miss my patients and felt that they would miss me at times, also. Many of them still keep in touch with the occasional phone call or e-mail.

TRANSFORMATION STEPS IN PHASE 4

Integration of Suffering

The transformation step in Phase 4 is the *integration* of patients' suffering as a meaningful part of their lives. The suffering is not simply *allowed* and *respected.* Nor are patients merely *compassionate* toward their suffering. In Phase 4, they have made this most rejected aspect of their experience an integral part of their lives.

Free Will, Daily Acts of Bravery

This integration is manifested in patients' freely choosing to live with all the difficulties inherent in their condition, hard though that is. This is a perpetual, repeated choice. They commit to constant bravery because assaults on their courage and good intentions occur every day. They cannot avoid pain or instances of social stigmatization. It is easy to tire of constantly having to maintain their worth in the face of indifference, dismissal, or outright malice. Even friends can in ignorance be hurtful. There is, moreover, a nearly inextinguishable fear most patients feel that by their sheer existence they are taxing their partners and families. It takes strength and faith and courage to assert otherwise, and that effort can sometimes seem impossible. Nonetheless, though they stumble, they also persist.

Societal Action, Creative Action

Phase 4 patients also demonstrate integration of their suffering by their commitment to social action. They not only reject society's rejection, but also actively work to change social attitudes and to protect and inform those who have only recently begun to suffer from their illness. Phase 4 patients further show their integration of suffering through their creative work. Such creativity points to their belief that even people in unpromising situations can add richness and substance to life (Axtell, 1999; Longmore, 1995; Pastio, 1995; Wade, 1994a, 1994b).

Living with Paradox

Phase 4 patients take on the difficult task of living with paradox. They find worth in endurance and exhibit faith in themselves and their future despite the chronicity and ambiguity of their situation (Albrecht & Devlieger, 1999; Larson, 1998; Schaefer, 1995).

Examples

The prior sections have detailed how all of the patients who achieved Phase 4 learned to integrate their suffering into full, meaningful lives. They all recognize that they make a daily effort to be brave. Even if they are the only ones to recognize it—and most realize that their significant supporters recognize it also—they can take pride in their courage. All the patients have incorporated some level of social action and creativity into their lives. All are aware of the paradox in which they dwell, but they have committed to living as fully as they can day by day despite the ambiguity and chronicity of their condition and despite the possibility, even likelihood, that they will suffer other crises in the future.

CLINICAL STANCE IN PHASE 4

Parallel Integration

At the same time their patients are seeking to integrate all the parts of their new lives, clinicians carry out a parallel process. They must not only integrate the suffering and the pain that they have witnessed and guided in their patients, but also process the countertransferential fear, suffering, and pain that patients have stimulated. They must integrate their own experiences, as well as help patients to integrate theirs. They come to recognize that their deep relationship with their patients, their commitment to the healing process, and their faith in the positive outcome are in themselves meaningful. The engagement of

PHASE 4
Checklist for Countertransference

_____ 1. Do you feel strongly attached to this patient?

_____ 2. Are you sad that you will no longer be seeing this patient on a regular basis?

_____ 3. Do you feel a sense of loss at the patient's leaving?

_____ 4. Are you proud of the patient?

_____ 5. Have you been able, with the patient, to *integrate* suffering into life?

_____ 6. Have you been able to help the patient understand the free will involved in his or her life and the daily acts of bravery necessary?

_____ 7. Have you encouraged both societal action and creative action?

_____ 8. Are you able to live with the paradox of a full, meaningful life in limiting illness?

_____ 9. Have you achieved a parallel integration as the patient has?

_____ 10. Are you able to let the patient go?

clinicians shines as a light in what can be very dark times and gives comfort and strength to patients when it is sorely needed.

Release

Clinicians also need to release their patients into the new lives they have constructed. They must come to recognize that they have helped their patients achieve insight and provided them with a variety of methods for dealing with difficulties in the future. They have validated their patients, advocated for them, made it possible for them to grieve, and supported them in their search for meaning. It is now time to let them go.

SPIRITUAL/PHILOSOPHICAL PERSPECTIVE IN PHASE 4

Increased Awareness on All Levels

Phase 4 patients are increasingly aware of meaning on all levels of their existence. Whereas the central search in Phase 3 was to answer their personal existential questions, they now seek to find meaning in all their activities. It is as though they took the exercises of Phase 2, where they analyzed what activities they carried out in each of the four activity areas, and applied a new measure to those activities. Now it is not the practical value of an activity that concerns them, but rather its overall place and meaning in their existence. Their heightened awareness makes patients demand more from everything

---

PHASE 4
Spiritual/Philosophical Perspective

Experience
    Increased awareness on all levels
    Meaning a never-ending search
    Bottom-line truth
    Living in the mystery

Clinical Action
    Support for authenticity

they do. They may have to live with pain and limitations, but they can insist that whatever they do will be meaningful.

Meaning a Never-Ending Search

The search for meaning continues throughout the lives of most seekers. Time and the events of life are constantly shaking up perceptions that once seemed sure and clear. All the questions will probably never be answered, but there is satisfaction in pursuing the process and experiencing brief moments of illumination.

Bottom-Line Truth

Truth or authenticity is the bottom line for patients experiencing what are really the transient periods of Phase 4.

Living in the Mystery

When patients are in that true place that has meaning, they can live in the mystery of a universe where very bad things can happen to good people, or even just ordinary people. Moments of complete integration come only periodically and often only briefly. The rest of the time patients, like most people who intentionally examine their lives and beliefs, struggle with the paradoxes of life and fight to fend off encroaching doubts, fears, and pains. Yet even here, in the battle itself, meaning and transcendence may be found.

Examples ————————————————————————————

Although each person's sense of meaning contained vastly different details, they all shared a deep belief that only those things to which they could authentically subscribe would be part of their bedrock beliefs. **Sophia**, **Everett**, **Christine**, and **Joshua** belonged to different Christian denominations, but none of the four acquiesced in all the beliefs their church articulated as doctrine. The same was probably true for **Father Stephen**, although as a sincere priest, he actively tried to make his beliefs congruent with those of his church. **Erin** and **Lewis** were both agnostics who found greater meaning in secular philosophical formulations or in the spiritual insights of non-Christian faiths such as Buddhism. Like the other five, however, they felt that true meaning in the world—and God if

PHASE 4
Checklist for Spiritual/Philosophical Perspective

_____ 1. Have you seen an increased awareness of meaning on all levels in the patient?

_____ 2. Have you supported authenticity above all in the patient's search for meaning?

_____ 3. Do you feel that the patient, and you, have developed the capability of living meaningful lives in the mystery of a universe where bad things can happen to good people?

he existed—occurred at those moments when two or more people were creating good for themselves or others. Each patient had experienced unmediated, undemanding, generous love and goodness from others. All had learned that they could offer this to others as well. All found in the moment where this happens the basic meaning for their lives.

See Table 7.1 for a summary of Phase 4.

Table 7.1 Phase 4: Integration

1. Course of Illness
Physical/behavioral domain
    Recovery stage (integration as cure)
    Improvement/plateau/relapse
Psychological domain
    Role/identify integration
    New "personal best"
    Continued emotional/spiritual/philosophical development
Social/interactive domain
    New/reintegrated supporters
    Alternative work/vocation activities

2. Identifying Characteristics
    Understanding of the phases
    Integration of pre and post crisis self
    Reconstructed roles and relationships
    Broadened sense of meaning
    Quest for full life

Clinical Goal
    Integration

Clinical Summary
    Integration

3. Assessment
Physical/behavioral domain
    Recognition that plateau, improvement, relapse all possible

(continued)

Table 7.1 *Continued*

Psychological domain
    Role and identity integration
    Maintenance review protocols
    Ongoing creative activity and meaning development
    Ongoing personal narrative and emotional development
    Integration assessment
Social/interactive domain
    Family, couples, friends maintenance protocols
    New and reintegrated friends
    Workplace review
    Alternative jobs/vocations

4. Treatment

Physical/behavioral domain
    Review of maintenance protocols
    Review of relapse/stabilization/integration cycle
    Transience of Phase 4
Psychological domain
    Maintenance of new self
    Free will
    Continued creative work and narrative
    Continued and broadened meaning development
Social/interactive domain
    Continued social action
    Recruitment and maintenance of "integrated supports"
    Workplace modification or work change

5. Countertransference

    Attachment
    Grief
    Loss
    Pride

Clinical Stance

    Integration of suffering
    Free will
    Daily acts of bravery
    Societal action
    Creative action
    Living with paradox
    Parallel integration
    Release

6. Spiritual/Philosophical Perspective

Experience
    Increased awareness on all levels
    Meaning a never-ending search
    Bottom-line truth
    Living in the mystery
Clinical action
    Support for authenticity

PART III

FUTURE DIRECTIONS

Chapter 8

A PARADIGM SHIFT

CHRONICITY AND AMBIGUITY

The Four-Phase Model attempts to shift the focus of the standard paradigm for the assessment and treatment of chronically ill individuals. Most obviously, it moves from a unidirectional, acute model of illness to a conception that encompasses the cyclic nature of chronic conditions. It incorporates ambiguity as an essential, irreducible aspect of chronic illness. It posits an integrated, meaningful life as the end sought in patient treatment, rather than a cure, which, by the definition of chronic illness, does not exist. This does not exclude the possibility that cures may be found for chronic conditions, nor does it suggest that physicians and patients disregard advances in medical understanding. If such advances lead to cures, however, the conditions become acute ones, which moves them out of the chronic illness category. Most people with chronic conditions will not experience cure; hence, they are better served by a paradigm that organizes itself around the chronicity and ambiguity that reflects their actual situation.

SYSTEMS INCLUSIVENESS

The Four-Phase Model is also characterized by a broad inclusiveness. It combines the following into one whole: a descriptive course of change where illness imposed the change, a narrative model, assessment and treatment methods, new countertransferential understandings and applications, patient and clinician spirituality or philosophy, and broad sociocultural factors and dynamics. It addresses from a systems perspective the total environment of a patient's life, including the physical, psychological, family and social, and employment systems. Although the patient's physical and psychological systems are discussed as separate categories, the model emphasizes the complete interpenetration of mind and body and addresses many confusions and misunderstandings that arise from misunderstandings about the mind-body connection. The model envisions the patient's life as an ecology in which all systems are related, and all need attention to bring the patient into the most healthy, viable condition possible. The model includes continuous discussion of the dynamic interaction between patients and clinicians. It addresses philosophic and spiritual issues as these manifest and evolve in both patients and clinicians. The model has an overarching humanistic character and is distinguished by the transformation steps—allowance of, compassion for, respect for, and integration of suffering.

DISTINCTIVE FEATURES OF THE FOUR-PHASE MODEL

Umbrella Framework

The model is an umbrella framework not unlike the TTM stage model (Prochaska, DiClemente, & Norcross, 1992; Prochaska & Velicer, 1997a, 1997b; Prochaska et al., 1994) in that it permits clinicians to continue to employ prior assessment and therapeutic techniques. The Four-Phase Model differs in several ways from the TTM model. The two most important, however, are that it includes the physical/behavioral and social/interactive domains as well as the psychological, and it addresses changes that are almost wholly imposed on the patient rather than intentional change. Adopting this model does not require clinicians to learn an entirely new battery of interventions, but to supplement those already in use with new techniques. The change in approach that the model seeks to accomplish is moving clinicians from a binary, acute concept of illness, where the patient is either sick and in need of treatment or else is well and not their concern, to a longitudinal, cyclical, chronic conception that considers illness manifesting continuously in different ways over time. The model provides clinicians with new vision of how patients experience their condition and how whatever interventions clinicians use affect patients.

Cyclic Nature of Chronic Illness

Although the model identifies distinct phases in the illness experience of patients, these phases do not follow an irreversible progression forward. Rather, the model acknowledges the cyclic pattern of the chronic illness experience and incorporates the concept that severe relapses, other illnesses, or non-illness-related crises may return patients temporarily to earlier phases. In this, too, it resembles other stage theories (Brownell et al., 1986; Donovan & Marlatt, 1988; Prochaska, DiClemente, & Norcross, 1992). The Four-Phase Model asserts that patients who make one thoughtful, reflective progression through all four phases will have the knowledge, understanding, and techniques for moving through the phases more quickly a subsequent time. They will also have deeply assimilated the concept that it is possible for them to achieve a better life even within the limitations of their situation, and even if that situation worsens. The TTM model also posits a cyclic, spiraling pattern where patients learn from their relapses, but implicit in the TTM model is the eventual end of the stage process (Prochaska, DiClemente, & Norcross, 1992). In the Four-Phase Model, patients who reach Phase 4 continue to maintain themselves in that phase indefinitely. It is an ongoing process.

Conceptual Dichotomies

The Four-Phase Model asserts that several conceptual dichotomies common to the health care profession and the culture at large are misleading and potentially harmful. They may cause patients unnecessary secondary and iatrogenic trauma, and they can skew assessments of patients' conditions. This can, in turn, lead to inadequate and sometimes even harmful treatments or interventions.

Ongoing Trauma

The model calls attention to varieties of trauma that can occur continuously as a part of the chronic illness experience. Common perceptions of trauma, even in the health care profession, tend to encompass only effects on the physical body and a degree of psychological response. The model teases out a much broader array of traumas that can actively affect the ability of chronic illness patients to respond to treatment and achieve illness integration.

Countertransference

The model employs countertransference as an element that clinicians can use to help them understand, assess, and treat chronic illness. How clinicians behave with their patients may have a profound effect on how patients respond to treatment. The model posits that a warm, egalitarian relationship helps clinicians make correct assessments and provide effective interventions. Those doing clinical work with chronically ill patients face strong challenges. To meet these challenges requires a true sense of vocation, an intense personal engagement, and an empathetic character (Erlen, 2002). Clinicians working within the Four-Phase framework must also commit to working as a team with all the different specialists whose care most chronically ill patients require.

Development of Meaning

Finally, the Four-Phase Model asserts that it is vitally important to the therapeutic process for patients to engage in an ongoing development of a personal sense of meaning in life. Prochaska and colleagues have noted that insight alone is not enough to create behavioral change. It requires both insight and action to create long-lasting behavioral change (Prochaska, DiClemente, & Norcross, 1992). The Four-Phase Model posits that the chronically ill need to develop two kinds of insight in addition to taking action. They need the psychological insight, which permits them to understand their condition and adjust their lives accordingly. But they also need to develop a meaningful philosophy or spirituality. Commentators on stage intentional theory have noted that behavioral change appears to occur sometimes because the personal meaning, personal construction, or functional significance of the behavior in question changes without the individual's apparently experiencing contemplation and action. For example, they noted moderately risky drinkers who experienced significant life changes, which caused them to change the behavior (Davidson, 1992; Orford, 1992). Could these observers in fact be observing aspects of meaning development as part of a change process separate and apart from intentional cognitive change?

This is not to say that the chronically ill who progress through to Phase 4 arrive at an unchanging, definitive interpretation of the universe, but rather that they consciously engage with issues of meaning and its application to their lives. What they strive to achieve is a kind of deep personal authenticity in all aspects of their lives, and they use some form of creativity or creative process to arrive at authenticity. As to meaning development, the model most particularly recognizes how inextricably soma and psyche are intertwined. The model makes the simultaneous treatment of both soma and psyche the core for achieving patients' integration of the illness experience.

The following sections consider each of the distinctive characteristics in more detail.

UMBRELLA PARADIGM

Use of Standard Assessments

Like other stage models, the Four-Phase Model does not present an exclusive form of assessment and treatment (Brownell, et al., 1986; Kanfer & Grimm, 1980; Prochaska, 1979; Prochaska, DiClemente, & Norcross, 1992). It is distinctive, however, in addressing all three systems—the physical, the psychological, and the social/interactive. The greatest difference in the model's approach to assessment and treatment is that it considers the physical and psychological domains as having equal importance with each other and with family and work-related issues. Often, clinicians concentrate on the physical and, to a certain extent, on the psychological status of their chronic illness patients but are much more cursory about social/interactive issues, probably because that system is not their primary area of expertise. Clinicians in any field tend to evaluate a situation from the perspective of their specialty, so unless their attention is consciously drawn to other domains, they may not consider important aspects of their patients' lives. Yet in actual experience, once patients have acquired methods for maintaining the best level of physical well-being they can, most chronic illness patients cite social and economic issues as causing them the greatest difficulties.

Use of Current Therapies

The model incorporates most therapies that clinicians currently use. The techniques of stress management and of posttraumatic stress disorder (PTSD) reduction and management, for example, are particularly useful with Phase 1 patients who need to reduce the chaos of their experience before they can move forward. Many aspects of cognitive-behavioral therapy work well, particularly with Phase 2 patients as they try to gain insight into their activities and change habits that undermine the level of health that they can maintain. A host of art therapy techniques are especially useful during Phase 3, and the well-known benefits of journaling contributes to the writing and rewriting of the illness narrative, which is a distinctive feature of therapy throughout the four phases.

Additional Tools

The Four-Phase Model combines standard assessment tools and current therapeutic methods with additional investigatory tools and interventions. It also covers the entire range of the patient's life experience, not only the patient's medicalized body or psyche. It considers the patient to be firmly set in a social, work, and cultural context, which deeply affects the manifestations of the patient's symptoms and the effectiveness of interventions. The model also frequently expands on existing interventions.

In Phase 2, for example, patients learn to inventory their activities. In the Four-Phase Model, they begin with common inventorying systems, but then go further. They not only identify what they do—often in greater detail than most inventories call for—but also keep track of how they feel and whether what they have done matches with what they want to do or feel that others want them to do. This expansion of data recording permits patients and clinicians to gain deeper insight into the ways particular activities affect symptoms and the patient's recovery time. It also enables patients to recognize how their own expectations and the expectations of others drive them to carry out activities they cannot sustain without debilitating exhaustion or relapses. The building of insight is even more important than activity modification because, without insight, patients can rarely maintain behavioral changes in the long term.

Personal Illness Narrative

Journaling and other writing activities are used in many therapies. The Four-Phase Model builds on this. It encourages patients to create their own illness narrative, which they then revise as they gain insight and understanding via other interventions. These narratives take into consideration patients' ever-shifting symptoms and their emotional responses, as well as detail patients' experiences with their closest intimates, their friends in the community, and their coworkers. The narratives include patients' growing perceptions of social attitudes and the subtle or obvious stigmas attached to those who are ill and, particularly, those who are ill with chronic conditions. The narratives also come to include patients' personal philosophies or spiritual insights, which patients begin consciously developing during Phases 2 and 3. Rewriting their own story enables patients to nurture self-esteem, understanding, and a profound sense of authenticity. They become emotionally stronger and more independent of trauma-inducing factors in the home, the community, the workplace, the health care establishment, and the culture at large.

Family Narratives

Although less formal—it is rarely written—clinicians also use narratives with families or partners. Encouraging these important intimates to reflect on how the patient's illness affects their lives and to speak about their own traumas and suffering helps teach them to recognize their own often-unconscious attitudes and expectations. In this fashion, clinicians can help family members deal with their own issues while simultaneously learning how to help create a supportive environment for the patient.

CYCLIC PATTERN OF CHRONIC ILLNESS

It cannot be stressed enough that the Four-Phase Model recognizes the cyclic nature of chronic illness. Patients learn as they progress through the phases that they are not on a path rising ever upwards to greater happiness, complete integration of their experience, and permanent transcendence of all suffering. What they can achieve is a way to live meaningfully in the present, knowing, among other things, that they have learned how to deal with serious difficulties and will probably be able to do so in the future. Many chronic diseases are progressive. Patients know that their situation is unlikely to get better or even to stay the same. Other syndromes are characterized by long periods of plateau punctuated by sharp relapses. Apart from the patient's initial chronic illness, life itself serves up many crises, both medical and otherwise. Much as patients may fear the future, and often with good reason, they also know they have gained powerful techniques for dealing with pain, suffering, and frustration, and they can call on these techniques during any crisis in the future.

CONCEPTUAL DICHOTOMIES

Body-Mind

Chapter 1 listed the principal conceptual dichotomies that can interfere with appropriate understanding, assessment, and treatment of chronically ill patients. Central among them is the ancient split between body and mind. Although it has become commonplace in the literature and discourse of medicine to acknowledge that soma and psyche are actually integrated systems, in practice, many people, both health care professionals and laypeople, consider them independent of each other and value them differently.

Disease-Illness

In addition, the most common approach in modern Western medicine is to treat "disease," which is understood as a specific physical impairment that interferes with proper functioning of the body. But "illness," which can be understood to encompass the effects that the condition produces in the psyche, social relations, and work life of patients, as well as the effects produced in their bodies, is a better conception. More and more conditions can be treated effectively only as illnesses, and, increasingly, it appears that even conditions long considered diseases might better be treated within the paradigm of illness.

Empirical-Clinical

In the health care profession, those who actually treat the ill—the clinicians—may have very little contact with those who research the causes and treatments of disease—the empiricists. Clinicians are likely to recognize the importance of factors such as work life or family relationships in symptom presentation and treatment reaction, yet they rarely have the time to examine the empirical information that might permit them to see meaningful relationships among variables. Empiricists tend to design their studies along well-defined somatic lines because these are scientifically measurable and quantifiable. Most data sets are not constructed to capture the shifting heterogeneous symptom experience of the chronically ill over time and body systems. Typically, research pursues etiology, course of illness, and outcome. Outcome, however, can be hard to define in chronic illnesses. Less research is dedicated to clinically useful comparisons of treatment and illness management in the chronically ill.

Professional-Personal

The same model that privileges the quantifiable has encouraged the concept that clinicians can separate the professional and the personal. Although many people now articulate that no professional practices without feeling emotional engagement or reaction to patients, this knowledge is frequently not translated into useful suggested behaviors. This model holds that it is desirable for clinicians to recognize their reactions, process them, and, preferably, use them to improve assessment and treatment. Otherwise, these emotions operate, but below the level of consciousness where they are potentially capable of doing harm to patients, their families, the health care profession, and even society in general. Failure to use processed emotional responses can also cause clinicians to miss important opportunities for improved patient treatment and for their own personal and professional development.

Clinician-Patient

When clinicians regard themselves as entirely objective professionals, this encourages a distinction between themselves and patients that extends far beyond issues of medical problem and medical solution. Patients, because they are scared, weak, suffering, and needy and thus obviously subjective about their experiences, become lesser creatures whose opinions, capabilities, and insights the healthy, objective clinicians can largely ignore. Wise clinicians recognize how arbitrary this relative stance is and behave accordingly. Wise patients realize that clinicians possess only specialized knowledge and not necessarily superior mental abilities or social status. Nonetheless, an underlying sense pervades society, and especially the health care setting, that clinicians are creatures set apart from nonprofessionals and certainly apart from patients.

Acute-Chronic

Until the latter part of the twentieth century, most people understood sickness within an acute model, in which there are clear causes, specific onsets, identifiable symptoms, specific treatments, and a cure or death. Now, even some acute diseases can be treated in such a way that patients survive for long periods of time. In addition, a whole host of seemingly nebulous chronic illnesses have arisen that were never before apparent to the profession. Some appear to have arisen because peo, le live longer, but many of these conditions affect young as well as older people. These diseases often do not have obvious, single causes, easily measured symptoms, or clear treatments, and patients are rarely cured. A new way of understanding illness is essential if the profession is to provide these chronically ill patients with effective help.

Illness as Anomaly, Illness as Normal

American culture tends to undermine new understandings of illness, however, because it regards illness as an anomaly, a deviation from the universal norm of health. This attitude misleads because illness (and death) is a constant in life, not an anomaly. Illness is not necessarily a constant in the life of any given individual, but it will occur in the lives of everyone and is already a constant in the lives of approximately 50% of the American public.

Cure-Integration

The acute model of illness that pervades both the health care profession and the culture at large tends to create an expectation of cure in both patients and medical practitioners. Failure to achieve cure seriously disturbs both patients and clinicians and, unfortunately, can lead to blaming the patient for the ongoing problem. Many conditions, however, will never be cured. Even some that may be cured eventually must be dealt with as chronic now. Successfully achieving the best quality of life for chronic patients requires a changed goal. Clinicians need to help patients integrate the illness experience so that it becomes a part—sometimes a significant part—but not the whole, of patients' continuing existence. In this respect, unlike other stage models (Brownell et al., 1986; Prochaska, DiClemente, & Norcross, 1992; Prochaska & Velicer, 1997a; Prochaska et al., 1994), chronic illness patients do not exit the Four-Phase process. Instead, their goal is to achieve Phase 4 and maintain themselves in it as much of the time as possible.

Health care professionals need to assume leadership in resolving these conceptual dichotomies. Their concerted action and their changes of attitude will gradually shift the general culture. I believe that if we are to achieve improvement in the effectiveness of treatment for chronic illness, the profession needs to alter its approach.

ONGOING TRAUMA

The Four-Phase Model draws attention throughout the phases to the many varieties of trauma that chronic illness patients can suffer. These may occur not solely at the onset of their illness, but for the rest of the course of illness and in all the patient's interactions—with family, friends, coworkers, health care professionals, and the culture as a whole. The trauma of illness onset may not necessarily be a sharp, distinctive event. Illness onset trauma can be subtle and build over time, with patients' knowing that something is wrong but being unable to pinpoint the problem for themselves, let alone a medical professional. Quite apart from their physical distress, patients can often suffer the additional trauma of believing they are going crazy if their illness is met with disbelief or skepticism. How patients' families, friends, and coworkers react to them, first as they are becoming sick, and later after their illness is identified, may cause repeated traumas. How society regards particular chronic illnesses may also cause patient trauma. As with any ill person, patients with chronic illness can have premorbid and comorbid traumas, which affect their experience of the chronic illness. In addition, more than other patients, the chronically ill are likely to suffer iatrogenic traumatization in part because of their repeated exposure to the health care system, but also because of the frustration that the often nebulous, cyclic, changing nature of their illnesses can generate in some clinicians. Moreover, the cumulative effect of multiple traumas over time results in the potential manifestation of symptoms from mild to severe. A growing body of literature is examining this phenomenon, which includes traumas believed to be suffered at a subclinical level. Finally, but as important, is the potential for vicarious traumatization of those around patients with chronic illness, including health care workers.

COUNTERTRANSFERENCE

The Four-Phase Model is atypical in that it actively involves clinician countertransference in each phase of the therapeutic process. The model not only
asks clinicians to note and process their personal feelings and reactions, both
good and bad, but asserts the usefulness of these countertransferential experiences in promoting improvement in the lives of patients.

Most obviously and directly, the model asserts that properly processed
countertransferential feelings can enhance the clinician-patient relationship,
the foundation on which the best hope for successful treatment rests
(T. Lewis et al., 2000). Trust and goodwill must suffuse the relationship. Patients are being asked to do difficult work and to have faith that the clinical
process will make their lives better even though little in their present existence seems to indicate that it will. Patients have to be able to rely on their clinicians. They have to like them. This cannot be a one-way street. Despite
their pains and distractions, or perhaps because of them, patients are intensely alert to the negative feelings in others. They have usually accumulated a good deal of experience in this regard. Clinicians will not elicit from
patients the authentic, honest reporting that is essential for developing management strategies if the clinicians are suppressing feelings of anger, disgust,
annoyance, boredom, or whatever. They will not have clear insight into patients' areas of difficulty if they are blinded by feelings of admiration at what
patients are enduring.

Clinical Work with the Chronically Ill as a Vocation

In a very real sense, clinicians must be "called" to their work. They must feel
deeply that it is important. They must also seek to establish egalitarian, caring, and generous relationships with patients. Because of the many challenges
of the work, practicing with chronic illness patients is much more a vocation
than simply an honorable way to earn a living.

Importance of Witnessing

It is hard to overestimate the importance of witnessing in the clinician's role,
which is one reason the vocational aspect of the work is so key. Witnessing in
and of itself performs an essential intervention in the lives of patients. Patients need to have their experiences heard and validated. Often, no one has

acknowledged their illness, suffering, disability, or discouragement before the clinician. Like Doctors Without Borders in the political world, who assert the existence of individual instances of famine, terror, and so on, clinicians recognize the reality of the patient's illness experience. But to be effective, the witnessing must be completely authentic, genuine, and engaged. The clinician must be completely present to the patient and must hear without comment or stifling of the patient's discourse. The clinician cannot be mentally elsewhere, planning later activities or processing his or her own issues. The clinician cannot mentally shut off the patient's confidences because they are tedious or disturbing or repetitive. Such reactions indicate serious countertransferential issues that require the clinician's immediate analysis and processing. No clinician should practice in a vacuum. All should have others with whom to discuss their problematic reactions.

Supervision and Mentoring

Because clinicians must simultaneously analyze their patients' information and their own countertransferential reactions, it is important for them to have good supervision or reliable mentors. Clinicians should never deal with all issues privately and independently. Some of their personal reactions may be easy to analyze and simple to transmute into enhancing emotional understanding. But other reactions may draw on difficult traumas in the clinician's own past, and these will require the attentive, caring hearing of a person whom the clinician trusts and values. Clinicians must bring to themselves the same generosity and open spirit that they bring to their patients, and they must seek out the support and guidance of trustworthy others.

Patients with Psychiatric Problems

Some patients have pronounced personality disorders in addition to their chronic illnesses, and the manifestations of these can have a negative impact on the clinician. The clinician needs to be able to focus on the chronic illness and the process of helping the patient to traverse the four phases successfully. It is, therefore, advisable to bring a psychologist or psychiatric social worker onto the patient's medical team if the primary clinician needs assistance. This clinician is then available to focus on the patient's specific psychiatric needs, just as the patient may have a cardiologist or rheumatologist overseeing management of specific physical symptoms.

Dislike of Patients

When clinicians find that they strongly dislike patients, should they continue to treat these people? It is not unusual for clinicians to have powerful negative feelings about new patients. They need to examine these feelings with great care to separate out what actually disgusts, angers, or frightens them. In many cases, it is the experiences that the patient is enduring, rather than anything that might be considered intrinsic to the patient. In such a case, clinicians can often find that their original disgust turns into a compelling desire to help. Some patients can be tiresomely whiny. Some are deceptive. Some are manipulative. With insight, clinicians can frequently come to see these behaviors as illness management strategies—often clever ones—developed in the hostile environment that preceded the patient's coming to the clinician. If this can help the clinician reach the patient, by recognizing, acknowledging, and even admiring the inventiveness of the strategy, a bond may be formed that will eventually permit development of more effective illness management.

It is always possible that despite clinicians' best efforts to analyze and resolve their countertransferential issues, they will not be able to connect positively with a patient. If it is simply not possible to establish a relationship, clinicians have an obligation to help the patient find alternative sources of treatment.

Closeness with Patients

On the other hand, the warmth and closeness that the Four-Phase Model encourages in the relationship between clinician and patient may come to resemble friendship, which can potentially create a different set of problems. Although the model promotes an open and egalitarian relationship between clinician and patient, it is not a friendship in the ordinary sense of the word. Clinicians process their countertransferential feelings, but they share these or any other personal material only selectively and only when it will be useful to the patient. The egalitarianism describes the clinician's stance, not the equal exchange of intimacies. Moreover, clinicians practice with the expectation—which they convey to their patients—that the patients will eventually leave the therapeutic situation and be in touch only occasionally, as it is appropriate, afterwards. Clinicians need to convey to their patients that their relationship is another kind of intimacy, with its own rules. It is not friendship, nor family affection, but a different situation in which the clinician gives and keeps counsel with the patient.

Payment for Services

Health maintenance organizations have created a new set of exigencies in the provision of clinical care. Those who work with the chronically ill must often argue for the value of their services with insurance companies, but they can frequently show that what they do is cost-effective in the long run. My clinical practice regularly receives reimbursement from HMOs for the services we provide. However, it is also likely that some patients will have to pay all or part of the clinician's fees themselves.

Many people—disproportionately large numbers of those with chronic illness—have no health insurance and are eligible for subsidized care, usually only in Phase 1 crises or because of addictions used to blunt their suffering. Nonetheless, even these public clinics could engage in phase assessment and treatment cost-effectively in the long run because it can take patients out of the repetitive crisis or crisis/containment loop. I am also a strong advocate of clinicians' performing limited but regular pro bono care in an attempt to reach the extensive population of patients who would otherwise receive little or no care.

NECESSITY FOR TEAMWORK

It is important to reiterate that the Four-Phase Model demands teamwork. Almost all chronic illness patients receive treatment from several different health care professionals, even though visits to some of these specialists occur only intermittently over long periods of time. The assessments and interventions of all the patient's health care professionals need coordination. Interventions recommended by a rheumatologist or cardiologist may have important implications for the patient's dentist, ophthalmologist, or physical therapist. Medications prescribed by one specialist may have side effects, which affect the patient in ways that worsen symptoms only another specialist will notice. Exercise or interventions recommended by one clinician may undermine or vitiate the recommendations of another. The coordinating clinician may know, for example, that the patient is emotionally drained by a level of treatment, which creates deficits that the prescribing physician does not know. Ultimately, the Four-Phase Model seeks to train patients themselves to become coordinators of their own health care.

MEANING DEVELOPMENT

Patients' development of meaning over the course of the phase process is central to achieving integration of the illness experience. It might be called the ultimate union of soma and psyche. But because of the orientation of modern scientific medicine, few clinicians engage their patients actively in meaning development. Although researchers are increasingly coming to recognize, and even measure, the importance of belief and meaning in the health of patients (Johnson-Taylor et al., 1995; Kahn, 1995; Schirm, 2002), many clinicians feel that issues of meaning are someone else's specialty. They believe it is inappropriate for them to intervene in this area.

The Search, Not the Content

The Four-Phase Model mitigates this dilemma by promoting the search for meaning rather than the discovery of any particular meaning content. There is no way, as a matter of fact, that clinicians could effectively promote content because the entire object of the search is for patients to discover what is uniquely authentic to them. Many philosophical or spiritual advisors claim the universal effectiveness of their beliefs, but such universality in itself misses the point. To be effective, the individual patient has to discover what is personally meaningful—and only after wide exploration. It has to be freely chosen and deeply compatible. Moreover, the search for meaning rarely achieves finality. Like all thinking people, patients are constantly approaching knowledge or insight or understanding, but moments of arrival are usually fleeting at best, just as transcendence of illness experience is usually transient.

Providing Resources

Because popular American culture promotes little except material goods and the pleasures to be derived from a healthy young life, clinicians can and should provide a wide variety of resources about meaning for patients to explore.

Often, when chronically ill patients come to clinicians, they have not given considerable thought to the issues of life, death, human purpose, and meaning. Even those who have participated in a religious tradition from childhood have often not given the substance of their professed beliefs much thought. For some people, the chronic illness is the first true test of how well the basic tenets of their religion meet their spiritual and existential needs. Many people in this culture are unaware of how other ancient, time-honored traditions regard pain, illness, suffering, disease, and death. Although these may not provide patients with answers, they give insight into the multiplicity of ways that individuals have used to deal with life's deep, pressing concerns. They also offer insights that patients may never have considered into what life means and what constitutes a meaningful life.

By the time meaning development becomes a significant part of treatment, clinicians should have great familiarity and a strong relationship with their patients. They should have a general sense of what might stimulate their thinking and what might appeal to them emotionally. Nor are the resources all obviously religious or philosophical. Folk and fairy tales, varieties of secular wisdom literature, selected items from the self-help genre, and biographies of great men and women can open patients' eyes to what is valuable and important.

PUBLIC POLICY AND CHRONIC ILLNESS

Public policy has not been a focus in this book, but policy considerations are of crucial importance and should be a topic of future research and analysis. Chronic illness must play an integral part in discussions of public policy concerning the country's health needs (Jason & Taylor, 2003; C. Lewis & Elnitsky, 1995; Lubkin & Larsen, 2002; Smith-Campbell, 2002). Although this book does not attempt to address specific policy issues or potential solutions, it does draw attention to many aspects of chronic illness that require the development of effective public policy. In addition, it is my belief that a phase approach to chronic illness could permit the most cost-effective management of it.

The sheer numbers of those with chronic conditions make it essential that chronic as well as acute conditions be understood as part of the nation's health care situation. As the population ages and once-deadly, acute illnesses have become chronic ones, the numbers will only grow (Lubkin & Larsen, 2002).

As reiterated previously, chronic illness has a profound effect on not only patients, but also their families, the communities in which they live, and their places of employment. The cost of managing a chronic illness often requires more resources at the very time that patients and their families have progressively fewer to expend. Moreover, a disproportionate number of those with chronic illnesses had little to begin with.

Health care costs already represent a significant portion of the nation's gross national product, and those costs are rising (Hardin, 2002). More and more people are not insured, and this number includes not only the poor or unemployed, but also working members of the middle class. With the ever-increasing costs of health insurance, employers are passing more of that expense on to their employees. The system is becoming increasingly dysfunctional. As a result, legislators, employers, insurance companies, patients, clinicians, and the public at large are clamoring for a different national health care policy to help solve a health care crisis that is not only national but also global.

Chronic illness must figure prominently in any new system because chronicity is an aspect of health care that is becoming more significant every year. The high cost of health care and the need for a comprehensive health plan make public policy considerations of the utmost importance to those with chronic illness and to the public in general (Hardin, 2002; C. Lewis & Elnitsky, 1995; Lubkin & Larsen, 2002).

RESEARCH CONSIDERATIONS

Increasingly research has been focusing on the issues associated with chronic illness in general, and not solely on individual conditions (Germino, 2002). I believe such research is highly desirable and necessary.

Heterogeneity in Chronic Illness

Multiple Physical Systems

Heterogeneity is probably the most salient factor in chronic illness. It manifests itself in three significant ways. First, chronic illnesses involve multiple body systems. Patient symptoms encompass pain or weakness in muscles, bones, and joints; they include gastrointestinal problems, neurological malfunctioning, vascular irregularities, urological problems, sleep dysfunctions, and so on. The study of chronic illness must, therefore, consider manifestations in several different systems at the same time.

Changing Symptom Manifestation

Second, the symptoms in any particular physical system fluctuate. It cannot simply be determined that a chronically ill person has low blood pressure or persistent fever or a rash or joint pain. On the contrary, the blood pressure may return to normal for a period, then drop precipitously again, rise moderately, return to normal, and sink again. In addition, the individual's activity level may affect the presentation and severity of symptoms.

Multiple Domains

In addition to various aspects of the patient's physical system, chronic illnesses also involve the patient's psychological and social/interactive systems. Such involvement is not unique to chronic illness, but it receives insufficient attention in the health care response to or research in chronic or acute conditions. Moreover, in chronic illness, the involvement of these other systems persists over time and significantly affects patient reporting, patient compliance, and, most importantly, patient experience of and coping with the illness (Berg et al., 2002; Schirm, 2002).

Usefulness of this Phase Model

The Four-Phase Model helps address the heterogeneity inherent in chronic illness. It addresses many of the issues associated with major life changes that are imposed on individuals rather than chosen. Unlike other stage behavioral models, it considers extensively the patient's physical/behavioral system and his or her social/interactive system, in addition to the psychological system. By identifying different capacities at different phases, it can help clinicians select interventions that may be appropriate and effective and avoid choosing treatments that, although useful at another time, may be counterproductive at this phase. It offers possible explanations for the conflicting findings in chronic illness research. It provides a framework for clinicians to measure qualitative differences in patient experience as they progress through the phases. Clinicians may find that divergent patient experiences are often best understood as a function of the phase a patient is in. And finally, patients may prove more compliant with various treatment options in one phase rather than another. This model has received some empirical validation, but I believe that like other models, its effectiveness makes it clinically useful while it undergoes further empirical examination (Heather, 1992; Stockwell, 1992).

Existent Empirical Research

The Four-Phase Model has been clinically applied to a variety of chronically ill populations, as well as to individuals suffering from posttraumatic stress syndrome and other psychological issues such as addictions and depression. It has been empirically tested with patients who have chronic fatigue syndrome (CFS).

Fennell Phase Inventory

To classify patients into phases, the Fennell Phase Inventory (Fennell, Jason, & Klein, 1998) was developed. This inventory includes four groups of five items, with each group representing aspects of the four different phases: crisis, stabilization, resolution, and integration. Each of the 20 statements expresses a sentiment that people in the appropriate phase agree with more strongly than they do with other items in the inventory that represent phases these individuals are not experiencing.

The Fennell Inventory has been empirically tested several times with CFS patients. The initial study (Jason, Fennell, et al., 1999) performed factor analysis on the responses of 400 participants who self-reported that physicians had diagnosed them with CFS. The crisis items loaded together, as did the integration items, which offered support for the convergent and discriminant validity of these subdomains. Stabilization and resolution items loaded together. Hence, their convergent validity was supported, but their discriminant validity was not. In a subsequent study using data from the original study (Jason, Fennell, et al., 2000), a cluster analysis identified a distinction between all four phases, including the stabilization and resolution phases.

In a subsequent study, Jason, Fricano, and their colleagues (2000) examined 65 participants who had been diagnosed with CFS by a specialist according to the Fukuda et al. (1994) criteria. The study employed the Fennell Inventory, and again the 65 divided into the four phase groups. Because only one fell in the integration category, this group was not analyzed further. That only one individual was in the integration phase, however, was not surprising because it seems probable that most individuals in Phase 4 have taken charge of their own health care and see their own primary practitioners on an as-needed basis.

The 65 participants provided sociodemographic information and a description of their symptoms, and they were asked how long they had experienced CFS. They also completed a variety of measures in addition to the Fennell Inventory: the CFS Symptom Rating form, the CFS Severity Index, the Fatigue Severity Scale, the Medical Outcomes Scale SF-36 Health Survey, and the Illness Management Questionnaire.

The findings of this study support the earlier studies and supplement them by introducing measures of psychosocial functioning and coping as they relate to the four phases. The crisis group was characterized by more profound illness severity, greater symptom severity, greater fatigue, more psychological distress, and greater functional impairment compared with the other phases. They showed significantly lower coping skills and engaged in far less information seeking. The lower educational and occupational status of this group suggests the desirability of including a social/interactive component into the assessment and treatment of chronic illness. The stabilization group reflected some plateau or decrease in symptoms as well as an increasing adaptation to the illness. They used more strategies for accommodating to the illness and engaged in more information seeking than those in the crisis group, but less than those in the resolution group. Some of the resolution group experienced relapse or renewed escalation of symptoms, but they were better prepared psychologically to cope than were individuals in the crisis phase. Individuals in the resolution phase reported intermediate levels of impairment, which were higher than the stabilization group, but lower than the crisis group. Although they continued to struggle to integrate their pre- and postillness lives, these individuals were significantly more likely than individuals in the crisis group to use coping strategies and information seeking.

Most recently, a study in Belgium set out to replicate these earlier findings on the robustness of the Fennell Phase Model. In addition, the study sought to examine the stability and utility of the Fennell Phase Inventory and its utility in the development of treatment plans. Forty-four subjects were selected at a chronic fatigue syndrome clinic in Brussels from a pool of individuals presenting at the clinic for medical examinations to exclude other explanations for their excessive fatigue. The study results appear to capture the Fennell Model and support a distinction between the phases. The Fennell Phase Inventory was found valid and reliable in the Belgian sample, and the researchers determined that health promotion strategies, which influence both the individual and population, can be used within the phases to facilitate more appropriate treatment outcomes (Van Hoof et al., forthcoming-a, forthcoming-b).

The results of these studies suggest that clinicians can use the Fennell Phase Inventory as a way to differentiate the phases experienced by the patient and hence as a tool to enhance their assessment of patients' illness coping and adaptation and their progress in psychotherapy and health management.

Queries Raised about Past Research

Stabilization and Resolution as Separate Phases

The issue raised by the initial study as to whether stabilization and resolution were distinct phases seems to have been resolved in the subsequent studies described previously. Although overlap occurs between phases, individuals in resolution have grasped and acknowledged the concept of their illness as chronic, whereas individuals in stabilization are still seeking a cure. The improved coping skills of individuals in the resolution phase have also shown them to cope better than individuals in stabilization even though they may have more severe physical symptomatology.

Integration Is Primarily a Psychological Achievement

Another query arose because individuals in the integration group reported improved symptoms, whereas the model asserts that achievement of Phase 4 is largely a psychological adaptation. Should individuals be included in the integration group only if their physical symptoms are so much improved that they are not bothered by them? Does integration simply mean the individual is suffering fewer symptoms? I believe that individuals in Phase 4 may have improved symptomatology, they may have reached a stable plateau of symptoms, or they may have relapses or the experience of new symptoms. Their physical status is not the issue, but rather how they regard themselves, their overall lives, and their future. That the few individuals in integration who have participated in studies have experienced improved symptoms may possibly indicate a paucity of data. Bringing significant numbers of individuals who have achieved integration into formal studies will probably require concerted outreach because these people have tended to move on with their lives and are no longer living so intensely with their illness. The characteristics of the integration phase are largely social and psychological, but this will be shown empirically only when Phase 4 individuals with problematic symptoms also participate in studies.

Unique Knowledge

There has also been a logical query as to whether patients can return to earlier phases if passage out of the phase results from information or knowledge that patients acquire only once. Can patients reinhabit the prior state of ignorance? A look at the literature of stage-based intentional behavioral change, addiction, trauma, and 12-step programs shows that an individual may inhabit the paradoxical position of both having a unique instance of knowledge and reverting to former attitudes of denial and dysfunctional behaviors. Individuals do make a unique breakthrough when they recognize and acknowledge that they are alcoholics or drug addicts, for example. As anyone treating these populations knows, however, for individuals to maintain this insight is very difficult or even impossible without ongoing support and encouragement. The TTM model posits that individuals recycle many times before successfully completing their stage process (Prochaska, DiClemente, & Norcross, 1992; Prochaska et al., 1994). The authors of that model hold that insight alone is insufficient but needs to be tied to a readiness to take action (Prochaska, DiClemente, & Norcross, 1992). As Chapter 6 on Phase 3 emphasizes, maintenance of insight is a key treatment issue in Phase 3 because Phase 3 individuals experience the loss and grief that is inherent in acquiring the unique knowledge that they "can't go home again," that their illness is forever. People subjected to such profound loss and grief do not want to maintain an insight that causes the pain. It is extraordinarily easy for them to lose the insight and slip back into denial of the learned knowledge and dysfunctional behavior.

Nature of Meaning Acquisition

Similarly, *meaning* is not a single nugget of information or even a packet of nuggets acquired once. It is an ongoing process that must constantly respond to new events and extend over fresh areas. It helps the chronically ill to deal with the paradox in which they live, where they must maintain an awareness of their situation, which entails grief and loss, while continuing to lead lives that are as full as possible. Meaning is what helps to cope with the paradox, including even the possibility of improvement. The meaning that allows chronic illness patients to move from resolution to integration might be said to resemble a large spiritual territory, which they map out for themselves generally. There they feel at home, and they come to have fairly firm general attitudes about the nature of the landscape. But the specific typography of their spiritual geography changes as individuals acquire new experience and refine their current beliefs.

Barriers between Phases

Some analysts experience difficulty with the concept of distinct phases between which there are no impermeable boundaries, where an individual may progress through a phase, slide back, move forward again, and so forth. Conversely, if such movement is possible, can distinct phases be said to exist? Others have already addressed this issue to say that individuals can recycle many times through distinct stages that they identify in their model (Brownell et al., 1986; Prochaska, DiClemente, & Norcross, 1992; Prochaska et al., 1994). I agree with this concept. There are clear distinctions between the phases. Crisis is characterized by trauma, particularly of illness onset; stabilization, by making order from chaos and seeking behavior; resolution, by recognition that "you can't go home again" but the concomitant insight maintenance and development of meaning; and integration, by the functioning integration of the pre- and postillness self into a meaningful new identity and life. At the same time, movement back into earlier phases is possible because insight can be lost and trauma can be overwhelming.

Return to Earlier Phases after Achieving Phase 4

Some analysts question whether patients who have reached Phase 4, particularly if they have "transcended" their illness, can slide back into earlier phases. Transcendence does not relieve an individual of the human condition. Individuals who experience transcendence understand in a felt way the best they can be, and they attempt to remain in this state of being as much of the time as possible. But they are not immune from frustration or failures or periodic loss of faith. This has long been documented historically among those who have achieved significant spiritual transcendence.

Patients who successfully develop the insight and meaning that takes them into integration understand their situation of their current illness very well. As discussed earlier, however, few people remain steadfastly in Phase 4 because issues about meaning are constantly being tested in the real world of people's lives. Most patients, even concerning the illness they have processed, find themselves needing to work on problems of meaning repeatedly. Unlike stage models of intentional behavioral change such as the TTM model, which project the eventual exit from the stage process by individuals who have successfully progressed through their stages, the Four-Phase Model asserts that chronic illness patients must continue to maintain themselves in Phase 4 indefinitely. It is an ongoing process constantly subject to reverses. This ongoing character may reflect the continuing nature of integration as opposed to the "cure" of stage completion.

By far, the most common cause for return to earlier phases from Phase 4 is a totally new illness or completely extraneous event. The death of a spouse or other loved one, for example, is excruciatingly painful and shocking for any individual. It is often even more disruptive for a person with a chronic illness because the deceased is someone who had come to understand the ill person's special circumstances and had helped make it possible for the ill person to live reasonably well and fully. Such loss can easily produce Phase 1 crisis psychologically, but also physically because body and mind are so closely linked. It may also produce serious social or work crises.

Patients who have engaged in phase therapy can, when they regain a bit of balance, begin to contain their crisis on their own. They know what kind of help to seek in others. Once they have a chance to reflect, they can also begin to carry out the kinds of tasks that helped them stabilize in Phase 2. They know that Phase 3 resolution is possible, even if they need assistance getting there.

A new illness, a serious trauma, or even a relapse in the old illness that produces symptoms and pain totally unlike anything the patient has ever suffered before can also thrust the patient back into crisis. Pain and suffering cause misery in everyone, even patients who have thought about these issues intensely. Intense pain can obliterate almost any mental and emotional equipoise. But when patients are able to begin processing again—when their crisis or pain is sufficiently contained—they have an armory of techniques. Probably even more important, they have faith that they will be able to work their way to a better life again. Their faith comes from the proven effectiveness of their first journey.

Semantic Difficulties

Two terms used in descriptions of the Four-Phase Model seem to generate interpretive problems for some readers. One term is *transcendence,* that condition in Phase 4 individuals where their comprehension of their illness and their placement of it in a meaningful metaphysical or philosophical context allows them to live psychologically with illness without making it the only focus of their lives. Transcendence occurs, but it is not the defining characteristic of integration. Rather, it is a state of being that the most fortunate achieve only temporarily.

The other term is *allowance,* as in the allowance of suffering, the transformative step of Phase 1 (crisis). Some may take *allowance* to mean acceptance in the sense of welcoming or embracing. The term is meant to denote only acknowledgment of the reality of individual suffering and psychological recognition that suffering is happening to the individual. The term implies no welcome and no embrace of suffering, but merely conscious acknowledgement of its actual existence in the individual's life.

Potential Research Projects

Testing Phase Assessment Instruments

It is worthwhile noting again that most research has been dedicated to stage theories that address intentional change and focus on psychological processes. Little research has been done on the other forms of behavioral change and how they are similar to or different from the behavioral change models that have been tested (Prochaska, DiClemente, & Norcross, 1992). Testing the validity of stage theory is difficult. It is important to distinguish between true stage theory and continuum processes, and research designs differ greatly in their ability to do so (N. D. Weinstein et al., 1998). Given this complexity, attempts to demonstrate stage change can fail because the stages have not been identified or assessed properly, the barriers between stages have not been identified, and so on (N. D. Weinstein et al., 1998). It could be illuminating, therefore, to further investigate the Fennell Phase Inventory and other potential assessment instruments of imposed change. Would revisions of the Fennell Inventory items or the addition of new items produce a more efficacious instrument? Does having patients complete the inventory at different times during their illness provide new insight into the experience of chronic illness and thus insight into treatment concerns such as patient compliance? Are there different rates of progress and recycling through the phase process depending on the particular chronic illness a patient has? How do variables such as socioeconomic status affect progress through the phases? Do certain assessment tools work better than others? Do some psychometric assessment instruments provide additional useful data within the phase framework? Should some be used only at certain moments, for example, after the patient has arrived at a solid Phase 2 level of stability?

As an addendum to the Fennell Phase Inventory, it could be helpful to examine clinician attitudes toward chronic illness, their countertransferential reactions, their experience of the phase process, and so on, as well as those of patients.

Testing Intervention Techniques and Their Timing

Are some interventions more effective than others, and/or are they more effective in one phase rather than in another? Are some interventions ineffective in certain phases? Should clinicians put off some activities until patients reach certain levels of insight? It has been suggested that experimental studies of matched and mismatched interventions might provide better tests of stage ideas than the correlational designs that have dominated intentional stage research thus far. It has also been argued that sequence treatment matched to stage should, hypothetically, be the most effective protocols (Prochaska, DiClemente, & Norcross, 1992; Prochaska & Velicer, 1997a; Prochaska et al., 1994). Thus, I propose that in the psychological domain during Phase 1 (crisis), patients receive protocols and interventions that modify and manage trauma symptoms and sequelae. In Phase 2 (stabilization), they are able to learn activity modification and life restructuring. Attempting to teach life restructuring would be ineffective in the crisis phase and might discourage a patient in crisis from performing this necessary activity when he or she becomes capable of it in Phase 2. Similarly, in the physical domain, crisis patients may be unable to integrate physiological medical protocols such as physical therapy until they experience the stabilization of Phase 2. Again it is important to note that thus far, all the research on matched and mismatched interventions has examined intentional change models, not models addressing imposed change. Empiricists are still debating the results.

Pursuing designs intended to study matched and mismatched interventions by phase could result in more efficacious treatment of patients and their families and improvement in their subsequent quality of life. Obviously, the value of phase-matched protocols will also need to be assessed against standardized treatments.

Testing Systems Assessment and Treatment

Empirical work on the effectiveness of treating all patient systems—the social and work environments as well as the physical and psychological—might yield some very productive results. Investigations would test to determine the effectiveness and timeliness of interventions in each of the three domains in each phase. Clinicians' anecdotal evidence suggests that patients with chronic illness suffer most profoundly in the social and work worlds rather than their personal physical or psychological ones, especially once their initial Phase 1 crisis has passed. Because the current structure of health care underuses appropriate social worker and rehabilitation specialist support for these patients, it might be useful to measure whether assessments and interventions that helped patients in these areas from the start did not ultimately reduce medical costs.

Testing for the Function and Usefulness of Meaning Development

I believe that meaning development is an important aspect of successful adjustment for those who have experienced imposed change. There has been some empirical study related to meaning development and certain illnesses such as AIDS (Botha, 1996), and I believe this could be a very fruitful arena of investigation for any ongoing, that is, chronic, condition.

Testing of Phase and Trauma

Studies that consider the experience of trauma, grief, and illness through the phases might also prove clinically helpful and fruitful. The entire concept of trauma and its definition are currently undergoing reexamination because studies of the manifestations of trauma and its effects have been seen as more pervasive than was once thought (Fullilove et al., 1992; Scott & Stradling, 1994; Turner & Lloyd, 1995). There is evidence that accumulated experiences of trauma or adversity produce a cumulative traumatic effect and that this can happen even when some of the experiences are subclinical in nature (Blank, 1993; Vrana & Lauterbach, 1994).

Testing the Function and Usefulness of Countertransference

How does the relationship established between clinician and patient correlate with phase placement and intervention effectiveness? Is it determinate of intervention effectiveness? Commentators have noted that the emotions and motivations of others play a role in treatment (Orford, 1992; Stockwell, 1992). They have pointed out that in the intentional stage model analysis, these issues apply not only to clinicians but also to others who may influence the patient. Both clinicians and these others may be at the "action" stage, but patients themselves may not be ready for action. This can make clinicians or others frustrated with the patient, which can set in motion a negative process that will not help the patient to move toward action. Research into the relationship between patients, clinicians, and significant lay others connected with the patients could improve treatment effectiveness significantly.

Health Care Teams

The great heterogeneity of chronic illness makes it almost certain that a cadre of doctors and other specialists will treat most chronic illness patients. A team approach using a phase framework, with all members informed about the assessments and interventions of the others, permits clinicians to address syndrome complexity. It also allows them to address the variability of symptoms in all the systems over time. It would be helpful to research how clinical teams are best constructed, who on the team serves best as team leader, and how information is best communicated among team members. It could be useful to investigate the efficacy of including social workers and rehabilitation specialists in the assessment and treatment of chronic illness patients because there are many indications that these health care specialists bring a much-needed systems and case management approach that could serve chronic illness patients very well (Remsburg & Carson, 2002). It would be useful to investigate the most cost-effective team arrangements.

Development of a Chronic Illness Data-Gathering Framework

A data-gathering framework that uses the Four-Phase Model might significantly help improve the study of chronic illness. As noted throughout this book, patients not only experience shifting symptoms of varying severity over the course of their chronic illness, but they also experience their symptoms differently in different phases. Individuals may also significantly affect their symptoms by their activity levels. Thus, there is significant heterogeneity in symptom presentation in chronic illness that current data collection methods may fail to capture.

Much data collection takes place in a binary system. The clinician notes whether the patient has the symptom (fever, swollen glands, fatigue, joint pain) or does not have the symptom. If data is collected on several different occasions—and often it is not—the information usually does not reveal anything about the severity of the symptom at each time of data collection, only whether the symptom was present or absent. Chronic illnesses are often characterized by symptoms that appear and disappear and fluctuate in intensity. When studies use a one-time, binary data collection system that collapses the responses of patients who are in different points of the time line of the illness or who are in different phases, the findings can be muddied. In some cases, this model of data collection can greatly complicate diagnosis or even lead to misdiagnosis (Friedberg & Jason, 1998).

Useful data collection would not only include regular assessments over time, but also rate symptom severity each time. It would also note other factors that affect symptom presentation and severity at the time of reporting. Patient activity levels can significantly affect symptoms. Patients who report a significant decline in impairment, for example, but little or no decline in symptoms, may be carrying out more activities than their illness will let them accomplish without causing them symptomatic problems.

The phase that patients are in also appears to affect how they experience symptoms (Jason, Fricano, et al., 2000; Van Hoof et al., forthcoming-a, forthcoming-b). It may be desirable to ask them to compare the severity now with the severity at, for example, illness onset or during the stabilization phase.

Data collection should also include how significant social others are reacting to the patient. Evidence strongly suggests that social factors have significant impact on patient coping and patient compliance with treatment protocols. It could help clinicians make more effective assessments and accomplish more effective interventions if they had better information about factors that affect coping, what circumstances support compliance, and when particular interventions are most likely to help.

Other Illness Populations

Clinically, the Four-Phase Model has been applied to a variety of chronic conditions in addition to CFS (for which it has undergone some empirical examination). I encourage empiricists to conduct studies on the applicability of the Four-Phase Model and the Fennell Phase Inventory to chronic illnesses such as MS, lupus, Sjogren's syndrome, scleroderma, fibromyalgia, as well as stroke survivors, cancer survivors, survivors with heart conditions, depression, posttraumatic stress disorder, AIDS-HIV, and so on. In addition, I believe the model should be examined for its effectiveness in treating addictions, situations involving intractable pain, postrape and abuse conditions, and bereavement.

Chronic Illness by Disease and Age Group

An awareness is emerging among health care providers that the age group of the patient seems to affect many aspects of living with chronic illness. Among young people, for example, developmental processes complicate learning to live with chronic illness. It would be useful to have empirical studies that examined developmental changes in conjunction with the phase process so that clinicians might intervene more successfully in the treatment of this population. Similarly, how do much older patients move through the phases? What is the experience of adults in their prime years, especially those with children? In addition, do different age groups move through the phases differently depending on the specific chronic illness?

Static and Dynamic Disabilities

Chronic illness has drawn attention to the fact that only a certain number of disabilities are static. Many more, and not all of them in chronic illness, are dynamic. Patients suffer greater or lesser disability over time. During one period, they may require a wheelchair, for example, but then arrive at periods when they can get along with only a cane or no aid whatsoever. How chronic illness patients experience disability can also change over time. This ebbing and flowing of dynamic disability among many chronically ill individuals offers a particularly rich and important field for study. There is added urgency to investigate these kinds of disabilities to interpret appropriately the Disabilities Act, which exists to protect individuals with disabilities.

Acute versus Chronic Illness

Finally, the different characteristics of acute as opposed to chronic illnesses suggest an extraordinarily important arena of study. Historically, the bulk of medical scientific investigation has pursued illness within the framework of acute disease, in which cure is the goal. This approach significantly obscures the care needs of the chronically ill and can distort understanding of the data relating to chronic illnesses. To develop appropriate scientific models for investigating individual chronic illnesses, it would certainly be useful to have empirical work on the distinctions between acute and chronic conditions.

Bibliography

Aberbach, D. (1989). Creativity and the survivor: The struggle for mastery. *International Review of Psycho-Analysis, 16*(3), 273–286.

Abrums, M. (2000). Jesus will fix it after awhile: Meanings and health. *Social Science and Medicine, 50*(1), 89–105.

Agnetti, G. (1997). Facing chronic illness within the family: A systems approach. *New Trends in Experimental and Clinical Psychiatry, 13*(2), 133–139.

Agnetti, G., & Young, J. (1993). Chronicity and the experiences of timelessness: An intervention model. *Family Systems Medicine, 11,* 67–81.

Ahles, T. A., Khan, S. A., Yunus, M. B., Spiegel, D. A., & Masi, A. T. (1991). Psychiatric status of patients with primary fibromyalgia, patients with rheumatoid arthritis, and subjects without pain: A blind comparison of *DSM-III* diagnoses. *American Journal of Psychiatry, 148*(12), 1721–1726.

Aiken, J. H. (1997). A citizens' AIDS task force: Overcoming obstacles. *Journal of Homosexuality, 32*(3/4), 145–167.

Akhtar, S. (1987). Schizoid personality disorder: A synthesis of developmental, dynamic and descriptive features. *American Journal of Psychotherapy, 41*(4), 499–518.

Albrecht, G. L., & Devlieger, P. J. (1999). The disability paradox: High quality of life against all odds. *Social Science and Medicine, 48*(8), 977–988.

Alexandris, A., & Vaslamatzis, G. (Eds.). (1993). *Counter-Transference: Theory, technique, teaching.* London: Karanc Books.

Allport, G. W., & Ross, J. M. (1967). Personal religious orientation and prejudice. *Journal of Personality and Social Psychology, 5*(4), 432–443.

Alonzo, A. A. (2000). The experience of chronic illness and posttraumatic stress disorder: The consequences of cumulative adversity. *Social Science and Medicine, 50,* 1475–1484.

Alonzo, A. A., & Reynolds, V. R. (1996). Emotions and care-seeking during acute myocardial infarction: A model for intervention. *International Journal of Sociology and Social Policy, 16*(9/10), 97–122.

Alter, C. L., Pelcovitz, D., Axelrod, A., Goldenberg, B., Harris, H., Meyers, B., et al. (1996). Identification of PTSD in cancer survivors. *Psychosomatic Medicine, 37*(2), 137–143.

Anderton, J. M., Elfert, H., & Lai, M. (1989). Ideology in the clinical context: Chronic illness, ethnicity and the discourse on normalization. *Sociology of Health and Illness, 11*(3), 253–278.

Armstrong, D. (1987). Theoretical tensions in biopsychosocial medicine. *Social Science and Medicine, 25*(11), 1213–1218.

Armstrong, D. (1990). Use of the genealogical method in the exploration of chronic illness: A research note. *Social Science and Medicine, 30*(11), 1225–1227.

Aronoff, M., & Gunter, V. (1991). *It's hard to keep a good town down. Local recovery efforts in the aftermath of toxic contamination.* Washington, DC: American Sociological Association.

Asmundson, G. J., Frombach, I., McQuaid, J., Pedrelli, P., Lenox, R., & Stein, M. B. (2000). Dimensionality of posttraumatic stress symptoms: A confirmatory factor analysis of *DSM-IV* symptom clusters and other symptom models. *Behavioral Research and Therapy, 38*(2), 203–214.

Auslander, G. K., & Gold, N. (1999). Disability terminology in the media: A comparison of newspaper reports in Canada and Israel. *Social Science and Medicine, 48,* 1395–1405.

Auslander, W. F., Thompson, S., Dreitzer, D., White, N., & Santiago, J. V. (1997). Disparity in glycemic control and adherence between African American and Caucasian youths with diabetes. *Diabetes Care, 20*(10), 1569–1575.

Ax, S., Gregg, V. H., & Jones, D. (1997). Chronic fatigue syndrome: Sufferers' evaluation of medical support. *Journal of the Royal Society of Medicine, 90,* 250–254.

Ax, S., Gregg, V. H., & Jones, D. (1998). Chronic fatigue syndrome: Illness attributions and perceptions of control. *Homeostasis, 39*(1/2), 44–51.

Axtell, S. (1999). Disabilities and chronic illness identity: Interviews with lesbians and bisexual women and their partners. *Journal of Gay, Lesbian, and Bisexual Identity, 4*(1), 53–72.

Ayers, S., & Pickering, A. D. (2001). Do women get posttraumatic stress disorder as a result of childbirth: A prospective study of incidence. *Birth, 28,* 111–118.

Baker, C., & Stern, P. N. (1993). Finding meaning in chronic illness as the key to self care. *Canadian Journal of Nursing Research, 25*(2), 23–36.

Baldwin, B. A. (1978). A paradigm for the classification of emotional crises: Implications for crisis intervention. *American Journal of Orthopsychiatry, 48*(3), 538–551.

Ballweg, M. (1997). Blaming the victim: The psychologizing of endometriosis. *Obstetrics and Gynecology Clinics of North America, 24*(2), 441–453.

Banks, J., & Prior, L. (2001). Doing things with illness: The micro politics of the CFS clinic. *Social Science and Medicine, 52,* 11–23.

Barnett, P. B. (1998). Clinical communication and managed care. *Medical Group Management Journal, 45*(4), 60–66.

Barshay, J. (1993). Another strand of our diversity: Some thoughts from a feminist therapist with severe chronic illness. In M. E. Millmuth & L. Holcomb (Eds.), *Women with disabilities: Found voices* (pp. 159–169). Binghamton, NY: Hayworth Press.

Bartley, M., & Owen, C. (1996). Relation between socioeconomic status, employment, and health during economic change, 1973–93. *British Medical Journal, 313,* 445–449.

Bates, D. W., Schmitt, W., Buchwald, D., Ware, N. C., Lee, J., Thoyer, E., et al. (1993). Prevalence of fatigue and chronic fatigue syndrome in a primary care practice. *Archives of Internal Medicine, 153,* 2759–2765.

Bates, M. S. (1990). A critical perspective on coronary artery disease and coronary bypass surgery. *Social Science and Medicine, 30*(20), 249–260.

Bates, M. S., & Rankin-Hill, L. (1994). Control, culture and chronic pain. *Social Science and Medicine, 39*(5), 629–645.

Bates, M. S., Rankin-Hill, L., & Sanchez-Ayendez, M. (1997). The effects of the cultural context of health care on treatment of and response to chronic pain and illness. *Social Science and Medicine, 45*(9), 1433–1447.

Baumann, A. O., Deber, R. B., Silverman, B. E., & Mallette, C. M. (1998). Who cares? Who cures? The ongoing debate in the provision of health care. *Journal of Advanced Nursing, 28*(5), 1040–1045.

Baumann, S. L. (1997). Contrasting two approaches in a community-based nursing practice with older adults: The medical model and Parse's nursing theory. *Nursing Science Quarterly, 10*(3), 124–130.

Beardslee, W. R., Versage, E. M., & Gladstone, T. G. (1998). Children of affectively ill parents: A review of the past 10 years. *Journal of the American Academy of Child and Adolescent Psychiatry, 37*(11), 1134–1141.

Bedell, G. (2000). Daily life for eight urban gay men with HIV/AIDS. *American Journal of Occupational Therapy, 54*(2), 197–206.

Belza, B. L., Henke, C. J., Yelin, E. H., Epstein, W. V., & Gilliss, C. L. (1993). Correlates of fatigue in older adults with rheumatoid arthritis. *Nursing Research, 42,* 93–99.

Bendelow, G. A., & Williams, S. J. (1995). Transcending the dualism: Toward a sociology of pain. *Sociology of Health and Illness, 17*(2), 139–165.

Benet, A. (1996). A portrait of chronic illness: Inspecting the canvas, reframing the issues. *American Behavioral Scientist, 39*(6), 767–776.

Bennett, R. M. (1993). Fibromyalgia and the facts: Sense or nonsense. *Rheumatic Disease Clinics of North America, 19*(1), 45–59.

Bennett, R. M. (1999). Emerging concepts in the neurobiology of chronic pain: Evidence of abnormal sensory processing in fibromyalgia. *Mayo Clinic Proceedings, 74*(4), 385–398.

Berg, J., Evangelista, L. S., & Dunbar-Jacob, J. M. (2002). Compliance. In I. Lubkin & P. D. Larsen (Eds.), *Chronic illness: Impact and interventions* (5th ed., pp. 203–232). Sudbury, MA: Jones and Bartlett.

Berger, K. S., & Thompson, R. A. (1995). *The developing person through childhood and adolescence.* New York: Worth.

Berger, P. L. (1999). *Redeeming laughter: The comic dimension of human experience.* New York: Walter de Gruyter.

Bergquist, S., & Neuberger, G. B. (2002). Altered mobility and fatigue. In I. Lubkin & P. D. Larsen (Eds.), *Chronic illness: Impact and interventions* (5th ed., pp. 147–177). Sudbury, MA: Jones and Bartlett.

Berwick, D. M. (1989). Sounding board continuous improvement as an ideal in health care. *New England Journal of Medicine, 320*(1), 53–56.

Bezard, E., Imbert, C., & Gross, C. E. (1998). Experimental models of Parkinson's disease: From the static to the dynamic. *Review of Neuroscience, 9*(2), 71–90.

Biordi, D. (2002). Social isolation. In I. Lubkin & P. D. Larsen (Eds.), *Chronic illness: Impact and interventions* (5th ed., pp. 119–146). Sudbury, MA: Jones and Bartlett.

Blalock, S. J., DeVellis, R. F., Giorgino, K. B., DeVellis, B. M., Gold, D. T., Dooley, M. A., et al. (1996). Osteoporosis prevention in premenopausal women: Using a stage model approach to examine the predictors of behavior. *Health Psychology, 15,* 84–93.

Blank, A. S. (1993). The longitudinal course of posttraumatic stress disorders. In J. R. Davidson & E. B. Foa (Eds.), *Posttraumatic stress disorder: DSM-IV and beyond* (pp. 3–22). Washington, DC: American Psychiatric Press.

Bloom, A. (1996, Fall). Suggestions for filing CFIDS LTD claims. *CFIDS Chronicle.*

Blum, R. W., Potthoff, S. F., & Resnick, M. D. (1997). The impact of chronic conditions on Native American adolescents. *Families, Systems and Health, 15*(3), 275–282.

Blumenthal, D., Campbell, E. G., Causino, N., & Louis, K. S. (1996). Participation of life-science faculty in research relationships with industry. *New England Journal of Medicine, 335*(23), 1734–1739.

Bose, J. (1995). Trauma, depression, and mourning. *Contemporary Psychoanalysis, 31*(3), 399–407.

Botha, L. F. H. (1996). Posttraumatic stress disorder and illness behavior in HIV+ patients. *Psychological Reports, 79,* 843–845.

Boyer, B. A., Leman, C. J., Shipley, T. E., Jr., McBrearty, J., Quint, A., & Goren, E. (1996). Discordance between physician and patient perceptions in the treatment of diabetes mellitus: A pilot study of the relationship to adherence and glycemic control. *Diabetes Educator, 22*(5), 493–499.

Boyer, K. M. (1999). Disability benefits: What is the Social Security Administration thinking? *Journal of Medical Practice Management, 14*(6), 297–300.

Bradley, L. A. (1989). Cognitive-behavioral therapy for primary fibromyalgia. *Journal of Rheumatology, 16,* 131–136.

Bradley, L. A., & Alberts, K. R. (1999). Psychological and behavioral approaches to pain management for patients with rheumatic disease. *Rheumatic Disease Clinics of North America, 25*(1), 215–233.

Brink, S. (2000). To get top care, get pushy. If your health plan won't send you to a leading hospital, seek allies. *U.S. News and World Report, 129*(3), 72–73.

Brody, J. E. (2000, August 1). Fibromyalgia: Real illness, real answers. *The New York Times Company* (Health & Fitness), p. 8.

Brown, J. W. (1999). Neuropsychology and the self-concept. *Journal of Nervous Mental Disorders, 187*(3), 131–141.

Brown, L. (1991). Laughter: The best medicine. *Canadian Journal of Medical Radiation Technology, 22*(3), 127–129.

Brownell, K. D., Marlatt, G. A., Lichtenstein, E., & Wilson, G. T. (1986). Understanding and preventing relapse. *American Psychologist, 41*(7), 765–782.

Buchwald, D., Pascualy, R., Bombardier, C., & Kith, P. (1994). Sleep disorders in patients with chronic fatigue syndrome. *Clinical Infectious Diseases, 18* (Suppl. 1), S68–S72.

Bull, M., & Jervis, L. (1997). Strategies used by chronically ill older women and their caregiving daughters in managing posthospital care. *Journal of Advanced Nursing, 25,* 541–547.

Burckhardt, C. S. (1987). Coping strategies of the chronically ill. *Nursing Clinics of North America, 22*(3), 543–550.

Burckhardt, C. S., Woods, S. L., Schultz, A. A., & Ziebarth, D. M. (1989). Quality of life of adults with chronic illness: A psychometric study. *Research in Nursing and Health, 12,* 347–354.

Burke, M. D. (1990). Estimating the clinical usefulness of diagnostic tests. *American Journal of Clinical Pathology, 94*(5), 663–664.

Burton, D. (1995). Agency maze. In I. Lubkin (Ed.), *Chronic illness: Impact and interventions* (3rd ed., pp. 459–480). Boston: Jones and Bartlett.

Butler, R. N. (1996). Palliative medicine: Providing care when cure is not possible. *Geriatrics, 51*(5), 33–44.

Byrd, W. M., Clayton, L. A., & Kitchen, K. (1994). African American physicians' view on health reform: Results of a survey. *Journal of the National Medical Association, 86*(3), 191–199.

Caggiano, A. P., Jr., Weisfeld, N. E., Palace, F. M., & Klein, P. G. (1997). New HMO regulations protect patients as never before. *New Jersey Medicine, 94*(4), 25–32.

Cameron, K., & Gregor, F. (1987). Chronic illness and compliance. *Journal of Advanced Nursing, 12,* 671–676.

Campbell, E. G., Louis, K. S., & Blumenthal, D. (1998). Looking a gift horse in the mouth: Corporate gifts supporting life sciences research. *Journal of the American Medical Association, 279*(13), 995–999.

Canam, C., & Acorn, S. (1999). Quality of life for family care givers with people with chronic health problems. *Rehabilitative Nursing, 24*(5), 192–196, 200.

Cannon, C. A., & Cavanaugh, J. C. (1998). Chronic illness in the context of marriage: A systems perspective of stress and coping in chronic obstructive pulmonary disease. *Families, Systems and Health, 16*(4), 401–418.

Carbone, L. (1999). An interdisciplinary approach to the rehabilitation of open-heart surgical patients. *Rehabilitation Nursing, 24*(2), 55–61.

Carrasquillo, O., Himmelstein, D. U., Woolhandler, S., & Bor, D. H. (1999). Trends in health insurance coverage, 1989–1997. *International Journal of Health Services, 29*(3), 467–483.

Carter, B., & McGoldrick, M. (Eds.). (1988). *The changing family life cycle: A framework for family therapy* (2nd ed.). New York: Gardner Press.

Casey, M. (1999). Physicians still seeking a cure. *Medical Data International.* Available from http://www.medicaldata.com.

Chin, P. A. (2002). Change agent. In I. Lubkin & P. D. Larsen (Eds.), *Chronic illness: Impact and interventions* (5th ed., pp. 313–336). Sudbury, MA: Jones and Bartlett.

Chodoff, P. (1982). Therapy of hysterical personality disorders. *Current Psychiatric Theory, 21,* 59–65.

Christiansen, C. H. (1999). Defining lives: Occupation as identity: An essay on competence, coherence, and the creation of meaning. *American Journal of Occupational Therapy, 53*(6), 547–558.

Chuengsatiansup, K. (1999). Sense, symbol, and soma: Illness experience in the soundscape of the everyday life. *Culture, Medicine and Psychiatry, 23*(3), 273–301.

Clark, M. L., & Gioro, S. (1998). Nurses, indirect trauma, and prevention. *Image: Journal of Nursing Scholarship, 31*(1), 85–87.

Clarke, A. (1994). What is a chronic disease? The effects of a re-definition in HIV and AIDS. *Social Science and Medicine, 39*(4), 591–597.

Clifford, J. C. (1993). Successful management of chronic pain syndrome. *Canadian Family Physician, 39,* 549–559.

Coderch, J. (1991). Comments on the treatment of a narcissistic patient. *International Journal of Psychoanalysis, 72*(Pt. 3), 393–401.

Coles, N. (1984). Sinners in the hands of an angry utilitarian. In J. P. Kay (-Shuttleworth): The moral and physical condition of the working classes employed in the cotton manufacture in Manchester. (1832). *Bulletin of Research in the Humanities, 86*(4), 453–488.

Collicott, P., Gage, J., Oblath, R., & Opelka, F. (1996). In their own words: Surgeons representatives discuss legislative and regulatory issues: Part II. *Bulletin of the American College of Surgeons, 81*(10), 22–31.

Collins, H. M. (1994). Dissecting surgery: Forms of life depersonalized. *Social Studies of Science, 24,* 311–333.

Cooksey, E., & Brown, P. (1998). Spinning on its axes: *DSM* and the social construction of psychiatric diagnosis. *International Journal of Health Services, 28*(3), 525–554.

Cooper, M. C. (1990). Chronic illness and nursing's ethical challenge. *Holistic Nursing Practice, 5*(1), 10–16.

Cordova, M. J., Studts, J., Hann, D. M., Jacobsen, P. B., & Andrykowski, M. A. (2000). Symptom structure of PTSD following breast cancer. *Journal of Traumatic Stress, 13*(2), 301–319.

Counselman, E. F., & Alonso, A. (1993). The ill therapist: Therapists' reaction to personal illness and its impact on psychotherapy. *American Journal of Therapy, 47*(4), 591–603.

Craft, C. A. (1999). A conceptual model of feminine hardiness. *Holistic Nursing Practice, 13*(3), 25–34.

Cuijpers, P. (1998). Prevention of depression in chronic general medical disorders: A pilot study. *Psychological Reports, 82,* 735–738.

Cullen, J. (1998). The needle and the damage done: Research, action research, and the organizational and social construction of health in the "information society." *Human Relations, 51*(12), 1543–1564.

Cutcliffe, J. R. (1998). Hope, counseling and complicated bereavement reactions. *Journal of Advanced Nursing, 28*(4), 754–761.

Davidson, R. (1992). The Prochaska and DiClemente models: Reply to the debate. *British Journal of Addiction, 87,* 833–835.

DeVeaugh-Geiss, J. (1993). Diagnosis and treatment of obsessive compulsive disorder. *Annual Review of Medicine, 44,* 53–61.

DiClemente, C. C. (1991). Motivational interviewing and the stages of change. In W. R. Miller & S. Rollnick (Eds.), *Motivational interviewing: Preparing people for change* (pp. 191–202). New York: Guilford Press.

DiMatteo, M. R. (1998). The role of the physician in the emerging health care environment. *Western Journal of Medicine, 168,* 328–333.

Dixon, T. L., & Linz, D. (2000). Race and the misrepresentation of victimization on local television news. *Communications Research, 27*(5), 547–573.

Doherty, W. J., & Colangelo, N. (1984). The family FIRO model: A modest proposal for organizing family treatment. *Journal of Marital and Family Therapy, 10*(1), 19–29.

Doherty, W. J., Colangelo, N., & Hovander, D. (1991). Priority setting in family change and clinical practice: The family FIRO model. *Family Practice, 30,* 227–240.

Doherty, W. J., McDaniel, W. J., & Hepworth, J. (1994). Medical family therapy: An emerging arena for family therapy. *Association for Family Therapy, 16,* 31–46.

Dohrenwend, B. P. (2000, March). The role of adversity and stress in psychopathology: Some evidence and its implications for theory and research. *Journal of Health and Social Behavior, 41,* 1–19.

Donovan, D. M., & Marlatt, G. A. (Eds.). (1988). *Assessment of addictive behaviors: Behavioral, cognitive and physiological procedures.* New York: Guilford Press.

Do Rozario, L. (1997). Spirituality in the lives of people with disability and chronic illness: A creative paradigm of wholeness and reconstitution. *Disability and Rehabilitation, 19*(10), 427–434.

Drench, M. E. (1994). Changes in body image secondary to disease and injury. *Rehabilitation Nursing, 19*(1), 31–36.

Druss, B. C., Schlesinger, M., Thomas, T., & Allen, H. (2000). Chronic illness and plan satisfaction under managed care. *Health Affairs, 19*(1), 203–209.

Durana, C. (1998). The use of touch in psychotherapy: Ethical and clinical guidelines. *Psychotherapy: Theory, Research, Practice and Training, 35*(2), 269–280.

Durban, J., Lazar, R., & Ofer, G. (1993). The cracked container, the containing crack: Chronic illness—its effect on the therapist and the therapeutic process. *International Journal of Psycho-Analysis, 74,* 705–713.

Dyson, J., Cobb, M., & Forman, D. (1997). The meaning of spirituality: A literature review. *Journal of Advanced Nursing, 26*(6), 1183–1188.

Edwards, G. M. (1993). Art therapy with HIV-positive patients: Hardiness, creativity and meaning. *Arts in Psychotherapy, 20*(4), 325–333.

Elliot, C. M. (1996). Through a glass darkly: Chronic illness in the therapist. *Clinical Social Work Journal, 24*(1), 21–34.

Emanuel, L. (1995). On being a doctor: The privilege and the pain. *Annals of Internal Medicine, 122,* 797–798.

Engel, G. L. (1977). The need for a new medical model: A challenge for biomedicine. *Science, 196,* 129–136.

Engel, G. L. (1980). The clinical application of the biopsychosocial model. *American Journal of Psychiatry, 137*(5), 535–544.

Epstein, R., Quill, T. E., & McWhinney, I. R. (1999). Somatization reconsidered: Incorporating the patient's experience of illness. *Archives of Internal Medicine, 159,* 215–222.

Erikson, E. H. (1959). Identity and the life cycle: Selected papers. *Psychological Issues, 1,* 50–100.

Erlen, J. A. (2002). Ethics in chronic illness. In I. Lubkin & P. D. Larsen (Eds.), *Chronic illness: Impact and interventions* (5th ed., pp. 407–429). Sudbury, MA: Jones and Bartlett.

Faison, K. J., Faria, S. H., & Frank, D. (1999). Caregivers of chronically ill elderly: Perceived burden. *Journal of Community Health Nursing, 16*(4), 243–253.

Falicov, C. J. (Ed.). (1988). *Family development and the impact of a child's chronic illness* (pp. 293–309). New York: Guilford Press.

Federal Register. (1999a). *Food and Drug Administration Modernization Act of 1997* (List of documents issued by the Food and Drug Administration that apply to medical devices regulated by the Center for Biologics Evaluation and Research; Food and Drug Administration), 64 (79), 20312–20313.

Federal Register. (1999b). *Social Security Ruling, SSR 99–2p; Titles II and XVI* Evaluating Cases Involving Chronic Fatigue Syndromes (CFS), 64 (83), 23380–23384.

Fennell, P. A. (1993, Summer). A systematic, four-stage progressive model for mapping the CFIDS experience. *CFIDS Chronicle,* 40–46.

Fennell, P. A. (1995a). CFS sociocultural influences and trauma: Clinical considerations. *Journal of Chronic Fatigue Syndrome, 1*(3/4), 159–173.

Fennell, P. A. (1995b). The four progressive stages of the CFS experience: A coping tool for patients. *Journal of Chronic Fatigue Syndrome, 1*(3/4), 69–79.

Fennell, P. A., Jason, L., & Klein, S. (1998). Capturing the different phases of the CFS illness. *CFIDS Chronicle, 11*(3), 3–16.

Fennell, P. A. (2001). *The chronic illness workbook: Strategies and solutions for taking back your life.* Oakland, CA: New Harbinger.

Fennell, P. A. (2003a). A four-phase approach to understanding chronic fatigue syndrome. In L. A. Jason, P. A. Fennell, & R. R. Taylor (Eds.), *The chronic fatigue syndrome handbook* (pp. 155–175). Hoboken, NJ: Wiley.

Fennell, P. A. (2003b). Phase-based interventions. In L. A. Jason, P. A. Fennell, & R. R. Taylor (Eds.), *The chronic fatigue syndrome handbook* (pp. 455–492). Hoboken, NJ: Wiley.

Fennell, P. A. (2003c). Sociocultural influences and trauma. In L. A. Jason, P. A. Fennell, & R. R. Taylor (Eds.), *The chronic fatigue syndrome handbook* (pp. 73–88). Hoboken, NJ: Wiley.

Fennell, P. A., Levine, P., & Uslan, D. (2001, January). *Applications for the practicing physician: A multidisciplinary approach.* American Association for Chronic Fatigue Syndrome (AACFS) Conference, Seattle, WA.

Figley, C. R. (1995). *Compassion fatigue.* New York: Brunner/Mazel.

Fisch, R. Z., & Tadmor, O. (1989, December 9). Iatrogenic posttraumatic stress disorder. *Lancet,* 1397.

Fisher, L., & Weihs, K. L. (2000). Can addressing family relationships improve outcomes in chronic disease? *Journal of Family Practice, 49*(6), 561–567.

Fishman, S. (2001, August 6). Doctor Feelbad. *New York, 34*(30), 20–25.

Flodberg, S. O., & Kahn, A. M. (1995). Sexuality. In I. Lubkin (Ed.), *Chronic illness: Impact and interventions* (3rd ed., pp. 144–167). Boston: Jones and Bartlett.

Fossati, A., Maffei, C., Battaglia, M., Bagneto, M., Donati, D., Fiorelli, M., et al. (2001). Latent class analysis of *DSM-IV* schizotypal personality disorder criteria in psychiatric patients. *Schizophrenia Bulletin, 27*(1), 59–71.

Foster, P. S., & Eisler, R. M. (2001). An integrative approach to the treatment of obsessive compulsive disorder. *Comprehensive Psychiatry, 42*(1), 24–31.

Fowler, J. W. (1982). *Stages of faith: The psychology of human development and the quest for meaning.* San Francisco: HarperSanFrancisco.

Frankl, V. E. (1983). Meaninglessness: A challenge of psychologists. In T. Millon (Ed.), *Theories of personalities and psychopathology* (3rd ed., pp. 256–263). New York: Holt, Rinehart and Winston.

Friedberg, F., & Jason, L. A. (1998). *Understanding chronic fatigue syndrome: An empirical guide to assessment and treatment.* Washington, DC: American Psychological Association.

Fries, J. F. (1998). Reducing the need and demand for medical services. *Psychosomatic Medicine, 60,* 140–142.

Frosch, J. (1990). Normal—abnormal—emotional health—emotional illness. *Psychiatric Journal of the University of Ottawa, 15*(1), 2–10.

Fugelli, P. (1998). Clinical practice: Between Aristotle and Cochrane. *Swiss Medical Weekly [Schweizerische Medizinsche Wochenschrift], 128,* 184–188.

Fukuda, K., Straus, S. E., Hickie, I., Sharpe, M. C., Dobbins, J. G., & Komaroff, A. (1994). The chronic fatigue syndrome: A comprehensive approach to its definition and study. *Annals of Internal Medicine, 121,* 953–959.

Fullilove, M. T., Lown, A., & Fullilove, R. E. (1992). Crack 'hos and skeezers: Traumatic experiences of women crack users. *Journal of Sex Research, 29*(2), 275–287.

Furst, G., Gerber, L. H., & Smith, C. (1985). *Rehabilitation through learning: Energy conservation and joint protection—a workbook for persons with rheumatoid arthritis.* Washington, DC: National Institute of Health.

Furst, G., Gerber, L. H., & Smith, C. (1997). *Energy conservation: A workbook for persons with fatigue.* Washington, DC: National Institute of Health.

Gallagher, R. M. (1999). Treatment planning in pain medicine integrating medical, physical and behavioral therapies. *Medical Clinics of North America, 83*(3), 823–849.

Gamsa, A. (1994). The role of psychological factors in chronic pain. II: A critical appraisal. *Pain, 57,* 17–29.

Gatchel, R. J., & Gardea, M. A. (1999). Their importance in predicting disability, response to treatment, and search for compensation. *Neurological Clinics of North America, 17*(1), 149–167.

Gawande, A. A., & Bates, D. W. (2000, February 22). The use of information technology in improving medical performance. Part III: Patient-support tools. *General Medicine Journal, 2*(1), E 12.

Germino, B. B. (2002). Research in chronic illness. In I. Lubkin & P. D. Larsen (Eds.), *Chronic illness: Impact and interventions* (5th ed., pp. 385–405). Sudbury, MA: Jones and Bartlett.

Gershuny, B. S., & Thayer, J. F. (1999). Relations among psychological trauma, dissociative phenomena, and trauma-related distress: A review and integration. *Clinical Psychology Review, 19*(5), 631–657.

Gignac, M. A. M., & Cott, C. (1998). A conceptual model of independence and dependence for adults with chronic physical illness and disability. *Social Science and Medicine, 47*(6), 739–753.

Gignac, M. A. M., Cott, C., & Badley, E. M. (2000). Adaptation to chronic illness and disability and its relationship to perceptions of independence and dependence. *Journals of Gerontology: Series B, Psychological Sciences and Social Sciences, 55,* 362–372.

Gilden, J. L., Hendryx, M. S., Clar, S., Casia, C., & Singh, S. P. (1992). Diabetes support groups improve health care of older diabetic patients. *Journal of the American Geriatrics Society, 40,* 147–150.

Glassner, B. (2000). Where meanings get constructed. *Contemporary Sociology, 29*(4), 590–594.

Goldberg, A. I. (1974). On the prognosis and treatment of narcissism. *Journal of American Psychoanalytic Association, 22*(2), 243–254.

Gordon, G. H., Baker, L., & Levinson, W. (1995). Physician-patient communication in managed care. *Western Journal of Medicine, 163,* 527–531.

Gore, M. J. (2000). Patient no longer? Consumers want to move into health care driver's seat. *Medicine and Health, 54*(20), 1–4.

Gorgievski-Duijvesteijn, M., Steensma, H., & TeBrake, E. (1998). Protestant work ethic as a moderator of mental and physical well-being. *Psychological Reports, 83*(3), 1043–1050.

Gournay, K. (1998). Obsessive compulsive disorder: Nature and treatment. *Nursing Standard, 13*(10), 46–52.

Granello, D. H., Pauley, P. S., & Carmichael, A. (1999). Special issue: The role of the media in mental health—theory and research—relationship of the media to attitudes toward people with mental illness. *Journal of Humanistic Education and Development, 38*(2), 98–111.

Greenberg, M., & Wartenberg, D. (1990). Risk perception understanding mass media coverage of disease clusters. *American Journal of Epidemiology, 132*(1), S192–S195.

Greer, S., Morris, T., & Pettingdale, K. W. (1979). Psychological response to breast cancer: Effect on outcome. *Lancet, 70,* 785–787.

Gulick, E. (1991). Reliability and validity of the Work Assessment Scale for persons with multiple sclerosis. *Nursing Research, 40,* 107–112.

Gunderson, J. G., & Zanarini, M. C. (1987). Current overview of the borderline diagnosis. *Journal of Clinical Psychiatry, 48,* 5–14.

Halkitis, P. N., & Dooha, S. M. (1998). The perceptions and experience of managed care by HIV-positive individuals in New York City. *AIDS Public Policy Journal, 13*(2), 75–84.

Hall, J. A., Stein, T. S., Roter, D. L., & Rieser, N. (1999). Inaccuracies in physicians' perceptions of their patients. *Medical Care, 37*(11), 1164–1168.

Hampton, M. R., & Frombach, J. (2000). Women's experience of traumatic stress in cancer treatment. *Health Care for Women International, 21,* 67–76.

Hanson, G. (2000). Victimhood for all. Ever wonder why everyone is claiming to be a victim? *Insight, 16*(1), 16.

Harder, S. D., Kelly, P., & Dunkelblau, E. (1997). Patient-physician communication: A selective literature review. *Journal of Oncology Management, 6*(4), 279–283.

Hardin, S. R. (2002). Financial impact. In I. Lubkin & P. D. Larsen (Eds.), *Chronic illness: Impact and interventions* (5th ed., pp. 471–490). Sudbury, MA: Jones and Bartlett.

Harvard Mental Health Letter. (2000). *General review: Antisocial Personality—Part I.* Cambridge, MA: Harvard Health.

Harvard Mental Health Letter. (2001). *General review: Antisocial Personality—Part II.* Cambridge, MA: Harvard Health.

Hassed, C. (2001). How humor keeps you well. *Australian Family Physician, 30*(1), 25–28.

Hastings Center Report. (2000, January/February). *Alternative and complementary medicine: What's a doctor to do?* 47–48.

Hatcher, R. L. (1973). Insight and self-observation. *Journal of American Psychoanalytical Association, 21*(2), 377–398.

Hayes, V. E. (1997). Families and children's chronic conditions: Knowledge development and methodological considerations. *Scholarly Inquiry for Nursing Practice: An International Journal, 11*(4), 259–291.

Heather, N. (1992). Addictive disorders are essentially motivational problems. *British Journal of Addiction, 87,* 828–830.

Heijmans, M., & de Ridder, D. (1998). Assessing illness representations of chronic illness: Explorations of their disease-specific nature. *Journal of Behavioral Medicine, 21*(5), 485–503.

Heinzer, M. M. (1998). Health promotion during childhood chronic illness: A paradox facing society. *Holistic Nursing Practice, 12*(2), 8–16.

Hellstrom, O., Bullington, J., Karlsson, G., Lindqvist, P., & Mattson, B. (1999). A phenomenological study of fibromyalgia: Patient perspectives. *Scandinavian Journal of Primary Health Care, 17*(1), 11–16.

Helseth, L. D. (1999). Primary care physicians' perceptions of diabetes management: A balancing act. *Journal of Family Practice, 48*(1), 37–42.

Henderson, P. A. (1997). Psychosocial adjustment of adult cancer survivors: Their needs and counselors' interventions. *Journal of Counseling and Development, 75,* 188–194.

Henly, S. J., Tyree, E., Lindsey, D. L., Lambeth, S. O., & Burd, C. M. (1998). Innovative perspectives on health services for vulnerable rural populations. *Family and Community Health, 21*(1), 22–31.

Herman, J. L. (1999). Complex PTSD: A syndrome in survivors of prolonged and repeated trauma. In M. J. Horowitz (Ed.), *Essential papers on post traumatic stress disorder* (pp. 82–98). New York: New York University Press.

Hinojosa, J., & Kramer, P. (1997). Statement—fundamental concepts of occupational therapy: Occupation, purposeful activity, and function. *American Journal of Occupational Therapy, 51*(10), 864–866.

Hinrichsen, G. A., Revenson, T. A., & Shinn, M. (1985). Does self-help help? An empirical investigation of scoliosis peer support groups. *Journal of Social Issues, 41*(1), 65–87.

Hirschauer, S. (1991). The manufacture of bodies in surgery. *Social Studies of Science, 21,* 279–319.

Hoffman, C., Rice, D., & Sung, H. (1996). Persons with chronic conditions: Their prevalence and costs. *Journal of the American Medical Association, 276,* 1473–1479.

Holm-Hadulla, R. (1996). The creative aspect of dynamic psychotherapy: Parallels between the construction of experienced reality in the literary and the psychotherapeutic process. *American Journal of Psychotherapy, 50*(3), 360–369.

Horowitz, M. H. (1987). Some notes on insight and its failures. *Psychoanalytic Quarterly, 56*(1), 177–196.

Horowitz, M. J. (1997). The psychotherapy for histrionic personality disorder. *Journal of Psychotherapy Practice and Research, 6*(2), 93–104.

Hoult, J. (1998). Silencing the victim: The politics of discrediting child abuse survivors. *Ethics and Behavior, 8*(2), 125.

Houser, R., & Chace, A. (1993). Job satisfaction of people with disabilities placed through a project with industry. *Journal of Rehabilitation, 59,* 45–48.

Howard, B. S., & Howard, J. R. (1997). Occupation as spiritual activity. *American Journal of Occupational Therapy, 51*(3), 181–185.

Howe, E. G. (1995). At the bedside: Transforming or vampiric? When care-providers share their subjective realities with their patients. *Journal of Clinical Ethics, 6*(2), 98–111.

Hummel, F. I. (2002). Advocacy. In I. Lubkin & P. D. Larsen (Eds.), *Chronic illness: Impact and interventions* (5th ed., pp. 359–383). Sudbury, MA: Jones and Bartlett.

Humphreys, K. (1997, Spring). Individual and social benefits of mutual aid self-help groups. *Social Policy,* 12–19.

Inui, T. S. (1998). Establishing the doctor patient relationship: Science, art, or competence? *Swiss Medical Weekly [Schweizerische Medizinsche Wochenschrift], 128*(7), 225–230.

Irvine, A. A., Phillips, E. K., Fisher, M., & Cloonan, P. (1989). Out of the Ivory Tower: The value of collaborative research. *Home Health Care Services Quarterly, 10*(3/4), 117–130.

Ivanoff, A., Robinson, E. A. R., & Blythe, B. J. (1987). Empirical clinical practice from a feminist perspective. *Social Work, 32*(5), 417–422.

Jacoby, M. B., Sullivan, T., & Warren, E. (2001). Rethinking debates over health care financing: Evidence from the bankruptcy courts. *New York University Law Review, 76*(2).

Jason, L. A., Fennell, P. A., Klein, S., Fricano, G., Halpert, J., & Taylor, R. R. (1999). An investigation of the different phases of the CFS illness. *Journal of Chronic Fatigue Syndrome, 5*(3/4), 35–54.

Jason, L. A., Fennell, P. A., & Taylor, R. R. (2003). *The chronic fatigue syndrome handbook.* Hoboken, NJ: Wiley.

Jason, L. A., Fennell, P. A., Taylor, R. R., Fricano, G., & Halpert, J. A. (2000). An empirical verification of the Fennell Phases of the CFS illness. *Journal of Chronic Fatigue Syndrome, 6*(1), 47–56.

Jason, L. A., Fricano, G., Taylor, R. R., Halpert, J., Fennell, P. A., Klein, S., et al. (2000, December). Chronic fatigue syndrome: An examination of the phases. *Journal of Clinical Psychology,* 1497–1508.

Jason, L. A., Richman, J. A., Friedberg, F., Wagner, L., Taylor, R. R., & Jordan, K. M. (1997). Politics, science, and the emergence of a new disease: The case of chronic fatigue syndrome. *American Psychologist, 52*(9), 973–983.

Jason, L. A., & Taylor, R. R. (2003). Community-based interventions. In L. A. Jason, P. A. Fennell, & R. R. Taylor (Eds.), *The chronic fatigue syndrome handbook* (pp. 726–754). Hoboken, NJ: Wiley.

Jeffrey, J. E. & Lubkin, I. M. (2002). Chronic pain. In I. Lubkin & P. D. Larsen (Eds.), *Chronic illness: Impact and interventions* (5th ed., pp. 77–118). Sudbury, MA: Jones and Bartlett.

Jennings, J. L. (1985). The fallacious origin of the mind-body problem: A reconsideration of Descartes' method and results. *Journal of Mind and Behavior, 6*(3), 357–372.

Jobst, K. A., Shostak, D., & Whitehouse, P. J. (1999). Diseases of meaning, manifestations of health, and metaphor. *Journal of Alternative Complementary Medicine, 5*(6), 495–502.

Johnson-Taylor, E., Jones, P., & Burns, M. (1995). Quality of life. In I. Lubkin (Ed.), *Chronic illness: Impact and interventions* (3rd ed., pp. 193–212). Boston: Jones and Bartlett.

Jordan, K. D., Mayer, T. G., & Gatchel, R. J. (1998). Should extended disability be an exclusion criterion for tertiary rehabilitation? *Spine, 23*(19), 2110–2116.

Joung, I. M. A., van de Mheen, H. D., Stronks, K., van Poppel, F. W. A., & Mackenbach, J. P. (1998). A longitudinal study of health selection in marital transitions. *Social Science and Medicine, 46*(3), 425–435.

Jung, C. (1990). *Collected works of Carl Jung*. Princeton, NJ: Princeton University Press.

Kahn, A. M. (1995). Coping with fear and grieving. In I. Lubkin (Ed.), *Chronic illness: Impact and interventions* (3rd ed., pp. 241–260). Boston: Jones and Bartlett.

Kane, R. L. (1996). Health perceptions real and imagined. *American Behavioral Scientist, 39*(6), 707–716.

Kanfer, F. H., & Grimm, L. G. (1980). Managing clinical change: A process model of therapy. *Behavior Modification, 4*(4), 419–444.

Kauffman, J. (1994). Dissociative functions in the normal mourning process. *Journal of Death and Dying, 28*(1), 31–38.

Keefe, F. (2001). Pain and spirituality. *Journal of Pain, 2,* 101–110.

Kelly, E. W. (1995). Spirituality and religion. *Counseling and psychotherapy: Diversity in theory and practice.* Alexandria, VA: American Counseling Association.

Kelner, M., & Wellman, B. (1997). Health care and consumer choice: Medical and alternative therapies. *Social Science and Medicine, 45*(2), 203–212.

King, M. L., Jr. (1986). *A testament of hope: The essential writings and speeches of Martin Luther King, Jr.* New York: HarperCollins.

Kirkwood, W. G., & Brown, D. (1995). Public communication about the causes of disease: The rhetoric of responsibility. *Journal of Communication, 45,* 55–76.

Kirmayer, L. J., Robbins, L. J., & Paris, J. (1994). Somatoform disorders: Personality and the social matrix of somatic disease. *Journal of Abnormal Psychology, 103*(1), 125–136.

Kissane, D. W. (2000). Psychospiritual and existential distress: The challenge for palliative care. *Australian Family Physician, 29*(11), 1022–1025.

Kitzinger, J. (1990). Audience understanding of AIDS media messages: A discussion of methods. *Sociology of Health and Illness, 12*(3), 319.

Klein, R., & Schermer, V. (2000). *Group psychotherapy for psychological trauma.* New York: Guilford Press.

Kohlberg, L. (1959). *Stages in the development of moral thought and action.* New York: Holt.

Kohlberg, L. (1981). *The philosophy of moral development.* San Francisco: Harper & Row.

Kohler, K., Schweikert-Stary, M. T., & Lubkin, I. (1995). Altered mobility. In I. Lubkin (Ed.), *Chronic illness: Impact and interventions* (3rd ed., pp. 117–142). Boston: Jones and Bartlett.

Komaroff, A. L., Fogioli, L. R., Doolittle, T. H., Gandek, B., Gleit, M. A., Guerriero, R. J., et al. (1996). Health status in patients with chronic fatigue syndrome and in general population and disease comparison groups. *American Journal of Medicine, 101,* 281–290.

Kontz, M. M. (1989). Compliance redefined and implications for home care. *Holistic Nurse Practice, 3*(2), 54–64.

Korn, D. (2000). Medical information privacy and the conduct of biomedical research. *Academic Medicine, 75*(10), 963–968.

Kornfield, J. (1993). *A Path with Heart.* New York: Bantam Books.

Korszun, A. (2000). Sleep and circadian rhythm disorders in fibromyalgia. *Current Rheumatology Reports, 2*(2), 124–130.

Kraft, C. A. (1999). A conceptual model of feminine hardiness. *Holistic Nursing Practice, 13*(3), 25–34.

Krippner, S., & Welsh, P. (1992). *Spiritual dimensions of healing: From native shamanism to contemporary health care.* New York: Irvington.

Krupp, L. B. (1989). The Fatigue Severity Scale: Application to patients with multiple sclerosis and systemic lupus erythematosis. *Archives of Neurology, 46,* 1121–1123.

Krupp, L. B., & Mendleson, W. B. (1990). Sleep disorders in chronic fatigue syndrome. In J. Horne (Ed.), *Sleep '90* (pp. 261–263). Bochum, Germany: Pontenagel Press.

Kübler-Ross, E. (1969). *On death and dying.* New York: Macmillan.

Kwoh, C. K., O'Connor, G. T., Regan-Smith, M. G., Olmstead, E. M., Brown, L. A., & Burnett, J. B. (1992). Concordance between clinician and patient assessment of physical and mental health status. *Journal of Rheumatology, 19*(7), 1031–1037.

Lambert, C. E., & Lambert, V. A. (1999). Psychological hardiness: State of the science. *Holistic Nursing Practice, 13*(3), 11.

Landro, L. (2000, July 7). National group goes to battle for patients fighting their insurers. *Wall Street Journal*, p. B1.

Lang, F. (1990). Resident behaviors during observed pelvic examinations. *Family Medicine, 20,* 153–155.

Larson, E. (1998). Reframing the meaning of disability of families: The embrace of paradox. *Social Science and Medicine, 47*(7), 865–875.

Lazare, A. (1987). Shame and humiliation in the medical encounter. *Archives of Internal Medicine, 147,* 1653–1658.

Lee, A. (1998). Seamless health care for chronic disease in a dual health care system: Managed care and the role of family physicians. *Journal of Management in Medicine, 12*(6), 398–405.

Leveille, S. G. (1998). Preventing disability and managing chronic illness in frail older adults: A randomizing trial of a community based partnership with primary care. *Journal of the American Geriatric Society, 46*(10), 1191–1198.

Levine, S. (1979). *A gradual awakening.* New York: Doubleday.

Levinson, W., Gorawara-Bhat, R., Dueck, R., Egener, B., Kao, A., Kerr, C., et al. (1999). Resolving disagreement in the patient-physician relationship: Tools of improving communication in managed care. *Journal of the American Medical Association, 282*(15), 1477–1483.

Lewis, C., & Elnitsky, C. (1995). Social/health policy. In I. Lubkin (Ed.), *Chronic illness: Impact and interventions* (3rd ed., pp. 507–527). Boston: Jones and Bartlett.

Lewis, J. (1999). Status passages: The experience of HIV-positive gay men. *Journal of Homosexuality, 37*(3), 87–115.

Lewis, P., & Lubkin, I. (2002). Illness roles. In I. Lubkin & P. D. Larsen (Eds.), *Chronic illness: Impact and interventions* (5th ed., pp. 25–52). Sudbury, MA: Jones and Bartlett.

Lewis, T., Amini, F., & Lannon, R. (2000). *A general theory of love.* New York: Random House.

Lindy, J. D., Grace, M. C., & Green, B. L. (1981). Survivors: Outreach to a reluctant population. *American Journal of Orthopsychiatry, 51*(3), 468–478.

Lindy, J. D., Green, B. L., & Grace, M. C. (1987). The stressor criterion and posttraumatic stress disorder. *Journal of Mental and Nervous Disease, 175,* 269–272.

Loewe, R., Schwartzman, J., Freeman, J., Quinn, L., & Zuckerman, S. (1998). Doctor talk and diabetes: Toward an analysis of the clinical construction of chronic illness. *Social Science and Medicine, 47*(9), 1267–1276.

Longmore, P. K. (1995, September/October). The second phase: From disability rights to disability culture. *Disability Rag and Resource,* 4–11.

Low, J. (1999). The concept of hardiness: Persistent problems, persistent appeal. *Holistic Nursing Practice, 13*(3), 20–24.

Lubkin, I. M., & Larsen, P. D. (2002a). *Chronic illness: Impact and interventions* (5th ed.). Sudbury, MA: Jones and Bartlett.

Lubkin, I. M., & Larsen, P. D. (2002a). What is chronicity? In I. Lubkin & P. D. Larsen (Eds.), *Chronic illness: Impact and interventions* (5th ed., pp. 3–24). Sudbury, MA: Jones and Bartlett.

Lutgendorf, S. K., Antoni, M. H., Ironson, G. E., Klimas, N. K., Patarca, R., & Fletcher, M. A. (1995). Physical symptoms of chronic fatigue syndrome are exacerbated by the stress of Hurricane Andrew. *Psychosomatic Medicine, 57,* 310–323.

Macintyre, S., Ford, G., & Hunt, K. (1999). Do women "over-report" morbidity? Men's and women's responses to structured prompting on a standard question on long standing illness. *Social Science and Medicine, 48,* 89–98.

Magid, C. S. (2000). Pain, suffering, and meaning. *Journal of the American Medical Association, 283*(1), 114.

Maines, D. R. (2000). The social construction of meaning. *Contemporary Sociology, 29*(4), 577–584.

Managed health care Aetna implodes. (1997, October 4). *Economist,* p. 69.

Mandela, N. (1994). *A long walk to freedom: The autobiography of Nelson Mandela.* Boston: Little, Brown.

Marbach, J. J. (1999). Medically unexplained chronic orofacial pain. *Medical Clinics of North America, 83*(3), 691–710.

Marbach, J. J., Lennon, M. C., Link, B. G., & Dohrenwend, B. P. (1990). Losing face: Sources of stigma as perceived by chronic facial pain patients. *Journal of Behavioral Medicine, 13*(6), 583–604.

Martin, C. A. (2000). Putting patients first: Integrating hospital design and care. *Lancet, 356*(9228), 518.

Matsakis, A. (1992). *I can't get over it: A handbook for trauma survivors.* Oakland, CA: New Harbinger.

Mattoon, M. A. (1985). *Jungian psychology in perspective.* New York: Free Press.

Mayer, T. G. (1999). Rehabilitation: What do we do with the chronic patient? *Neurologic Clinics of North America, 17*(1), 131–147.

McCahill, M. E. (1995). Somatoform and related disorders: Delivery of diagnosis as first step. *American Family Physician, 52*(1), 193–203.

McCahon, C. P. & Larsen, P. D. (2002). Client and family education. In I. Lubkin & P. D. Larsen (Eds.), *Chronic illness: Impact and interventions* (5th ed., pp. 337–358). Sudbury, MA: Jones and Bartlett.

McGorry, R. W., Webster, B. S., Snook, S. H., & Hsiang, S. M. (2000). The relationship between pain intensity, disability, and the episodic nature of chronic and recurrent low back pain. *Spine, 25*(7), 834–841.

McHorney, C. A., Ware, J. E., Lu, J. F., & Sherbourne, C. D. (1994). The MOS 36-item short-form health survey (SF-36). III: Tests of data quality, scaling assumptions, and reliability across diverse patient groups. *Medical Care, 32,* 40–66.

McHorney, C. A., Ware, J. E., & Raczek, A. E. (1993). The MOS 36-item short form health survey (SF-36). II: Psychometric and clinical test of validity in measuring physical and mental health constructs. *Medical Care, 31,* 247–263.

McReynolds, C. J. (1998). Human immunodeficiency virus (HIV) disease: Shifting focus toward the chronic, long-term illness paradigm for rehabilitation practitioners. *Journal of Vocational Rehabilitation, 10,* 231–240.

Mechanic, D., & Schlesinger, M. (1996). The impact of managed care on patients' trust in medical care and their physicians. *Journal of the American Medical Association, 275*(21), 1693–1697.

Mercer, R. J. (1989). Response to life-span development: A review of theory and practice for families with chronically ill members. *Scholarly Inquiry for Nursing Practice:An International Journal, 3*(1), 23–27.

Mezey, G., & Robbins, I. (2001, September 8). Usefulness and validity of posttraumatic stress disorder as a psychiatric category. *British Medical Journal, 323,* 561–563.

Michael, S. R. (1996). Integrating chronic illness into one's life: A phenomenological inquiry. *Journal of Holistic Nursing, 14*(3), 251–267.

Mitrani, J. (1993). Deficiency and envy: Some factors impacting the analytic mind from listening to interpretation. *International Journal of Psycho-Analysis, 74,* 689–704.

Morrison, J. (1989). Histrionic personality disorder in women with somatization disorder. *Psychosomatics, 30*(4), 433–437.

Morse, J. M. (1997). Responding to threats to integrity of self. *Advances in Nursing Science, 19*(4), 21–36.

Nash, K., & Kramer, K. D. (1993). Self-help for sickle cell disease in African American communities. *Journal of Applied Behavioral Science, 29,* 202–215.

National Institute of Health Technology Assessment Panel. (1996). Integration of behavioral and relaxation approaches into the treatment of chronic pain and insomnia. *Journal of the American Medical Association, 276*(4), 313–318.

Neimeyer, R. A. (2000). Searching for the meaning of meaning: Grief therapy and the process of reconstruction. *Death Studies, 24*(6), 541–558.

Neimeyer, R. A., & Levitt, H. (2001). Coping and coherence: A narrative perspective on resilience. In K. Dobson (Ed.), *Handbook of cognitive behavioral psychotherapies* (2nd ed., pp. 393–430). New York: Guilford Press.

Nelson, E. C., Splaine, M. E., Batalden, P. B., & Plume, S. K. (1998). Building measurement and data collection into medical practice. *Annals of Internal Medicine, 128,* 460–466.

Neuberger, G., & Woods, C. T. (1995). Alternative modalities. In I. Lubkin (Ed.), *Chronic illness: Impact and interventions* (3rd ed., pp. 396–415). Boston: Jones and Bartlett.

Newby, N. M. (1996). Chronic illness and the family life-cycle. *Journal of Advanced Nursing, 23,* 786–791.

Newcomer, L. N. (2000). Shifting power: Is the consumer next? *Physician Executive, 26*(6), 18–19, 22–23.

Nicassio, P. M., & Smith, T. W. (Eds.). (1995). *Managing chronic illness: A biopsychosocial perspective.* Washington, DC: American Psychological Association.

Nisbet, L. A., & McQueen, V. D. (1993). Anti-permissive attitudes to lifestyle associated with AIDS. *Social Science and Medicine, 36*(7), 893–901.

Nochi, M. (2000). Reconstructing self-narratives in coping with traumatic brain injury. *Social Science and Medicine, 51*(12), 1795–1804.

Nouwen, H. J. M. (1972). *The wounded healer.* New York: Doubleday.

Olkin, R. (1999). *What psychotherapists should know about disability.* New York: Guilford Press.

Onega, L. L., & Larsen, P. D. (2002). Powerlessness. In I. Lubkin & P. D. Larsen (Eds.), *Chronic illness: Impact and interventions* (5th ed., pp. 297–310). Sudbury, MA: Jones and Bartlett.

O'Neill, D. P., & Kenny, E. K. (1998). Spirituality and chronic illness. *Image: Journal of Nursing Scholarship, 30*(3), 275–280.

Orford, J. (1992). Davidson's dilemma. *British Journal of Addiction, 87,* 832–833.

Parson, E. R. (1999). The voice in dissociation: A group model for helping victims integrate trauma representational memory. *Journal of Contemporary Psychotherapy, 29*(1), 19–38.

Pastio, D. (1995, September/October). Identifying with our culture ourselves. *Disability Rag and Resource,* 11.

Payne, I. R., Bergin, A. E., Bielema, K. A., & Jenkins, P. H. (1991). Review of religion and mental health: Prevention and the enhancement of psychosocial functioning. *Prevention in Human Services, 9*(2), 11–40.

Pearlman, L. A., & Saakvitne, K. W. (1995). *Trauma and the therapist.* New York: Norton.

Peck, M. S. (1987). *The different drum.* New York: Simon & Schuster.

Penninx, B., van Tilburg, T. G., Kriegsman, D., Boeke, A., Deeg, D., & van Eijk, J. (1999). Social network, social support, and loneliness in older persons with different chronic diseases. *Journal of Aging and Health, 11*(2), 151–168.

Perrig, W. J., & Grob, A. (Eds.). (2000). *The control of unwanted states and psychological health.* Mahwah, NJ: Erlbaum.

Perugi, G., Nassini, S., Socci, C., Lenzi, M., & Toni, C. (1999). Avoidant personality in social phobia and panic-agoraphobic disorder: A comparison. *Journal of Affective Disorders, 54*(3), 277–282.

Peters, D. (1995). Growth and development. In I. Lubkin (Ed.), *Chronic illness: Impact and interventions* (3rd ed., pp. 26–50). Boston: Jones and Bartlett.

Phukan, N. (1999, August 7–14). Class structure and social philosophy in health care. *Economic and Political Weekly,* 1688.

Piaget, J. (1952). *The origins of intelligence in children.* New York: International Universities Press.

Pilnick, A., & Hindmarsh, J. (1999). When you wake up, it'll be all over: Communication in the anesthetic room. *Symbolic Interaction, 22*(4), 345–360.

Plehn, K., Peterson, R., & Williams, D. (1998). Anxiety sensitivity: Its relationship to functional status in patients with chronic pain. *Journal of Occupational Rehabilitation, 8*(3), 213–222.

Pless, B., & Nolan, T. (1991). Revision, replication and neglect: Research on maladjustment in chronic illness. *Journal of Child Psychology, 32*(2), 347–365.

Polatajko, H. J. (2000). Dynamic performance analysis: A framework for understanding occupational performance. *American Journal of Occupational Therapy, 54*(1), 65–72.

Prigerson, H. G., Shear, M. K., Frank, E., Beery, L. C., Silberman, R., Prigerson, J., et al. (1997). Traumatic grief: A case of loss-induced trauma. *American Journal of Psychiatry, 154*(7), 1003–1009.

Primeau, L. A. (1996). Work and leisure: Transcending the dichotomy. *American Journal of Occupational Therapy, 50*(7), 569–577.

Prochaska, J. O. (1979). *Systems of psychotherapy: A transtheoretical analysis.* Homewood, IL: Dorsey Press.

Prochaska, J. O., DiClemente, C. C., & Norcross, J. C. (1992). In search of how people change: Applications to addictive behavior. *American Psychologist, 47*(9), 1102–1114.

Prochaska, J. O., DiClemente, C. C., Velicer, W. F., & Rossi, J. S. (1992). Criticisms and concerns of the transtheoretical model in light of research. *British Journal of Addiction, 87,* 825–835.

Prochaska, J. O., Norcross, J. C., & DiClemente, C. C. (1994). The Transtheoretical Model of Change and HIV prevention: A review. *Health Education Quarterly, 21*(4), 471–486.

Prochaska, J. O., & Velicer, W. F. (1997a). Misinterpretations and misapplications of the Transtheoretical Model. *American Journal of Health Promotion, 12*(1), 11–12.

Prochaska, J. O., & Velicer, W. F. (1997b). The Transtheoretical Model of Health Behavior Change. *American Journal of Health Promotion, 12*(1), 38–48.

Prochaska, J. O., Velicer, W. F., Fava, J. L., Rossi, J. S., & Tsoh, J. Y. (2001). Evaluating a population-based recruitment approach and a stage-based expert system interpretation of smoking cessation. *Addictive Behaviors, 26*(4), 583–602.

Pulver, S. E. (1992). Psychic change: Insight or relationship? *International Journal of Psychoanalysis, 73*(Pt. 2), 199–208.

Quality Assurance Project. (1990). Treatment outlines for paranoid, schizotypal and schizoid personality disorders. *Australian and New Zealand Journal of Psychiatry, 24*(3), 339–350.

Rakowski, W., Dube, C., Marcus, B. H., Prochaska, J. O., Velicer, W. F., & Abrams, D. B. (1992). Assessing elements of women's decisions about mammography. *Health Psychology, 11,* 111–118.

Rankin, S., & Weekes, D. P. (1989). Life-span development: A review of theory and practice for families with chronically ill members. *Scholarly Inquiry for Nursing Practice: An International Journal, 3*(1), 3–22.

Rauber, C. (1998). Evolution or extinction? Experts say HMOs must reinvent themselves if they are to survive [Cover story]. *Modern Health Care,* p. 36.

Rebeiro, K. L., & Polgar, J. M. (1999). Enabling occupational performance optimal experiences in theory. *Canadian Journal of Occupational Therapy, 66*(1), 14–22.

Register, C. (1987). *The chronic illness experience: Embracing the imperfect life.* Center City, MN: Hazelton.

Rehm, R. S. (1999). Religious faith in Mexican-American families dealing with chronic childhood illness. *Image: Journal of Nursing Scholarship, 31*(1), 33–38.

Reis, S., Hermoni, D., Borkan, J. M., & Biderman, A. (1999). A new look at low back complaints in primary care. *Journal of Family Practice, 48*(4), 299–303.

Reiss, D., Gonzalez, S., & Kramer, N. (1986). Family process, chronic illness, and death: On the weakness of strong bonds. *Archives of General Psychiatry, 43,* 795–804.

Reissman, F. (2000). A demand-side cure for the chronic illness crisis. *Social Policy,* 14–19.

Relt, M. V. (1997). Illuminating meaning and transforming issues of spirituality in HIV disease and AIDS. *Holistic Nursing Practice, 12*(1), 1–8.

Remsburg, R. E., & Carson, B. (2002). Rehabilitation. In I. Lubkin & P. D. Larsen (Eds.), *Chronic illness: Impact and interventions* (5th ed., pp. 455–583). Sudbury, MA: Jones and Bartlett.

Rest, J. R. (1973). The hierarchical nature of moral judgment: A study of patterns of comprehension and preferences of moral stages. *Journal of Personality, 41*(1), 86–109.

Rettew, D. C. (2000). Avoidant personality disorder, generalized social phobia, and shyness: Putting the personality back into personality disorders. *Harvard Review of Psychiatry, 8*(6), 283–289.

Richards, P. S., & Bergin, A. E. (1997). *A spiritual strategy for counseling and psychotherapy.* Washington, DC: American Psychological Association.

Ridson, C., & Edey, L. (1999). Human doctoring: Bringing authenticity to our care. *Academic Medicine, 74*(8), 896–899.

Riska, E. (2000). The rise and fall of Type A man. *Social Science and Medicine, 51*(11), 1665–1674.

Roberts, F. (2000). The interactional construction of asymmetry: The medical agenda as a resource for delaying response to patient questions. *Sociological Quarterly, 41*(1), 151–170.

Robins, L. N., Helzer, J., Cottler, L., & Goldring, E. (1989). National Institute of Mental Health Diagnostic Interview Schedule, Version Three Revised. DIS-III-R. St. Louis, MO: Department of Psychiatry, Washington University School of Medicine.

Robinson, I. (1990). Personal narratives, social careers and medical courses: Analyzing life trajectories in autobiographies of people with multiple sclerosis. *Social Science and Medicine, 30*(11), 1173–1186.

Roblin, D. W., Juhn, P. I., Preston, B. J., & Della Penna, R. (1999). A low-cost approach to perspective identification of impending high cost outcomes. *Medical Care, 37*(11), 1155–1163.

Rodning, C. B. (1988). Humor and healing: A creative process. *Pharos: Alpha Omega Alpha Honor Medical Society, 51*(3), 38–40.

Roessler, R. T., & Rumrill, P., Jr. (1998). Reducing workplace barriers to enhance job satisfaction: An important postemployment service for employees with chronic illness. *Journal of Vocational Rehabilitation, 10*, 219–229.

Roessler, R. T., & Sumner, G. (1997). Employer opinions about accommodating employees with chronic illness. *Journal of Applied Rehabilitation Counseling, 28*(3), 29–34.

Rolland, J. S. (1984). Toward a psychosocial typology of chronic and life-threatening illness. *Family Systems Medicine, 2*(3), 245–261.

Rolland, J. S. (1987). Chronic illness and the life cycle: A conceptual framework. *Family Process, 26,* 203–221.

Rolland, J. S. (1994). *Families, illness, and disability: An interactive treatment model.* New York: Basic Books.

Rood, R. P. (1996). Patient and physician responsibility in the treatment of chronic illness. *American Behavioral Scientist, 39*(6), 729–751.

Rosenbaum, D. E. (2000). Ideas and trends: Swallow hard; What if there is no cure for health care's ills? [Week in Review Desk]. *The New York Times,* Sec 4, p. 1.

Rosenberg, M., & Molho, P. (1998). Nonviolent (empathic) communication for health care providers. *Haemophilia, 4,* 335–340.

Rosenberg, S. A. (1996). Sounding board secrecy in medical research. *New England Journal of Medicine, 334*(6), 392–394.

Rosman, B. L. (1988). Family development and the impact of a child's chronic illness. In C. J. Falicov (Ed.), *Family transitions: Continuity and change over the life cycle* (pp. 293–309). New York: Guilford Press.

Roter, D. L., Stewart, M., Putnam, S. M., Lipkin, M., Jr., Stiles, W., & Inui, T. S. (1997). Communication patterns of primary care physicians. *Journal of the American Medical Association, 277*(4), 350–356.

Rothman, D. J., & Edgar, H. (1991). AIDS, activism, and ethics. *Hospital Practice, 26*(7), 135–142.

Rovner, J. (1999). U.S. Senate passes patients' bill of rights. *Lancet, 354*(9175), 316.

Rumrill, P. D., Millington, M. J., Webb, J. M., & Cook, B. G. (1998). Employment expectations as a differential indicator of attitudes toward people with insulin-dependent diabetes mellitus. *Journal of Vocational Rehabilitation, 10,* 271–280.

Rutberg, M. P. (1999). Medical records confidentiality. *Neurologic Clinics, 17*(2), 307–313.

Ryynanen, O. P., Myllykanga, M., Kinnunen, J., & Takala, J. (1999). Attitudes to health care prioritization methods and criteria among nurses, doctors, politicians and the general public. *Social Science and Medicine, 49,* 1529–1539.

Safran, D. G., Rogers, W. H., Tarlov, A. R., Inui, T., Taira, D., Montgomery, J. E., et al. (2000). Organizational and financial characteristics of health plans: Are they related to primary care performance? *Archives of Internal Medicine, 160,* 69–76.

Saigh, P. A., & Bremner, J. D. (Eds.). (1999). *Posttraumatic stress disorder: A comprehensive text.* Needham Heights, MA: Allyn & Bacon.

Salmon, P., Peters, S., & Stanley, I. M. (1999). Patients' perceptions of medical explanations for somatization disorders: Qualitative analysis. *British Medical Journal, 318,* 372–376.

Samra, C. (1985). Spiritual care: A time to laugh. *Journal of Christian Nursing, 2*(4), 15–19.

Satcher, J. (1992). Responding to employer concerns about the ADA and job applicants with disabilities. *Journal of Applied Rehabilitation Counseling, 23*(3), 37–40.

Satcher, J., & Hendren, G. R. (1991). Acceptance of the Americans with Disabilities Act of 1990 by persons preparing to enter the business field. *Journal of Applied Rehabilitation Counseling, 22*(2), 15–18.

Saylor, C., Yoder, M., & Mann, R. J. (2002). Stigma. In I. Lubkin & P. D. Larsen (Eds.), *Chronic illness: Impact and interventions* (5th ed., pp. 53–76). Sudbury, MA: Jones and Bartlett.

Scambler, G., & Hopkins, A. (1990). Generating a model of epileptic stigma: The role of qualitative analysis. *Social Science and Medicine, 30*(11), 1187–1194.

Schaefer, K. M. (1995). Women living in paradox: Loss and discovery in chronic illness. *Holistic Nursing Practice, 9*(3), 63–74.

Schelling, G., Stoll, C., Haller, M., Briegel, J., Manert, W., Bullinger, M., et al. (1998). Health-related quality of life and posttraumatic stress disorder in survivors of the acute respiratory disease syndrome. *Critical Care Medicine, 26*(4), 651–659.

Schiller, N. G., Crystal, S., & Lewellen, D. (1994). Risky business: The cultural construction of AIDS risk groups. *Social Science and Medicine, 38*(10), 1337–1346.

Schirm, V. (2002). Quality of life. In I. Lubkin & P. D. Larsen (Eds.), *Chronic illness: Impact and interventions* (5th ed., pp. 181–201). Sudbury, MA: Jones and Bartlett.

Schlesinger, M., Druss, B., & Thomas, T. (1999). No exit? The effect of health status on dissatisfaction and disenrollment from health plans. *Health Services Research, 34*(2), 547–579.

Schwartz-Salant, N., & Stein, M. (Eds.). (1995). *Transference countertransference*. Wilmette, IL: Chiron.

Scott, M. J., & Stradling, S. G. (1994). Posttraumatic stress disorder without the trauma. *British Journal of Clinical Psychology, 33,* 71–74.

Scotton, B. W., Chinen, A. B., & Battista, J. (Eds.). (1996). *Textbook of transpersonal psychiatry and psychology.* New York: HarperCollins.

Selby, J. V. (1997). Linking automated databases for research in managed care settings. *Annals of Internal Medicine, 127*(8, Pt. 2), 719–724.

Shafranske, E. P., & Gorsuch, R. L. (1984). Factors associated with the perception of spirituality in psychotherapy. *Journal of Transpersonal Psychology, 16*(2), 231–241.

Shalev, A. Y., Schrieber, S., & Galai, T. (1993). Posttraumatic stress disorder following medical events. *British Journal of Clinical Psychology, 32,* 247–253.

Siegel, K., Raveis, V. H., & Karus, D. (1997). Illness-related support and negative network interactions: Effects on HIV-infected men's depressive symptomatology. *American Journal of Community Psychology, 25*(3), 395–420.

Siever, L. J., & Gunderson, J. G. (1983). The search for a schizotypal personality: Historical origins and current status. *Comprehensive Psychiatry, 24*(3), 199–212.

Silbermann, L. (1967). Reflections on working through and insight. *Israeli Annals of Psychiatry and Related Disciplines, 5*(1), 53–60.

Singer, M. (1994). The politics of AIDS. *Social Science and Medicine, 38*(10), 1321–1324.

Singer, M. (1995). Beyond the Ivory Tower: Critical praxis in medical anthropology. *Medical Anthropology Quarterly, 9*(1), 80–106.

Small, S., & Lamb, M. (1999). Fatigue in chronic illness: The experience of individuals with chronic obstructive pulmonary disease and with asthma. *Journal of Advanced Nursing, 30*(2), 469–478.

Smith, I. K. (2001). Executive physical. There's a whole battery of new high-tech scans for those who can afford them. Are they worth it? *Time, 15*(3), 6.

Smith, M. Y., Redd, W. H., Peyser, C., & Vogl, D. (1999). Posttraumatic stress disorder in cancer: A review. *Psycho-Oncology, 8*(6), 521–537.

Smith-Campbell, B. (2002). Politics and policy. In I. Lubkin & P. D. Larsen (Eds.), *Chronic illness: Impact and interventions* (5th ed., pp. 491–511). Sudbury, MA: Jones and Bartlett.

Soliman, H. H. (1995). Rural communities' responses to the Great Flood of 1993: A tale of two cities. *Human Services in the Rural Environment, 19*(1), 36–41.

Starfield, B., Wray, C., Hess, K., Gross, R., Birk, P., & D'Lugoff, B. (1981). The influence of patient-practitioner agreement on outcome of care. *American Journal of Public Health, 71*(2), 127–130.

Stein, M. (1996). *Practicing wholeness.* New York: Continuum International Publishing.

Stephens, W. M. (1989). Six ways to guarantee denial of your patient's Social Security disability benefits. *Journal of the Tennessee Medical Association, 2*(5), 273.

Stephenson, A., Collerton, J., & White, P. (1996). Teaching medical students about long-term illness. *Academic Medicine, 71*(5), 549–550.

Stewart, E. C. (1995). The feeling edge of culture. *Journal of Social Distress and the Homeless, 4*(3), 163–202.

Stieg, R. L., Lippe, P., & Shepard, T. A. (1999). Roadblocks to effective pain treatment. *Medical Clinics of North America, 83*(3), 809–821.

Stockwell, T. (1992). Models of change, heavenly bodies and *weltanschaungs. British Journal of Addiction, 87,* 830–832.

Stoll, C., Schelling, G., Goetz, A. E., Kilger, E., Bayer, A., Kapfhammer, H. P., et al. (2000). Health-related quality of life and posttraumatic stress disorder in patients after cardiac surgery and intensive care treatment. *Journal of Thoracic and Cardiovascular Surgery, 120*(3), 505–512.

Stuart, S., & Noyes, R., Jr. (1999). Attachment and interpersonal communication in somatization. *Psychosomatics, 40*(1), 34–43.

Sugarek, N. J., Dyo, R., & Holmes, B. (1988). Locus of control and beliefs about cancer in a multiethnic clinic population. *Oncology Nursing Forum, 15*(4), 481–486.

Sumner, C. H. (1998). Recognizing and responding to spiritual distress. *American Journal of Nursing, 98*(1), 26–30.

Sumner, G. (1995). *Project alliance: A guide to job retention for people with chronic illness and their employers.* New York: National Multiple Sclerosis Society.

Sutton, S. R. (1997). Transtheoretical model of behavior change. In A. Baum, S. Newman, J. Weinman, R. West, & C. McManus (Eds.), *Cambridge handbook of psychology, health and medicine* (pp. 180–183). Cambridge, MA: Cambridge University Press.

Sweet, S. (1998). The effect of a natural disaster on social cohesion: A longitudinal study. *International Journal of Mass Emergencies and Disasters, 16*(3), 321–331.

Swenson, R. M. (1988). Plagues, history and AIDS. *American Scholar, 57,* 183–200.

Tait, R. C., Chibnall, J. T., & Richardson, W. D. (1990). Litigation and employment status: Effects on patients with chronic pain. *Pain, 43,* 37–46.

Tallandini, M. A. (1999). The dread of integration: Integrative process in a chronically ill borderline patient. *Psychoanalytic Study of the Child, 54,* 289–315.

Taylor, P. J. (1986). Psychopaths and their treatment. *Journal of the Royal Society of Medicine, 79*(12), 693–695.

Taylor, R. R., Friedberg, F., & Jason, L. A. (2001). *A clinicians guide to understanding controversial illnesses: Chronic fatigue syndrome, fibromyalgia, and multiple chemical sensitivities.* Sarasota, FL: Professional Resource Press.

Taylor, R. R., & Jason, L. A. (2002). Chronic fatigue, abuse-related traumatization, and psychiatric disorders in community-based sample. *Social Science and Medicine, 55*(2), 247–256.

Thomasma, D. C., & McElhinney, T. K. (1990). Ethical concerns about AIDS. *Pharos: Alpha Omega Alpha Honor Medical Society, 53*(2), 7–11.

Thorne, S., & Patterson, B. (1998). Shifting images of chronic illness. *Image: Journal of Nursing Scholarship, 30*(2), 173–178.

Thorne, S. E. (1990). Constructive noncompliance in chronic illness. *Holistic Nursing Practice, 5*(1), 62–69.

Thornton, J. (1998). We're all wackos: A new model of health. *International Journal of Sociology and Social Policy, 18*(9/10), 119–125.

Travis, S. S., & Piercy, K. (2002). Family caregivers. In I. Lubkin & P. D. Larsen (Eds.), *Chronic illness: Impact and interventions* (5th ed., pp. 233–260). Sudbury, MA: Jones and Bartlett.

Turk, D. C., & Rudy, T. E. (1991). Neglected topics in the treatment of chronic pain patients: Relapse, noncompliance, and adherence enhancement. *Pain, 44,* 5–28.

Turk, D. C., Rudy, T. E., & Stieg, R. L. (1988). The disability determination dilemma: Toward a multiaxial solution. *Pain, 34*(3), 217–229.

Turner, R. J., & Lloyd, D. A. (1995, December). Lifetime traumas and mental health: The significance of cumulative adversity. *Journal of Health and Social Behavior, 36,* 360–376.

Twombly, R. (2001). Posttraumatic stress disorder in childhood cancer survivors: How common is it? *Journal of the National Cancer Institute, 93*(4), 262–263.

Vacha, J. (1985). German constitutional doctrine in the 1920's and 1930's and pitfalls of the contemporary conception of normality in biology and medicine. *Journal of Medical Philosophy, 10*(4), 339–367.

van der Kolk, B. A., McFarlane, A. E., & Weisaeth, L. (Eds.). (1996). *Traumatic stress: The effects of overwhelming stress on mind, body and society.* New York: Guilford Press.

van der Wardt, E. M., Taal, E., Rasker, J. J., & Wiegman, O. (1999). Media coverage of chronic disease in the Netherlands. *Seminars in Arthritis and Rheumatism, 28*(5), 333–341.

van Eijk, J., & de Haan, M. (1998). Care for the chronically ill: The future role of health care professionals and their patients. *Patient Education and Counseling, 35,* 233–240.

Van Hoof, E., Coomins, D., Cluydts, R., & de Meirleir, K. (forthcoming-a). *Fennell phases: Toward a management program for patients with chronic fatigue syndrome.*

Van Hoof, E., Coomins, D., Cluydts, R., & de Meirleir, K. (forthcoming-b). *Psychological management of CFS by the Fennell Phases.*

Van Mens-Verhulst, J., & Bensing, J. (1998). Distinguishing between chronic and nonchronic fatigue: The role of gender and age. *Social Science and Medicine, 47*(5), 621–634.

Vaughan, M. (1994). Healing and curing: Issues in the social history and anthropology of medicine in Africa. *Social History of Medicine, 7*(2), 283–295.

Vrana, S., & Lauterbach, D. (1994). Prevalence of traumatic events and post-traumatic psychological symptoms in a nonclinical sample of college students. *Journal of Traumatic Stress, 7,* 289–302.

Wade, C. M. (1994a, November/December). Creating a disability aesthetic in the arts. *Disability Rag and Resource,* 29–31.

Wade, C. M. (1994b, September/October). Identity. *Disability Rag and Resource,* 32–36.

Wagner, E. H., Glasgow, R. E., Davis, C., Bonomi, A. E., Provost, L., McCulloch, D., et al. (2001). Quality improvement in chronic illness care: A collaborative approach. *Joint Commission Journal on Quality Improvement, 27*(2), 63–80.

Wallander, J. L., & Varni, J. W. (1998). Effects of pediatric chronic physical disorder on child and family adjustment. *Journal of Child Psychology, 39*(1), 29–46.

Walter, T. (2000). Grief narratives: The role of medicine in the policing of grief. *Anthropology and Medicine, 7*(1), 97–114.

Ware, N. C. (1998). Sociosomatics and illness course in chronic fatigue syndrome. *Psychosomatic Medicine, 60,* 394–401.

Ware, N. C. (1999). Toward a model of social course in chronic illness: The example of chronic fatigue syndrome. *Culture, Medicine and Psychiatry, 23,* 303–331.

Ware, N. C., & Kleinman, A. (1992). Culture and somatic experience: The social course of illness in neurasthenia and chronic fatigue syndrome. *Psychosomatic Medicine, 54,* 546–560.

Ware, N. C., Lachicotte, W. S., Kirschner, S., Cortes, D., & Good, B. (2000). Clinician experiences of managed mental health care: A rereading of the threat. *Medical Anthropology Quarterly, 14*(1), 2–27.

Warren, E., Sullivan, T., & Jacoby, M. B. (2000, May). Medical problems and bankruptcy filings. *Norton's Bankruptcy Advisor.*

Weber, D. O. (1997). The empowered consumer: New demands for access, information and services are changing the face of health care delivery. *Health Forum Journal, 40*(5), 20–33.

Weinstein, N. D., Rothman, A. J., & Sutton, S. R. (1998). Stage theories of health behavior: Conceptual and methodological issues. *Health Psychology, 17,* 290–299.

Weinstein, S. M., Laux, L. F., Thornby, J. I., Lorimor, R. J., Thorpe, D. M., & Merrill, J. M. (2000). Medical students' attitudes toward pain and the use of opioid analgesics: Implications for changing medical school curriculum. *Southern Medical Journal, 93*(5), 472–478.

Weissman, D. E. (1997). Consultation in palliative medicine. *Archives of Internal Medicine, 157,* 733–737.

Weissman, D. E., & Dahl, J. L. (1990). Attitudes about cancer pain: A survey of Wisconsin's first year medical students. *Journal of Pain Symptom Management, 5,* 345–349.

Weissman, D. E., & Griffie, J. (1998). Integration of palliative medicine at the medical college of Wisconsin 1990–1996. *Journal of Pain and Symptom Management, 15*(3), 195–201.

Wellard, S. (1998). Construction of chronic illness. *International Journal of Nursing Studies, 35,* 49–55.

Wells, S. M. (1998). *A delicate balance: Living successfully with chronic illness.* New York: Plenum Press.

White, N., & Lubkin, I. (1995). Illness trajectory. In I. Lubkin (Ed.), *Chronic illness: Impact and interventions* (3rd ed., pp. 51–73). Boston: Jones and Bartlett.

Willan, P. L., & Humpherson, J. R. (1999). Concepts of variation and normality in morphology: Important issues at risk of neglect in modern undergraduate medical courses. *Clinical Anatomy, 12*(3), 186–190.

Willems, D. (2000). Managing one's body using self-management techniques: Practicing autonomy. *Theoretical Medicine and Bioethics, 21*(1), 23–38.

Wilson, A. (2000). On the history of disease-concepts: The case of pleurisy. *History of Science, 38*(3), 271–319.

Wilson, J. P., & Lindy, J. D. (Eds.). (1994). *Countertransference in the treatment of PTSD*. New York: Guilford Press.

Wilson, T., & Holt, T. (2001, September). Complexity science: Complexity and clinical care. *British Medical Journal, 323,* 685–688.

Witztum, E., Dasberg, H., & Bleich, A. (1986). Use of a metaphor in the treatment of combat-induced posttraumatic stress disorder. *American Journal of Psychotherapy, 40*(3), 457–465.

Woodgate, R. L. (1998). Adolescents' perspective of chronic illness: It's hard. *Journal of Pediatric Nursing, 13*(4), 210–223.

Woods, N. F., Haberman, M. R., & Packard, N. J. (1993). Demands of illness and individual, dyadic, and family adaptation in chronic illness. *Western Journal of Nursing Research, 15*(1), 10–30.

Woodward, B. (1995). The computer-based patient record and confidentiality. *New England Journal of Medicine, 333*(21), 1419–1422.

World Health Report. (2000). *Health Systems: Improving performance.* Retrieved from http://www.who.int/whr/2000/en/report.htm.

Yates, S. (2001). Finding your funny bone: Incorporating your humor into medical practice. *Australian Family Physician, 30*(1), 22–24.

Yeheskel, A., Biderman, A., Borkan, J. M., & Herman, J. (2000). A course for teaching patient-centered medicine to family medicine residents. *Academic Medicine, 75*(5), 494–497.

Yehuda, R., & McFarlane, A. C. (1999). Conflict between current knowledge about posttraumatic stress disorder and its original conceptual basis. In M. J. Horowitz (Ed.), *Essential papers on post traumatic stress disorder* (pp. 41–60). New York: New York University Press.

Yen, S., & Shea, M. (2001). Recent development in research of trauma and personality disorders. *Current Psychiatry Reports, 3*(1), 52–58.

Young, J. (1994). The loss of time in chronic systems. An intervention model for working with longer term conditions. *Australian and New Zealand Journal of Family Therapy, 15,* 73–80.

Zimmerman, M., & Mattia, J. I. (1999). Is posttraumatic stress disorder underdiagnosed in routine clinical settings? *Journal of Nervous and Mental Disorders, 187*(7), 420–428.

Author Index

Subject Index